THE DUCTUS ARTERIOSUS

PLATE I

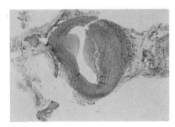 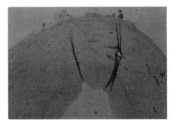

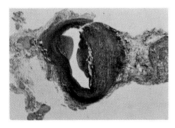 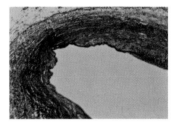

THE
DUCTUS
ARTERIOSUS

By

DONALD E. CASSELS, M.D.

Professor of Pediatrics (*Pediatric Cardiology*)
University of Chicago Pritzker School of Medicine
Director, Pediatric Cardiology, Wyler Children's Hospital
The University of Chicago Hospitals and Clinics
The University of Chicago, Chicago, Illinois

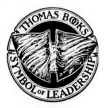

CHARLES C THOMAS • PUBLISHER
Springfield • Illinois • U.S.A.

Published and Distributed Throughout the World by
CHARLES   C   THOMAS   •   PUBLISHER
BANNERSTONE HOUSE
301-327 East Lawrence Avenue, Springfield, Illinois, U.S.A.

©*1973, by* CHARLES C THOMAS • PUBLISHER
ISBN 0-398-02720-X
Library of Congress Catalog Card Number: 72-92163

This Book is Dedicated to
ISABELLA COLLINS CASSELS
MY WIFE

PREFACE

The Purpose of This Monograph is to consider available information related to the ductus arteriosus, to review the present status of the ductus as a clinical problem and to present modern concepts of pathology and hemodynamics. Some new material related to innervation and aortic flows are included. The chapter index appropriately describes the contents.

The historical section was a source of concern. Originally I tried to verify quotations used, but this proved impossible. A number of translations and quotations were used and acknowledgement is made to the review of K. J. Franklin in the Annals of Science, Vol. 5, 1941-1947 entitled "A Survey of the Growth of Knowledge About Certain Parts of the Foetal Cardiovascular Apparatus, and About the Foetal Circulation: In Man and Some Other Mammals. Part I. Galen to Harvey." A review of the Galen references was made by John Sharp of the University of Texas, El Paso.

The work of Maude Abbott and Helen Taussig have not received adequate recognition in this volume, nor the surgical innovations and triumphs of Drs. Robert Gross and Willis Potts. Unfortunately most of those responsible for making Pediatric Cardiology and Surgery viable and responsible specialties have not been mentioned.

Others would have organized or presented this subject differently. It was very tempting to devote a larger section to the ductus in the newborn and to the very large literature related to the increasingly sophisticated studies of physiological closure. This problem alone could be the subject of a monograph, especially if comparative physiology, pharmacology and ultrastructure were considered.

However, the thrust of this book has been more toward consideration and discussion of patency and the related clinical problems. Drs. Otto Thilenius and Rene Arcilla furnished hemodynamic data, suggestions and comments. Surgical colleagues, Dr. Peter Moulder and Dr. Robert Replogle, gave anatomical description, pictures, explanation and most important, biopsy specimens. Drs. Replogle and Chung Lin did the aortic flow studies during surgery. Dr. Francis Strauss, Department of Pathology, has been kind and cooperative, and Dr. Klaus Ranniger, Department of Radiology, furnished x-rays and lucid discussion. Studies on the catecholamine content of the patent ductus arteriosus were done by Dr. Robert Y. Moore in his laboratory. This study will be reported in more detail in a separate publication.

It should be noted that Dr. Mildred Stahlman, friend and consultant in newborn physiology for many years, gave me material used in discussion of the ductus in hyaline membrane disease. She is credited with all of the dye curves, and the discussion probably represents at least some of her views.

This volume would not have been completed without the industry and loyalty of Jacqueline Lax technician and bibliographer who has received substantial support from the Children's Research Foundation, Inc. Mrs. Michaeleen Wallig has been more of an editorial assistant than a secretary and I am especially grateful for her wisdom and persistance. I am indebted to those mentioned and to many others who have been of assistance.

This work was supported in part by USPHS Training Grant 5 T01 HL05851-03 and by grants NS-05002 and HD-04583 from the National Institutes of Health, USPHS.

DONALD E. CASSELS

CONTENTS

THE DUCTUS ARTERIOSUS

One

INTRODUCTION

P REPARATION AND CONSIDERATION OF THIS MONOGRAPH has
extended over twenty years. It began with a review of the world
literature on the subject in what was then The Surgeon Generals
Library, and the Index Catalogue of the Library of the Surgeon
Generals Office furnished the references to the early literature.
The unique facilities available in the old building are recalled
with some nostalgia. Lunchtime meant a pleasant break at the
cafeteria in the Mellon Art Gallery (The National Art Gallery)
where the line formed next to Audubon prints. Such a literature
review was limited by some language barriers but was accelerated
by the numerical restriction of papers on the subject of the ductus
arteriosus.

Some milestones in ductus studies have occurred during the
period of interest in this problem. The paper of Kennedy and Clark
(1) was a source of admiration and discussion in the Obstetric
and Pediatric Departments. Surgical closure of the ductus by
Gross (2) had occurred just before this in 1938. The association
of rubella infection and patency was reported in 1941 (3), and
diagnosis and even quantitative assessment could be done after
the clinical application of cardiac catheterization by Cournand
and Ranges (4) and especially in congenital heart disease as shown
by Cournand, Baldwin and Himmelstein (5).

Sophisticated physiological studies of the fetal and neonatal circulation accented the details of functional closure of the newborn
ductus in animals, especially the lamb, and in similar problems in
the newborn.

The study of patency was hindered by the lack of an experi-

3

mental model in animals or man. There was no way to maintain persistent patency in animals and no way to recognize early in infants which ductus might not close. Orderly study of conditions associated with or conceivably causing nonclosure is not possible.

The dilemma of patency results in a confrontation:

1. Is functional closure a requisite for anatomical closure and is increased oxygen or ductus constriction necessary for tissue proliferation and anatomical closure.

2. Are prenatal changes present in the vessel, as noted by some, an indication that the anatomic details of closure are initiated before birth and completed after birth.

Hornblad (6) asserts that late prenatally the ductal morphology does not change, and the structure of the wall is indistinguishable from that of newborns. There was no evidence of (a) intimal proliferation or intimal mounds and (b) there was a rounded lumen with a smooth inner surface lined with a single layer of flat endothelial cells. During physiological closure functional anatomical closure occurs. But Hornblad concludes that if high arterial oxygen was the cause of closure in those animals where closure takes place almost instantaneously this would require functioning respiratory-oxygenation almost instantly, within a few seconds.

Sciacca and Condorelli (7) asserted that morphological studies in guinea pigs showed that involution of the ductus begins on the fortieth day of fetal life and sometimes reaches an advanced stage at term. Their hemodynamic studies indicated blood flow through the lungs was increased and the size of the ductus greatly diminished. They concluded, on the basis of extensive studies in the guinea pig, that involution of the ductus was an intrinsic process independent of functional changes occurring at birth, such as oxygen induced constriction.

Jones, Barrow and Wheat (8) did an ultrastructural evaluation of the closure of the ductus in rats. In preparations done with care to eliminate fixation artifacts, they found morphological characteristics described by others using light microscopy.

With the electron microscope the differences between the structure of the aorta and pulmonary artery were striking. In the prenatal ductus the endothelium projected conspicuously into the lumen and there were large vacuoles in the subendothelial space, apparently preliminary to the sloughing and necrosis appearing in the central endothelial cells of the closed ductus.

A feature of this study was the finding of smooth muscle cells extending through the internal elastic membrane and interdigitating between the subendothelial space and the media with many elastic lamellae intermingled or split. This is similar to the muscle cell extensions found in the obliteration of small pulmonary arteries in pulmonary hypertension noted by Hatt, et al. (9) and Esterly, Glagov and Ferguson (10).

Differences in ultrastructure of the ductus from that of the aorta and pulmonary artery which they believed to be preparation for closure were; (a) subendothelial vacuolization, (b) extension of smooth muscle cells through the internal elastic membrane, (c) interruption of elastic lamellae and (d) distended endoplasmic reticulum. Their Figure 4 is shown by permission.

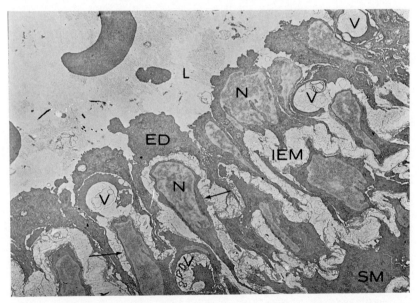

Figure 1. The predelivery ductus arteriosus of the rat demonstrates projection of endothelial cells through the internal elastic membrane (arrows), broken elastic lamellae by the interdigitating muscle cell processes and vacuoles in the subendothelial space (magnification x 6000). L = lumen; V = vacuoles; ED = endothelial cell; N = nucleus; SM = smooth muscle cell; IEM = internal elastic membrane.
From Jones, M., Barrow, M.V. and Wheat, M.W.: *Surg, 66*:891, 1969.

These changes were believed compatible with the view that

closure of the ductus is an active process underway before birth of the fetus.

And so the matter stands. There are numerous studies which tend to endorse either point of view.

Whatever the conclusion further studies of the ductus may warrant it is clear that in the human the intrinsic drive toward closure is very great and usually successful. This effort toward closure is so great that an attempt to prolong patency in the lamb by inserting a plastic tube in the ductus was unsuccessful. (Prec, unpublished (11)). The very strong effort to close merely extrudes the small tube.

<h1 style="text-align:center">REFERENCES</h1>

1. Kennedy, J.A. and Clark, S.L.: Observations on the ductus arteriosus of the guinea pig in relation to its method of closure. *Anat Rec, 79*:349, 1941.
2. Gross, R.E. and Hubbard, J.P.: Surgical ligation of patent ductus arteriosus; report of first successful case. *JAMA, 112*:729, 1939.
3. Gregg, N. McA.: Congenital cataract following German measles in the mother. *Trans Ophthalmol Soc Aust, 3*:35, 1941.
4. Cournand, A. and Ranges, H.S.: Catherization of the right auricle in man. *Proc Soc Exper Biol Med, 46*:462, 1941.
5. Cournand, A., Baldwin, J.S. and Himmelstein, A.: *Cardiac Catheterization in Congenital Heart Disease*. Published by the *Commonwealth Fund*, 1949.
6. Hornblad, P.Y.: Experimental studies on closure of the ductus arteriosus utilizing whole-body freezing. *Acta Paediatr Scand, Suppl 190*, 1969.
7. Sciacca, A. and Condorelli, M.: Involution of the ductus arteriosus: A morphological and experimental study, with a critical review of the literature. *Bibl Cardiol* Suppl of *Cardiol Fas 10*, 1960.
8. Jones, M., Barrow, M.V. and Wheat, M.W.: An ultrastructural evaluation of the closure of the ductus arteriosus in rats. *Surgery 66*:891, 1969.
9. Hatt, P.Y., Rouiller, Ch. and Grosgogeat, Y.: Les ultrastructures pulmonaires et le régime de la petite circulation. *Pathol Biol, 7/5-6*: 515, 1959.
10. Esterly, J.A., Glagov, S. and Ferguson, D.J.: Morphogenesis of intimal obliterative hyperplasia of small arteries in experimental pulmonary hypertension. *Am J Pathol, 52*:325, 1968.
11. Prec, K.J.: Unpublished work. 1957.

Two

THE DUCTUS ARTERIOSUS PROBLEM

THE DUCTUS ARTERIOSUS REMAINS A PHYSIOLOGICAL ANA-CHRONISM in spite of decades of unremitting study. These studies become increasingly sophisticated in concept and execution as laboratory facilities improve. Blood gases, drugs and hemodynamic status that dilate blood vessels and diminish resistance in the lungs constrict and reduce the lumen of the ductus. And procedures or environment that diminish pulmonary efficiency often augment ductus lumen.

Morbidity and mortality from isolated patent ductus arteriosus continue to be a facet of medicine not fully appreciated. A prospective study (1) which was a joint venture of the Perinatal Branch, National Institute of Neurological Diseases and Blindness and eleven cooperating centers included 56,109 births and 457 instances of heart disease.

Statistics related to ventricular septal defect and patent ductus arteriosus have been abstracted from Table 6, *Frequencies of Specific Lesions by Outcome.*

	Total	Stillbirth	Live Births Neonatal deaths	Infant deaths	Childhood deaths	Survivors
VSD	133	9	9	5	1	109
PDA (Isolated)	35	—	1	10	1	23

Disregarding stillbirths, which could not be reasonably attributed to an associated ventricular septal defect, there were only fifteen deaths associated with this lesion. This is in striking contrast to

7

patent ductus arteriosus, with twelve deaths in the thirty-five instances of the identified lesion. Nearly one-third died, with ten deaths in the infant group. If some of the surprising mortality followed surgery, the disease must have been life threatening without surgery.

In a retrospective study of mortality from congenital cardiovascular disease in Oregon (2) 390 deaths with congenital heart disease as the primary or underlying cause of death or coexisting and possibly contributing to death were tabulated for the period 1957 through 1961. These statistics were derived from death certificates supplemented by a review of birth certificates, clinical records of 97.5 percent and autopsy reports in 78 percent.

Abstracting their Table 6, to compare ventricular septal defect and patent ductus arteriosus occurring as isolated lesions, again patent ductus arteriosus in the first year was a threat to life.

		Under one year
VSD—single lesion	36	21
PDA—single lesion	26	22

Deaths recorded in the Department of Public Health, State of Illinois as caused by patent ductus arteriosus are shown in Table I. (3).

TABLE I

DEATHS DUE TO PATENT DUCTUS ARTERIOSUS
RECORDED IN THE DEPARTMENT OF PUBLIC HEALTH, STATE OF ILLINOIS

Years	1963	1964	1965	1966	1967	1968	1969	1970
Under 7 days	10	3	9	3	10	5	4	5
7 to 28 days	2	5	3	1		6	2	3
28 days to 1 year	10	1	10	7	9		5	4
1 to 15 years			4	1		1		2
15 to 65 years	2	3	1	3	2	5	3	1

In another survey of cardiovascular anomalies in 6,053 infants (4) the incidence was 0.6 percent in infants who survived for more than one month and 7.7 percent in infants who were stillborn or died within the first month. Isolated patent ductus arteriosus was considered as possibly normal for the first six months. There were five proven cases and one case of aneurysm of the ductus in a neonate in twenty-seven cases of congenital heart disease, and a total of fifty including the group with disease but without proven diagnosis.

The overall incidence was sixty in 6,053 infants or 0.83 percent; in stillborn over 500 gm, 5.4 percent; in neonatal deaths, 10.2 percent and in live born who survived over one month, 0.6 percent.

There were five (or six) cases of disease, an incidence of congenital heart disease of 10 percent, accepting as patent ductus arteriosus only in those after six months of age. This reduction would seem to denigrate the severely ill at two to six months of age and diminish the apparent incidence.

The study of heart disease in the first year of life from the University of Minnesota Hospitals is probably representative of the problem (5).

This was a study of 1,584 infants referred for suspicion of heart

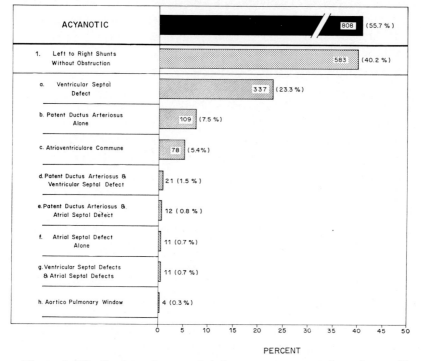

PERCENT

Figure 2. Distribution of types of defects among acyanotic patients with congenital heart disease.

From Eliot, R.S., Anderson, R.C., Adams, P., Jr. and Edwards, J.E.: *The Heart And Circulation In The Newborn And Infant.* New York, Grune & Stratton, Inc., 1966, p. 243.

disease of whom 1,456 or 91.7 percent had confirmed heart disease. Acyanotic heart disease, including both shunts and/or obstruction composed of 55.7 percent of the number and cyanotic congenital heart disease with shunts and/or obstruction 38.4 percent.

The distribution of defects in the category of acyanotic with left to right shunts without obstruction is shown in Figure 2. As in most surveys of incidence, ventricular septal defect was the most common single lesion, or 23.3 percent of those with heart disease. Isolated patent ductus arteriosus was next with 7.5 percent of those with heart disease. The association of the two was 1.5 percent of the total.

It was noted that the six most common types of congenital heart disease composed 71 percent of all heart disease in the first year of life and that the majority of these were correctible surgically.

If the general incidence of congenital heart disease is 6 per 1,000 live births and the incidence of isolated patent ductus arteriosus is 7.5 percent of those with heart disease, the occurrence of patent ductus arteriosus in the first year of life should be about 0.045 percent.

Gardiner and Keith (6) report the incidence of patent ductus arteriosus in school children as one in 3 to 4,000. However, this reflects survivors of the lesion occurring in infancy and in an age when diagnosis is more obvious. If the first year is included, as is necessary in a congenital lesion, the incidence is possibly about one in 2 or 3,000.

The usual clinical manifestations in preschool or early school age children suggest a benign lesion and do not encourage aggres-

TABLE II

THE IMPROVEMENT IN MORTALITY WHICH OCCURRED
FOLLOWING INSTITUTION OF AN
AGGRESSIVE DIAGNOSTIC AND SURGICAL REGIME

	Treated medically Mortality No. rate (%)		Treated surgically Mortality No. rate (%)		Inadequate diagnosis Error No. (%)		Total cases	Total mortality rate (%)
"Conservative" period	41	98	—	—	25	61	41	98
"Radical" period	4	100	31	6	3	9	35	17
Total	41	98	31	6	28	37	76	61

(From Pate, J.W. and Ainger, L.W.: Surgery, 53:811, 1963)

sive diagnosis and surgical repair in either the early infancy group or the early pulmonary hypertension group.

An improvement in mortality was noted by Pate and Ainger (7) when an aggressive approach to treatment of the symptomatic patent ductus in infancy was undertaken. The contrast between conservative management and an aggressive diagnostic and surgical regime is furnished by their table (Table II).

The ductus arteriosus problem in the infant is somewhat analogous to the appendicitis problem, where there has been little change in mortality in ten to twenty years.

The clinical patent ductus arteriosus problem has three major categories:

> I. In the infant under six months or under one year.
>
> II. The clinical group manifested by little distress, left aorta to pulmonary artery shunt with a diagnostic murmur and typical ancillary clinical or laboratory findings. These patients are readily diagnosed, and surgical mortality is usually restricted to complications that should not happen. Routine referral for operation is customary.
>
> III. Those with severe pulmonary hypertension pulmonary pressures are considered in relation to (a) age and (b) systemic pressure. The near systemic pressure under two years is probably operable, but the same relation at ten years probably is not.

The incidence of I and II have been estimated, but the incidence of III is more subtle. Although the subject is somewhat controversial, this group would become almost extinct with aggressive diagnostic and therapeutic measures in I and II.

This monograph is concerned almost exclusively with the ductus arteriosus as an isolated lesion. This vessel associated with other cardiovascular malformations will be considered in detail in a subsequent publication.

REFERENCES

1. Mitchell, S.C., Korones, S.B. and Berendes, H.W.: Congenital heart disease in 56,109 births, incidence and natural history. *Circulation,* *43*:323, 1971.
2. Menashe, V.D., Osterud, H.T. and Griswold, H.E.: Mortality from congenital cardiovascular disease in Oregon. *Pediatrics, 40*:334, 1967.

3. Communication from the Department of Public Health, State of Illinois.
4. Richards, M.R., Merritt, K.K., Samuels, M.H. and Langmann, A.G.: Congenital malformations of the cardiovascular system in a series of 6,053 infants. *Pediatrics 15*:12, 1955.
5. Eliot, R.S. Anderson, R.C., Adams, P., Jr. and Edwards, J.E.: Heart Disease in the First Year of Life. In Cassels, D.E. (ed.): *The Heart and Circulation in the Newborn and Infant.* New York, Grune & Stratton, Inc., 1966, p. 243.
6. Gardiner, J.H. and Keith, J.D.: Prevalence of heart disease in Toronto children, 1948-1949. Cardiac Registry, *Pediatrics 7*:713, 1951.
7. Pate, J.W. and Ainger, L.W.: Aggressive approach to malignant patent ductus arteriosus. *Surgery, 53*:811, 1963.

Three

HISTORICAL

G~ALEN~ (1) WROTE:

In this matter we have reason to admire the provisions of nature. For so long as the lung has only to be nourished and grow, it is supplied simply with blood, but when it is ready to take on an active motion, its tissue becomes lighter and capable of expansion and compression by the movements of the chest. On that account the vena cava in the foetus communicates by an opening with the arteria venalis. As this latter vessel thus performs for the lung the office of a vein *its companion must need at this time serve the purpose of an artery, and it is consequently made to communicate with the aorta.* As these two vessels are situated a little distance apart, *their communication is effected by means of a third smaller one which forms a junction with each.* A

The ductus arterious was identified.

The fetal anatomical channels are described, and he comments on their closure:

so far, no doubt, we have much to admire these contrivances of nature; but what surpasses them all is the way in which the foramen (ovale) not long afterwards become occluded. For soon after birth, either within a day or two, or, in some animals, after four or five days or a little longer, you will find the membrane at the foramen coalescing, but not yet fully adherent. Looking at the same place in the adult animal, you would say there never had been a time when it was open; and, on the other hand, in a fetus, before or immediatly after birth, when this membrane is attached, so to speak, only by its root, the rest of it hanging free in the vascular cavity, you would hardly believe in its ever becoming agglutinated. In like manner *the connecting vessel between the aorta and the vena arterialis,* while all other parts of the body increase in size, *not only stops growing but*

13

actually diminishes, becoming after a time completely shriveled and solidified. (The ligamentum arteriosum.) A

He later again referred to the postnatal obliteration of the fetal channels:

and it seems to me a much greater thing for her (Nature) to destroy what she has made because it has ceased to be useful than to have made something for the fetus beyond what she made for fully formed animals. B

The anatomical closure of the ductus arteriosus was recorded.

However, implications of knowledge of function cannot be inferred from the passages since Galen did not know that blood flowed through the vessels, and he could not speculate why nature should destroy what ceased to be useful since he assumed passage of blood from the right ventricle to the left ventricle through pores in the interventricular septum.

And so the matter stood for 1,300 years, while anatomy and medicine worked in the shadow of Galen's system of medicine, the Opera Omnia of A D 200.

Vesalius (2) (1514 to 1564) did not describe fetal channels in his anatomy atlas which introduced modern anatomy. He was criticized for this omission by Fallopio and by Rota (Franklin). He later (1564) stated the pulmonary artery and the aorta opened into each other without an intermediate vessel. He may, therefore, have seen an example of what is currently called the *window ductus.*

Gabrielle Fallopius (3) (1523 to 1562) noted the ductus arteriosus was of large size. This was the first description of the ductus since Galen.

Giulio Aranzi (4) extended Galen's account of the fetal circulatory anatomy and speculated upon function, but neither adult nor fetal circulation was understood at this time.

Leonardo Botallus (5) stated he had found a new way for blood to enter the left ventricle. The curious fate of the eponym *ductus Botalli* is of interest for Botallus rediscovered the foramen ovale, and at no time did he mention the ductus arteriosus. Franklin (6) traced the subsequent fate and distortion of the description.

Fabricius (7) descriptions and illustrations contain the components of the fetal circulation, the first illustration of the ductus arteriosus.

Guilio Casserio (8) contained the first illustration of the ligamentum arteriosum.

Carcano (9) gave an account of the fetal channels and stated the ductus arteriosus arises from the aorta and goes obliquely to where the pulmonary artery (called the *artery like vein* by these anatomists) divides into two, so that it appears to divide into three branches. He found variable times of closure of fetal channels, but in adult animals closure was complete.

In the meantime Servetus (10) and Colombo (11) had described the flow of blood through the lungs. Inspection of the interventricular septum had convinced Servetus that the supposition of Galen that blood passed to the left ventricle through pores in the ventricular septum was incorrect.

This is the end of the older era of circulatory speculation and scattered anatomical studies and the beginning of the modern era of experimental cardiovascular physiology. While this study is concerned with the ductus arteriosus, general concepts of the fetal circulation cannot be ignored. Nowhere are there concepts more lucid than in William Harvey, "Exercitatio anatomica de motu Cordis et Sanguinis in animalibus" (12). In Chapter VI, "the Way by Which the Blood Passes from the Vena Cavae to the Arteries, or from the Right Ventricle of the Heart to the Left", he says (Leake translation) (13):

> It is well known by all anatomists that the four blood vessels belonging to the heart, the vena cava, pulmonary artery, pulmonary vein, and aorta, are connected differently in the fetus than in the adult.

He then described the foramen ovale and the flow of venous blood to the left atrium and the ventricle and comes to a consideration of the ductus arteriosus:

> Another junction is by the pulmonary artery where it divides into two branches after leaving the right ventricle. It is like a third trunk added to these two, a sort of arterial canal passing obliquely toward and perforating the aorta . . . This canal gradually shrinks after birth and is finally obliterated like the umbilical vessels.
> There is no membrane in this arterial canal to impede the movement of the blood in either direction. At the entrance of the pulmonary artery, from which this canal extends, there are three sigmoid valves opening outwards, so the blood flows easily from the right ventricle into this vessel and the aorta, but by closing tightly they prevent any

back flow from the arteries or lungs into the right ventricle. Thus, when the heart contracts in the embryo, there is reason to believe the blood is continually propelled through this way from the right ventricle to aorta.

In embryos, then, while the lungs are as inert and motionless as though not present, Nature uses for transmitting blood the two ventricles of the heart as if they were one. The situation is the same in embryos with lungs, while the lungs are not used, as in those animals themselves without lungs . . .

In the more perfect warm-blooded adult animals, as man, the blood passes from the right ventricle of the heart through the pulmonary artery to the lungs, from there through the pulmonary vein into the left auricle, and then into the left ventricle, First, I shall show how this may be so, and then that it is so.

His thesis was that the blood circulated repetitiously, and he could prove it.

The ductus arteriosus had been described as a fetal channel and its change into a ligament without a lumen was known. But Harvey placed the ductus in its proper place in a coherent system of fetal circulation, asserting the fetal channels allowed a common ventricular ejection:

the heart, in its beat, forces the blood through the wide open passages from the vena cava to the aorta through the two ventricles. The right ventricle, receiving blood from its auricle, propels it through the pulmonary artery and its continuation, called the ductus arteriosus, to the aorta. At the same time, the left ventricle contracts and sends into the aorta the blood which, received from the beat of its auricle, has come through the foramen ovale from the vena cava.

He perceived that the ductus in the fetus does not bring blood from the aorta to the lungs *for their nourishment* as had been postulaated previously, but that the right ventricle pumps blood through the ductus to the aorta, bypassing the lungs, which were *motionless and useless.*

Carcano and Harvey made observations on the time of closure of the ductus, but the problem of closure continues to be a proper subject for study.

Following Harvey, the fetal channels have been studied continuously since this early demonstration of their purpose in the fetus. Many aspects of the fetal circulation remain debatable, and the cause of closure and especially the reason for persistent patency of the ductus arteriosus remains a subject of investigation and speculation, although partial explanations are becoming available.

It is difficult to abstract subsequent consideration of the ductus from general discussions of the fetal channels since the fetal circulation, or at least the immediate cardiac part of it, was so closely associated with the problem of the blood flow in the superior and inferior vena cavae in relation to the foramen ovale. The anatomical basis for the modern concepts of the distribution of the caval flows are related to the publications of Wolff (14), Kilian (15), and Von Haller (16) and Sabatier (17). Although the Sabatier publication was in 1791, the views expressed are strangely modern:

> all the blood that the trunk of the inferior cava received, instead of stopping in the right auricle, as in the adult, passes entire into the left through the foramen ovale, the superior edge of which is so arranged that nothing can mix with the blood of the superior cava; so that it is really with the left auricle that the inferior cava is continued.

There has been much speculation and some controversy concerning caval flows. This concerns the ductus problem in that blood which does not go through the foramen ovale and into the left atrium and left ventricle goes into the pulmonary artery and this flow then divides in variable proportions for flow to the lungs and. for flow through the ductus arteriosus into the descending aorta. Both of these flows control or at least influence strongly the blood flow to the placenta. The investigation of Windle and Becker (18) and the angiocardiographic studies of Barclay, Franklin and Pritchard (19) in the lamb were augmented by the studies of Lind and Wegelius (20). Shunts from the right atrium to the left atrium were demonstrated in the newborn by opacification via superior and inferior vena cavae. Injection from below demonstrated this in all cases. Opacification from above, however, sometimes showed. this shunt. The early investigator, Mery (21), believed he had proven the passage of blood from the left atrium to the right. If there is a large left to right shunt through a patent ductus arteriosus in early infancy a large left atrial to right is sometimes seen during angiocardiography. Since this anomalous atrial shunt disappears after ductus closure it is presumed that the left atrium can be so distended that the foramen ovale is incompetent.

Pohlman (22) made a list of the theories of the fetal circulation, and published his own findings which were based upon experiment and observation rather than speculation and polemic discussion. The original ideas are perhaps compressed into too neat a form but serve as a summary of the problem as it appeared in 1909:

1. The theory of Galen (1) and Harvey (12). This indicated the foramen ovale was a communication between two atria and mixed superior and inferior caval blood passed from the right atrium to the left.

2. The theory of Mery (21). He asserted blood passed from the left atrium to the right.

3. The theory of Wolff (14). He stated the foramen ovale did not communicate between the two atria, but connected the left opening of the inferior vena cava to the left atrium and the right opening of the inferior vena cava with the right atrium. He had shown that the orifice of the inferior cava bifurcated upon the free edge of the septum which divided the caval stream.

4. The theory of Von Haller (16) and Sabatier (17). This was the rather rigid idea of the crossed caval circulation, that the foramen ovale did not connect the two atria and all of the blood from the inferior vena cava flowed to the left atrium. The blood from the superior vena cava went to the right atrium.

The ideas were concerned chiefly with the relation of caval flows to the foramen ovale.

5. Kilian (15), however, believed all of the blood of the left ventricle went to the head and the upper extremities through the arch of the aorta and its brances, and all of the blood from the right ventricle went to the lungs, ductus and descending aorta through the pulmonary artery. The aorta functioned therefore as two parts, an upper and lower. These were connected by the pars communicans, the aorta between the left subclavian artery and the origin of the ductus, now called the isthmus. This did not carry blood during fetal life.

There is rather uniformly a narrowing of the aorta in this area in the fetus and newborn, and the flow through the isthmus may be diminished, but there is no evidence that it is absent. Modern studies in the lamb put about one-third to one-quarter of the aortic arch flow through the isthmus.

6. Ziegenspeck (23) also speculated upon hemodynamics and stated the blood flow through the superior vena cava was equal to the return through the pulmonary veins and the isthmus of the aorta carried the same amount of blood as the ductus arteriosus, each carried one-half the contents of the left and right ventricle.

Pohlman (22) applied for the first time the techniques of experiment to the problem of the fetal circulation. He injected starch granules into the venous flow at different sites and determined (a) direct pressures of the right and left ventricle, and (b) he determined the differential distribution of the starch granules. He believed he demonstrated:

1. The capacity of the right and left ventricles was equal.
2. The pressure in the right and left ventricle was equal.
3. The blood entering the heart through the superior and inferior vena cava mixed in the right atrium.
4. The foramen ovale communicated between the right and left atrium.
5. Mixed blood in sufficient quantity passed from the right atrium to the left atrium through the foramen ovale to substitute for the deficient pulmonary return.
6. The pulmonary return through the pulmonary veins was relatively small in amount and did not exceed one-fifth of the capacity of the ventricle.
7. The ductus arteriosus carried more blood than the descending aortic arch, probably in the ratio of 4 to 3.
8. The descending aorta was under lower resistance because of its connection with the placenta.
9. No artery in the fetus contained pure arterial blood—all contained mixed arterial and venous blood.

Direct investigation of the active fetal circulation replaced discussion based upon deduction from anatomical measurements or injection of the circulatory pathways in the dead fetus.

Kellogg (24) extended these experiments and found that material injected into either the umbilical vein or the superior vena cava appeared at the same time in both ventricles, a clear indication that under the conditions of the experiment there was mixing of caval flows in the right atrium.

An injection technique more refined than the use of particulate substances was applied to the problem of the ductus flow by Everett and Johnson (25). The radio isotope, radioactive phosphorus, P_{32}, which is easily detected and susceptible of quantitation was used. The distribution of blood from the pulmonary artery to the left branch of the pulmonary artery and to the aorta was studied in eleven fetal subjects and twenty-one newborn pups. The ages ranged from one week prepartum to three weeks postpartum. The pulmonary trunk was infused simultaneously from the left pulmonary artery and the aorta distal to the ductus before recirculation had occurred.

In the fetus the ratio of flow was about one to one. By nine hours postpartum a much larger proportion of the labelled blood went through the pulmonary artery and less through the ductus arteriosus. But the ductus continued to carry a small amount of blood, gradually decreasing until about fifteen days of age. Histological studies of closure agreed with the physiological findings.

The technique is a sensitive one, and it can be regretted that aortic injection above the ductus was not done to identify the aorta-pulmonary artery flow found in the human by catheterization of the pulmonary artery in the newborn period (26) and seen by dye curves when the proximal aorta is injected and the left atrium sampled.

Prec and Cassels (27) believed dye dilution curves in the newborn obtained by venous injection of Evans blue dye show right to left and left to right flow at the level of the ductus arteriosus at different times or in different patients, and suggested the ductus did not close at once in the human as in the lamb. This facet of the human fetal circulation is now generally accepted.

It was thought the discussion of the hemodynamics of the fetal circulation which had lasted several hundred years had been brought to a reasonable conclusion by the comprehensive studies of Barclay, Barcroft, Barron and Franklin (28-29). The results of these studies were reported in numerous publications and in the monographs Researches on Pre-Natal Life (30), and the Foetal Circulation (19). These studies on lambs were done with an intact placental circulation and with angiocardiography. Radiopaque material was injected into the umbilical veins, the femoral vein or the jugular vein.

In these studies all superior caval venous blood, now made radiopaque, passed through the right atrium, the right ventricle and into the pulmonary artery. Some went to the branches of the pulmonary artery and into the vascular channels of the lung, and there was a large flow through the ductus arteriosus into the descending aorta. The closure of the ductus was observed directly, or this was indicated by the absence of contrast material in the descending aorta. This occurred a few minutes after breathing was permitted and was considered to represent functional but not anatomical closure.

Interesting as these observations are, it is clear that is is not possible to say whether absence of blood flow through the ductus was related to an increase of pressure in the aorta and a dynamic obstruction to flow or if there was indeed a direct muscular sphincter action of the ductus itself as shown in the opacification study of Lind, Stern and Wegelius (31).

The flow from the umbilical vein or the lower vena cava divided, as had been demonstrated previously, into two parts, the larger flow going directly through the foramen ovale to the left heart, and a smaller amount passing directly into the right ventricle, the pulmonary artery and dividing into a portion for the lungs and a part for flow through the ductus into the descending aorta.

The fetal circulation, and especially pulmonary to aorta blood flow through the ductus arteriosus must really represent an unstable equilibrium, the controlling factors of which include volume flow, pressure and resistance in the (a) aortic arch above the ductus insertion and (b) the descending aorta below the ductus-aorta anastomosis.

The aortic arch flow includes the venous blood received chiefly from the inferior cava and umbilical vein, and a lesser and unknown but real amount returning from the lungs to the left atrium. The descending aorta flow includes the major pulmonary artery to aorta flow through the ductus and the unknown amount which flows across the narrowed isthmus just above the ductus-aorta connection. This area is narrow in the newborn, and it has been argued that this is so because the flow here is diminished. Average measurements in the human newborn may be aortic arch 0.7 to 0.8 cm, isthmus 0.5 cm and descending aorta 0.8 cm. But this narrowing may be an embryological remnant of the connection of the fourth branchial arch and the dorsal aorta, and flow across it will depend upon relative pressure and resistance above and below this aortic isthmus. It is not known whether in the human fetus there is a pressure gradient across this area. It is presumed there is not.

Below the ductus connection the aortic resistance is complex, and is made so by two completely different peripheral vascular areas involved: (a) that of the fetus below the iliac arteries and (b) the placenta with the umbilical arteries arising directly from these arteries. Presumably, in view of constant temperature and little movement, the fetal resistance is relatively fixed. Leg movement varies with fetal age, and the question of aortic runoff to this area must be considered. But the placental resistance must vary under the influence of uterine contraction and especially toward term with the development of arteriosclerosis and even infarction. No comparison between umbilical artery pressure in premature, term or post-term infants is available. Nor is it known whether interference with flow to the placenta can produce pressor substances for the fetus analogous to a similar circumstance in the kidney and conceivably in the lung.

This pressure is of great interest, since there must be nearly a common pressure in the placental system, the descending aorta, the ductus arteriosus and the pulmonary arteries. If this pressure becomes elevated, there results either (a) increased flow through the lungs or (b) pulmonary vasculature developing increased resistance to blood flow.

The inference is that if these pressures rise, overcompensation of resistance in the lung may be the origin of the small infant pulmonary hypertension when the ductus has persistent patency and would contribute to the origin of primary pulmonary hypertension.

REFERENCES

1. Galen: *Opera Omnia IV:243*. Kuhn Edition. A. Translation from Dalton, J.C.: *Doctrines of the Circulation*. Philadelphia, Lea's Son & Co., p. 68, 1884. B. Galen: On the Usefulness of the Parts of the Body. Translated from the Greek, with an Introduction and Commentary, Mary Tallmadge May, Vol. 1, Cornell University Press, p. 333, 1968.
2. Vesalius, A.: *De Humani Corporis Fabrica Libri Septem*. Basileae, ex officina Johannis Oporina, 1543.
3. Fallopius, G.: *Observationes Anatomicae*. To be found in Idem (1600). "Opera omnia, in unum congesta, and in medicinae studiosorum gratiam excusa. Francofurti apud haeredes Andreae Wecheli, Claud. Marnium and Jo. Aubrium, 1561.
4. Aranzi, Giulio Cesare: *De Humano Foetu Libellus*. 1564.
5. Botallus, Leonardo. Original not accessible. Reprinted as appendex Cp. 259-261 to Caecilius Folius (1641), with the description "Post libru de Catharro editum primo Parisiis apud Turrisanum." In via Jacobea,

in Bernadium. "Aldina Biblioteca Anno Saltis 1564 and Rursus Lugduni anno 1565". 1564.

6. Franklin, K.J.: A survey of the growth of knowledge about certain parts of the foetal cardiovascular apparatus, and about the foetal circulation, in man and some other mammals. Part I. Galen to Harvey. *Ann Sci,* 1941-47.

7. Fabricius, Hieronymus, ab Aquapendente (1600) — "De formato to foetu." Venetiis, Bolzetta, acc. to Capparoni.

8. Casserio, Giulio: *Tabulae Anatomicae LXXIIX, Omnes Novae Nec Ante Hac Visae.* 1627.

9. Carcano, Leone Grambattista: *Anatomici Libra II.* 1574.

10. Servetus, M.: *Christiani, Restitutio.* Facsimile of relevant passage in Osler, W. (1909). 1553.

11. Colombo, R.: *De Re Anatomica, Libra XV.* Venetiis, Ex typographia Nicholai Beuilacquae. 1559.

12. Harvey, William: *Exercitatio Anatomica de Motu Cordis et Sanguinis in Animalibus.* Francofurti, Sumptibus Gulielmi Fitzeri. 1628.

13. Harvey, William (translated by Chauncey Leake): *Anatomical Studies on the Motion of the Heart and Blood,* 3rd ed. Springfield, Thomas, 1941.

14. Wolff, C.F.: *De Foramine Ovali Ejusque in Dirigendo Sanguinis Motu.* Observ. novae, Nov. Comment. Scient. Petropolit XX. p. 357, 1778.

15. Kilian, H.F.: *Ueberden Kreislauf des Blutes im Kinde, Welches Noch Night Geathmet Hat.* Karlsruhe, 1826, p. 200.

16. Von Haller, A.: *Elementa Physiologiae Corporis Humani.*

17. Sabatier, R.B.: *Traite Complet D' anatomie.* Vol. II 1791, p. 493.

18. Windle, W.F. and Becker, R.F.: The course of the blood through the fetal heart. An experimental study in the cat and guinea pig. *Anat Rec, 77:*417, 1940.

19. Barclay, A.E., Franklin, K.J. and Pritchard, M.M.L.: *The Foetal Circulation.* Oxford, Blackwell Scientific Publication, 1944.

20. Lind, John and Wegelius, Carl: Human Fetal Circulation: Changes in the cardiovascular system at birth and disturbances in the postnatal closure of the foramen ovale and ductus arteriosus. In Symposium on Quantitative Biology *XIX:*109, 1954.

21. Mery, J.: Nouveau systeme de la circulation du sang par le trou ovale dans le foetus humain; avec les responses aux objections de MM. Duverney, Verheyen, Silvestre et Buissiere contre cette hypothese. Jean Boudot, Paris, 1700, p. 10, 1692.

22. Pohlman, August. The course of the blood flow to the heart of the fetal mammal with a note on the reptilian and anphibian circulations. *Anat Rec, 3:*75, 1909.

23. Ziegenspeck, R.: 1882. Welche Vuranderungen Erfahrt die Foetale Herzthatigxeit Regelmassig Durch die Geburt. In Inagidiss Jena. 1905. *Die Lehre Vonder Doggelt en Einmundung der Unteren Hoht-*

vene in die Vorhofe des Herzens. Samml. Kiln. Vortrage, Ser. XIV, Heft. II, No. 401.

24. Kellogg, H.B.: The course of blood flow through the fetal mammalian heart. *Am J Anat, 42*:443, 1928.

25. Everett, Newton B., Johnson, Robert T.: A study of the time of closure of the ductus arteriosus utilizing radio phosphorus. *Anat Rec, 106*:194, 1950. No. 94 of Papers of the Sixty Third Annual Session of the American Association of Anatomists.

26. Adams, F.H. and Lind, J.: Physiologic studies on the cardiovascular status of normal newborn infants. (With special reference to the ductus arteriosus.) *Pediatrics 19*:431, 1957.

27. Prec, K.J. and Cassels, D.E.: Dye dilution curves and cardiac output in newborn infants. *Circulation, 11*:789, 1955.

28. Barclay, A.E., Barcroft, J., Barron, D.H. and Franklin, K.J.: Closing of the ductus arteriosus. *J. Physiol, 93*:36, 1938.

29. Barclay, A.E., Barcroft, J., Barron, D.H. and Franklin, K.J.: A radiographic demonstration of the circulation through the heart in the adult and in the foetus, and the identification of the ductus arteriosus. *Br J Radiol, 12*:505, 1939.

30. Barcroft, Sir Joseph: *Researches On Prenatal Life.* Springfield, Thomas, 1947.

31. Lind, J., Stern, L. and Wegelius, Carl: *Human Foetal And Neonatal Circulation.* Springfield, Thomas, 1964.

Four

EMBRYOLOGY

I T IS CONVENTIONAL TO DESCRIBE THE DUCTUS ARTERIOSUS as the persistent terminal portion of the sixth branchial arch. For this purpose the figure of Rathke or some modification of it shows the form of the branchial arch system in mammalian embryos, and the portions which survive and are incorporated into the post-embryonal circulatory system, as in Figure 3. But the peculiar structure of the vessel, the unusual nature of its function in the fetus, and the interesting facets of its postfetal involution require a more substantial description of its origin. Consideration of these aspects of the ductus raise many questions. It is difficult to understand how this short vessel, a part of the branchial arch system, differs so in structure and function from the other derivatives of that system, or from any other part of the surviving vascular tree.

Its action and function almost suggests that as a part of the ever changing branchial system, its involution should be carried further, and not only obliteration but disappearance should be its fate; strangely it persisted too long, or curiously it does not resorb and disappear together. Certainly it retains embryonic drive and potentialities reminiscent of the branchial arches during their short active existence.

Since the ductus arteriosus is a derivative of the last, or sixth, or pulmonary arch, the pertinent embryology is related to (a) the formation of pulmonary arches and the pulmonary arteries and possible anomalies of formation and position of the ductus arteriosus and (b) a brief consideration of the possible anomalies of position when the left, fourth or aortic, arch is abnormally placed.

25

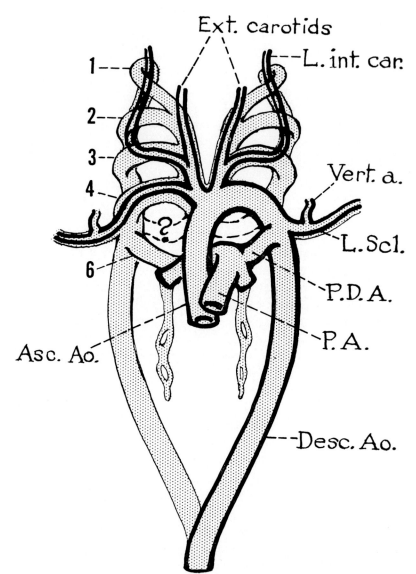

Figure 3. The embryonic branchial arch system, to indicate the origin of the normal arch and branches. The presence of a 5th arch is controversial. This is the usual schematic diagram.

The description of Congdon (1) has been followed relating to developmental aspects of the aortic arches. Paraphrase and some figures have been used, with permission.

The aortic arch system develops and changes during the time when the pharynx and its pouches develop in the area between the heart and the dorsal aorta and descend into the thorax. With this descent and concurrent changes in the pharynx, the blood flow channels from the heart to the dorsal aorta become displaced downward by the obliteration of the previously used upper arching vessels and the more or less simultaneous development of lower ones. Parts of the previous main flow vessels are retained to form auxiliary arteries from the new pathways to supply blood to the more anterior parts vacated by main vessels. This dropping out of upper arches occurs until the fourth is reached, part of which is then retained as the arterial channel to the dorsal aorta, either right or left, or rarely, both.

Older descriptions of the ductus arteriosus sometimes describe it as the terminal part of the fifth aortic arch rather than the current conventional sixth. This confusion is caused by debate concerning the presence or absence of a fifth arch. This is generally considered to be very transient and rudimentary if it is present at all. If there is no fifth arch, then the last arch may be called the fifth, the ductus representing the length of vessel from the left pulmonary artery to the juncture with the dorsal aorta. If there is a fifth, then the last arch or the ductus arch is called the sixth. A compromise is to omit reference to the possibility of a transient or rudimentary fifth, and use the conventional method of describing the pulmonary arch as the sixth. Peculiar arterial vessels from the arch which are difficult to place in the embryonic scheme of the arches are sometimes alluded to in the clinical literature as persistence of the fifth.

While the development and the subsequent history of the aortic arches will not be considered in detail except in regard to the sixth arch which is concerned with the ductus, a brief general outline of some of their characteristics is necessary since they also apply to the sixth. Congdon (1) points out the transformation of the arch system goes through two general phases, the branchial phase when the vessels resemble the pattern in lower vertebrates and is precursor of arteries supplying the gill system, and the postbranchial phase, when this system of arterial arches is replaced by the adult mammalian arterial system. The dissociation of the right sixth or pulmonary arch with the right aortic arch is considered the boundary between the two phases since this occurrence allows the formation of the pulmonary vascular system and separates the single circulation into a systemic and pulmonary circulation. The branchial phase lasts twenty-two days, and the main changes of the second phase lasts only fourteen days more. The period when the major congenital anomalies of the aortic arch system may occur is over about the time the mother realizes she is pregnant.

The aortic arches develop from a plexiform capillary net. Their central or arterial attachment is to an aortic sac, a vascular bulge just above the heart, and they terminate in the paired dorsal aorta. The plexus from which the pulmonary arch develops is not so restricted. The developing pulmonary arch may begin by independent extensions from the dorsal aorta and the aortic sac. A twig from the plexus originating at the aortic sac then passes to the pulmonary plexus on the trachea, the extension from the dorsal aorta joins this and completes the arch, and leaves the distal portion as the primitive pulmonary artery (2). In addition to arising first at its terminations the proximal end is plexiform in nature. The early development thus lends itself to two kinds of anomalies, (a) multiple channels, which can occur during the formation of vessels from a rudimentary network and (b) if the sprout from the dorsal aorta does not occur the ductus should be absent since this appears to represent the origin of the ductus and is the terminal part of the arch, the segment distal to the pulmonary artery. Further, it is easy to conceive other abnormalities of connections between the two vessels which go to form the pulmonary arch, stenosis at the site of the connection or abnormal dilatation at the origin of the dorsal twig from the aorta or from the ventral twig.

The sixth arch is more variable at its junction with the aorta, since it may be separated by an interval from the fourth arch or may be close to it or have a common upper end. The anatomical position of insertion into the adult aortic arch thus may be variable. It may be low on the arch, or it may be high on the arch. There is an embryological explanation for the peculiarities of anatomical position of the aortic insertion and hence abnormalities of the course of the ductus arteriosus which have been observed. It may well lie well below the origin of the subclavian, and have an almost horizontal position, or it may insert high on the aortic arch, even proximal to the left common carotid artery, although this is rare.

While it is not the purpose of this review to describe in detail the formation and disappearance of the branchial arch system, a few points should be emphasized. One is that the primitive left sub-clavian artery arises at a point below the fusion of the paired dorsal aortae, and moves upward along the left fourth arch until it passes the insertion of the left pulmonary arch, and hence the ductus arteriosus, and comes to lie above the ductus. But at one time the insertion of the ductus arteriosus lies well above the left subclavian. This anomaly of insertion is occasionally found in the human, frequently in association with stenosis or coarctation of the aorta below their junction. The forces which cause the subclavian to move upward along the arch are not clear, but presumably the movement is due to unequal growth of the side containing the vessel and the area opposite this (3). Since the left subclavian moves past the ductus insertion, it is possible for it to become fixed in this posi-tion should the process of movement be arrested, and thus the ductus sometimes inserts at the origin of the left subclavian artery. In this case, the area of the aorta between the subclavian and the insertion of the ductus, the isthmus of the aorta, does not exist. In one of the rare anatomical anomalies of the ductus the left sub-clavian artery forms a direct continuation of the ductus without having any attachment to the aorta. Presumably during its passage up the dorsal aorta this anomaly could arise if the subclavian had a more or less common insertion into the aorta at the level of the ductus and if the left aortic arch segments above and below this area disappear. The left subclavian is a direct continuation of the ductus. This usually occurs on the left and there is a right aortic arch. The aortic root segments involved have been described by Barry (3) (Fig. 4).

Congdon placed the beginning of the postbranchial phase of the arch system when the right pulmonary arch separated from the right dorsal aorta, thus releasing the vessel to partake in the formation of the pulmonary artery system. The proximal part of the sixth arch, the portion up to the point where the primitive pulmonary artery arises persists as the origin of the right pulmonary artery. The angle between this and the beginning pulmonary artery lessens. The pul-monary arches arise from the aortic sac close to the midsaggital

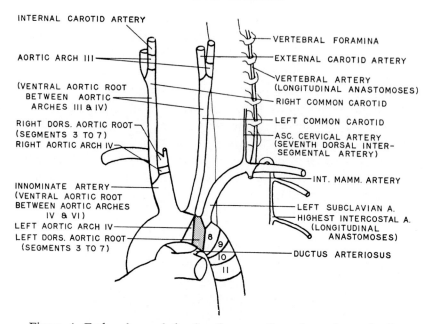

INTERNAL CAROTID ARTERY

AORTIC ARCH III

(VENTRAL AORTIC ROOT
  BETWEEN AORTIC
  ARCHES III & IV)

RIGHT DORS. AORTIC ROOT
(SEGMENTS 3 TO 7)
RIGHT AORTIC ARCH IV

INNOMINATE ARTERY
(VENTRAL AORTIC ROOT
BETWEEN AORTIC ARCHES
     IV & VI)
LEFT AORTIC ARCH IV
LEFT DORS. AORTIC ROOT
(SEGMENTS 3 TO 7)

VERTEBRAL FORAMINA

EXTERNAL CAROTID ARTERY

VERTEBRAL ARTERY
(LONGITUDINAL ANASTOMOSES)

RIGHT COMMON CAROTID

LEFT COMMON CAROTID

ASC. CERVICAL ARTERY
(SEVENTH DORSAL INTER-
  SEGMENTAL ARTERY)

INT. MAMM. ARTERY

LEFT SUBCLAVIAN A.
HIGHEST INTERCOSTAL A.
(LONGITUDINAL
  ANASTOMOSES)

DUCTUS ARTERIOSUS

Figure 4. Embryology of the fourth or aortic arch as shown by Barry
(3). The fourth left aortic root actually contributes only a part of the
arch.
Redrawn from Barry, A.: *Anat Rec, 111*:221, 1951.

plane, and a part of the sac containing their origins separates off,
giving a pulmonary trunk and its two branches. The pulmonary
trunk and the left pulmonary arch align, giving a relatively straight
pulmonary channel from the right ventricle to the aorta. The two
primitive pulmonary arteries approach each other, and at 40 mm
come off side by side, their length becoming shorter.

Table III, abstracted from Table II of Congdon relates fetal length, age and some events of fourth and sixth arches.

TABLE III

AORTIC-ARCH SYSTEM IN THE HUMAN EMBRYO

Length in mm	*Arches Present*	*Characteristic Features*
	(Just before establishment of fourth arch; estimated average length 4 mm; 31st day of development*)	
4	III, IV; pulmonary arches almost complete	
4	III, IV; one so-called fifth arch; pulmonary almost complete	Early formation of basilar artery
5	III, IV, and pulmonary arches	Late stage in formation of basilar artery. Splitting of aortic sac distinct. Unpaired aorta complete
6	III, IV, and pulmonary arches	
7	III, IV, two so-called fifth arches, and pulmonary arches	Subclavian artery surrounded by brachial plexus. Splitting of sac well marked. Islands at end of basilar artery.
8	III, IV, and pulmonary arches	Pulmonary and IV arches widely separated below.

*Estimates based on Mall's (1912) curve of length and age
(From Congdon, E.D. Extracted from Contributions to Embryology, No. 68 *14*:47, 1922.)

This is about the permanent organization of the pulmonary arterial system. There is a main trunk, with right and left pulmonary arteries, with a continuation from the left pulmonary artery, the ductus arteriosus, extending to the distal part of the dorsal aorta. A variety of possibilities exist between right and left aortic arches and a right or left ductus arteriosus.

Figures 5, 6, 7 and 8 selected from Congdon's monograph, illustrate the arch system in 5 mm, 14 mm and 18 mm embryos, as related to the fourth and sixth arches. In figures 5 and 6 the third arch has not yet changed, the fourth which will become the aorta is evident, but only the dorsal sprout of the sixth, the aortic origin of the subsequent ductus and a segment of the primitive pulmonary artery are present. The ventral sprout of the ductus arteriosus is not seen.

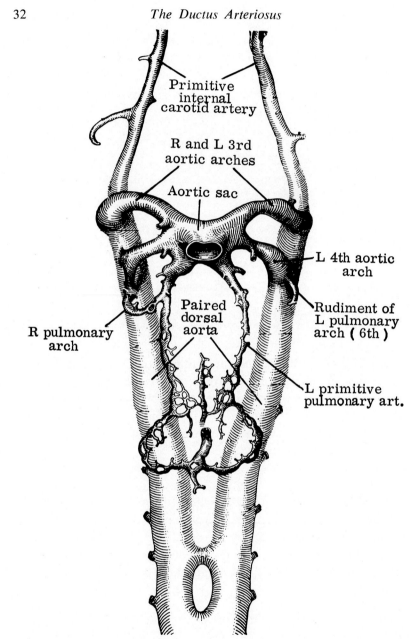

Figure 5. Ventral view of a 5 mm embryo. The third and fourth arches have reached maximum development. The dorsal and ventral sprouts of the pulmonary arch have nearly met. The primitive pulmonary arteries have considerable length.

From Congdon, E.D. Extracted from *Contr Embry,* no. 68 *14*:47, 1922. By courtesy of Carnegie Institution of Washington.

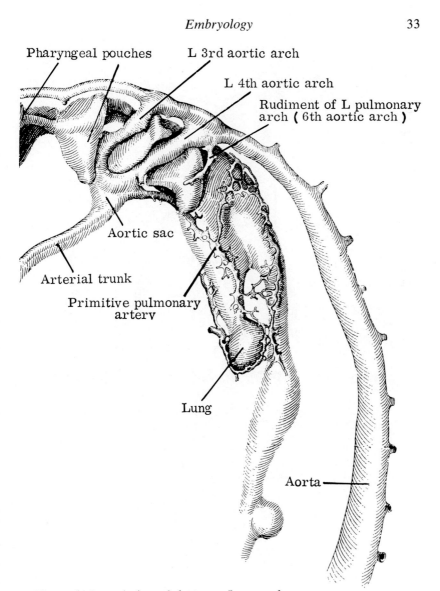

Pharyngeal pouches   L 3rd aortic arch

L 4th aortic arch

Rudiment of L pulmonary
arch (6th aortic arch)

Aortic sac

Arterial trunk

Primitive pulmonary
artery

Lung

Aorta

Figure 6. Lateral view of the same 5 mm embryo.
By courtesy of Carnegie Institution of Washington.
From Congdon, E.D. Extracted from *Contr Embry,* no. 68 *14*:47, 1922.

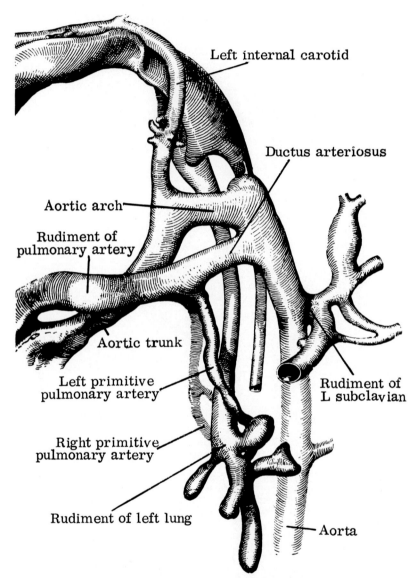

Figure 7. At 14 mm the general form of the definitive arch system is recognizable. The third arch has evolved into the carotid system. The 4th arch remains as a contribution to the adult aorta and the 6th arch exists as the primitive pulmonary artery and its continuation into the aorta, the ductus extension.

By courtesy of Carnegie Institution of Washington.

From Congdon, E.D. Extracted from *Contr Embry*, no. 68 *14*:47, 1922.

At 14 mm (Fig. 7) the general form of the definitive arch system is recognizable. The third arch as such has evolved into the carotid system. The fourth arch remains as a contribution to the adult aorta and the sixth arch exists as the primitive pulmonary artery and its continuation into the aorta, the ductus extension.

At 18 mm (Fig. 8) the adult arch system with a left aortic arch and ductus is nearly complete.

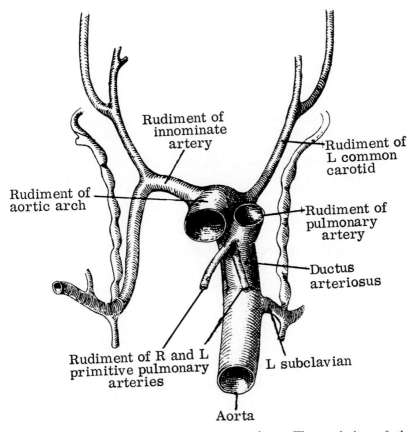

Rudiment of innominate artery

Rudiment of L common carotid

Rudiment of aortic arch

Rudiment of pulmonary artery

Ductus arteriosus

Rudiment of R and L primitive pulmonary arteries

L subclavian

Aorta

Figurt 8. Ventral view of an 18 mm embryo. The evolution of the arches has proceeded to a point where the adult arterial system is recognizable.

By Courtesy of Carnegie Institution of Washington.
From Congdon, E.D. Extracted from *Contr Embry*, no. 68 *14*:47, 1922.

Rychter (4) reviewed in detail the experimental morphology of the aortic arches and outlined sixty-two possible combinations in the chick embryo by eliminating specific aortic arches by clips. Of special interest were the studies related to suppression of the sixth right or left arch, to eliminate the ductus. Rychter (4) states he and Lemez found a constant disturbance in the ventricular septum after closure of both sixth right and sixth left arch. They studied the hemodynamic effect of suppression of both pulmonary arches by injecting dye into the right ventricle. This flowed into the pulmonary arteries, but in addition the left fourth arch became colored and the blood flow prevented its disappearance.

REFERENCES

1. Congdon, E.D.: Transformation of the aortic-arch system during the development of the human embryo. Extracted from Contributions to Embryology, No. 68 *14*:47, 1922.
2. Evans, H.M.: III. The Development of the Vascular System. In Keibel, Franz, and Mall, Franklin, P.: *Human Embryology*. Philadelphia, Lippincott, 1912, vol. II, p. 570.
3. Barry, A.: The aortic arch derivatives in the human adult. *Anat Rec, 111*:221, 1951.
4. Rychter, Z.: Experimental morphology of the aortic arches and the heart loop in chick embryos. *Adv Morphog, 2*:333, 1962.

Five

HISTOLOGY

It has been obvious to all observers that regardless of the immediate status of the ductus arteriosus after birth, its usual fate was transformation into an impervious ligament. With the advent of microscopy this process was studied in great detail by many investigators and these studies continue especially with the advent of histochemistry and electron microscopy. The considerable literature on this subject divided itself into three parts, the histology of the normal ductus prior to closure, the histological changes in the ductus tissue during the process of anatomical obliteration, and the state of the vessel walls after this process is more or less complete, for closure is never uniform throughout. There are few studies of the histology of persistent patency of the ductus arteriosus.

The ductus arteriosus had been considered similar to any other artery and even Rokitansky (1) found no histological difference between the aorta and the ductus. He believed closure resulted from direct adhesion and fusion of its walls without the mediation of the thrombus formation. As recently as 1902 Pfeiffer (2) reiterated this statement. This view was soon contradicted, and Langer (3) in 1857 usually is given credit for first describing the histological differences between the ductus and the aorta and pulmonary artery, although the muscular nature of the vessel had been mentioned previously.

Langer wrote as follows:

> I found significant differences, not only in mature, but even in 5 to 7 month fetuses. While the great vessels show sharply outlined fiber plates in their three distinctly delimited layers, especially in the media.

37

no such fibers can be demonstrated in the ductus. Here one sees only oblong nuclei concentrically arranged in close proximity. The concentric layers are interspersed with well defined groups of nuclei which apparently course longitudinally. The boundaries between the individual layers are somewhat obscured; otherwise the ductus walls have the same thickness as those of the aorta and pulmonary artery.

He noted proliferation of nuclei on the surface of the intima which gave a wrinkled appearance to the inner surface of the ductus. He stated that elastic tissue did not occur, but instead there was a kind of connective tissue which contained scattered short spindle-shaped cells. He observed that in longitudinal sections of the site of insertion of the ductus into the aorta and pulmonary artery the bundles of elastic fibers from the media of the arteries gradually wedged themselves into the ductus and contributed isolated loose fibers to the adventitia. He noted the caliber of the ductus corresponded to that of the pulmonary arteries,

> but its walls are so tensile that they dilate aneurysmally upon injection.

Langer stated postnatal changes did not become evident until the ninth day after birth when the proliferation on the wrinkled inner surface increased especially toward the middle so that the lumen took the shape of an hourglass. The longitudinal layers also proliferated so that on the fourteenth day the ductus was "barely pervious to a pin." In the third month connective tissue developed in the newly formed tissues.

He stated categorically these continued changes caused the ductus to shrink in length and thickness. Confirmation of change in length is difficult to find.

The studies of Langer (3) and especially the detailed histological description of Walkoff (4) in 1869 represent an important epoch in the anatomical description of the ductus arteriosus.

Because of the excellence of its illustrations and the general importance of this interesting 1869 medical document, it is summarized in some detail.

> I. On the basis of the studies by Walkoff of the ductus arteriosus in the newborn, the obliterating ductus and the ligamentum arteriosum, the author agreed with Langer that the ductus in fetal life and in the newborn differs histologically from the aorta and the pulmonary

artery by its loose structure and scarcity of elastic fibers.

II. A detailed description of the histology of the ductus is given, together with Walkoff's opinion of the factors entering into the process of obliteration. The histological aspects of the ductus at birth were outlined as follows:

In a Median section

1. Intima consists of

   a. epithelium (or endothelium)

   b. thin hyaline connective tissue enclosing oval nuclei and spindle-shaped elements interpreted as primordial connective and elastic tissue.

   c. a boundary of dense connective tissue and elastic fibers, corresponding to the fenestrated membrane in the great vessels, the internal elastic membrane.

2. Media

   a. elastic fiber plates and interstitial muscle cells are absent.

   b. there is an elastic network derived from elastic fiber bundles diffusing from aorta and pulmonary artery and containing longitudinally arranged cellular elements. In contrast to Langer who regarded these latter as nuclei. Walkoff considered these to be primordial elastic and connective tissue cells.

3. Adventitia—this does not differ from that of the aorta and pulmonary artery except that connective tissue exceeds elastic tissue.

4. At the ostia

The histology is similar to that toward the center of the ductus except that the walls of both ostia contain connective tissue and elastic fibers from the aorta and pulmonary artery. These enter the ductus in the form of thick bundles and then disperse toward the middle of the vessel.

III. Obliteration of the ductus is assumed to have three aspects.

1. Postnatal changes in the position of the ductus and the lungs which result from the onset of respiration and cause a sharp bend in the ductus and a slowed circulation.

2. Thrombosis is influenced by slower flow and contributes to obstruction of the lumen by *thrombus tissue.*

3. Histological changes are produced chiefly by proliferation of the epithelium and connective tissue layers of the intima and the longitudinal tracts of the media. It is these that cause the wrinkling of the surface of the intima.

IV. The obliterated ductus, now the ligamentum arteriosum, is characterized by:

1. Shrinking and reduction in size, both in length and diameter.

2. A strongly plicated but still recognizable intima.

3. Organized *thrombus tissue* filling the former lumen.

4. Taking over of the media by connective and elastic tissue.

5. An elastic network in the adventitia.

6. Strongly contracted ostia with a less plicated intima. The obliterated ostia may form small blind indentations, or a fine canal may persist in the ligamentum.

The histology of the fetal ductus and the histology of the process of obliteration became a popular subject for continental doctorate theses and for numerous papers in journals of most countries. In general, they agreed anatomical closure was brought about by proliferation of tissue in the substance of the intima and media, and following this proliferation the muscular nature of the media disappeared and was replaced by connective tissue. Modern descriptions are in essential agreement. It should be noted that the peculiar wrinkling of the intima which is a feature of the newborn ductus was described by Trew (5) in 1736.

The description of Gerard in 1900 (6) is completely modern in most respects. He concluded that in the first few days of life the internal layer alone participated in obliteration and in this layer only the connective tissue elements took part. Eminences or prominences are produced irregularly by proliferation of connective tissue and later elastic tissue multiplies. He coined the phrase *intimal mounds*. He said these endothelial prominences play the chief role in diminution and finally obliteration of the lumen, except that a permanent small central lumen is always found in restricted areas. By the end of the first year the convex summit of the mounds reach the opposite wall or each other and gradually unite. The process is tortuous with alternating areas of constriction.

Figure 9 demonstrates these intimal mounds very well. This is a longitudinal section of the ductus in a full term infant. Intimal proliferation rather than medial contraction seems to predominate.

The studies of Variot and Cailliau (7) in 1920, Melka (8) in 1926, Costa (9) in 1930 to 31, von Hayek (10) in 1935, Barnard (11) and Swensson (12) in 1939 and Jager and Wollenman (13) in 1942 may be taken as representative of current opinion.

It should be noted incidentally that Swensson (12) states that in the 35 cm fetus there is no difference in structure between the ductus and aorta. In the early fetal state there is no internal elastic membrane or it is difficult to stain, and this may form about the 10 mm fetal stage. The intima is thicker and according to Costa is

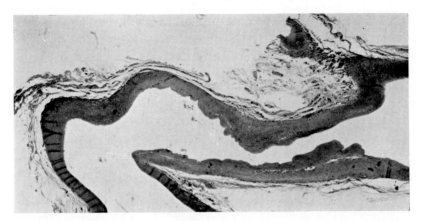

Figure 9. A longitudinal section of the ductus arteriosus in a full term newborn. The ductus extends from the aorta to the pulmonary artery. The intimal mounds of normal anatomical closure are quite evident and are present throughout the length of the ductus. There is considerable variation of the thickness of the intima which does not seem to be related to medial contraction. (H & E Stain X10.)

about one-third the width of the media of the ductus and about one-fifteenth as wide as the media of the aorta. In addition to being relatively thick, it is irregularly thickened by protuberances such as described by Gerard. These vary in number, thickness and length from location to location. They have been identified in the fetus of five to six months and are the active proliferating elements which contribute to the wrinkling of the inner surface of the vessel and the closure of the lumen.

This wrinkling which is so much a feature of the ductus in contrast to the smooth intima of other arteries certainly may be influenced by muscular contraction, as emphasized by Reynolds (14). But the histological studies have certainly identified the intimal and subintimal areas as important elements as the mechanism of anatomical obliteration.

In a three-month embryo the internal layer is a simple endothelial cellular layer with elongated nuclei. At four and one-half months the internal elastic layer has formed and a homogenous substance has formed above and below it. This stains poorly and contains numerous embryonic cells. Jager and Wollenman (13) note that at 28 cm or three months the thick internal elastic lamina was subendothelial except in several areas where low mounds projected into the lumen. These are described as composed of smooth muscle and moderate numbers of fine wavy underlying elastic lamina. Up to 45 cm the intimal mounds increased in size, with a greater tendency to fragmentation of the internal elastic membrane. At full term the mounds are larger and contain collagen. During closure of the ductus they increase in size, the collagen increases and fragmentation of the internal elastic membrane continues.

From one to three months of age obliteration was effected by increasing size of the mounds, with or without overlying caps of connective tissue.

The mounds contained more and more elastic tissue and increasing amounts of collagen. The smooth muscle fibers became less conspicuous and the internal lamina was often obscured by elastic fibers in the intima and media.

The size and time of appearance of the connective tissue caps, which projected into and diminished the lumen, were variable. They are generally considered to be subendothelial and to arise as an outgrowth of similar tissue in the mounds, but are differentiated from the mounds themselves by the absence of elastic fibers. Some of the time the expanding connective tissue caps appear to fuse. Rarely a thrombus occludes the lumen, and this organizes.

Variot and Cailliau (7) emphasize the appearance and gradual increase of poorly stained amorphous material in the intimal mounds, and state this substance does not take hyaline stain and is not fibrin. They describe the presence in it of proliferating embryonic cells and brilliant refractory globules which do not take fat stains. Barnard (11) called this substance edema. Others have emphasized this as a mucoid substance.

Since the advent of proper histological study, and especially since Langer and Walkoff, there has been general agreement on the muscular nature of the ductus arteriosus. There has been some discrepancy in the descriptions of the muscle fibers of the media.

The media is muscular even in the early embryo. At 28 cm, the media is loose and is composed of smooth muscle and fine wavy elastic fibers and the smooth muscle fibers are fusiform and contain an elongated nucleus (7). These fibers are inserted in a framework of loose supporting connective tissue. They have a different arrangement according to different authors. Just beneath the internal lamina the muscle fibers have an oblique or radial arrangement, while in the outer portion of the media they are circular, with a few longitudinal fibers (13). The media changes slowly with aging, the fibers thinning, the connective tissue framework increasing and the width of the media decreasing (7). From birth to three to four weeks the media becomes more cellular, the muscle fibers are reduced and it is invaded by elastic tissue. This invasion progresses and much connective tissue and fibroblasts are added. By about five months after birth the ductus approaches the elastic arterial type, except that it is losing its muscular nature by atrophy of muscle and the progressive formation of connective tissue and fibroblasts.

Some of the variation in descriptions of the course and direction of the muscle fibers in the middle layer are no doubt due to individual differences in the vessel and the point at which sections were made and possibly in the direction or obliquity of the section itself. Most frequently the muscle fibers have been described as primarily circular, especially by earlier authors, but some emphasized the longitudinal structure of the muscle. Melka described three layers in the media, while Costa reported the inner two thirds of the media had a circular muscle layer while the outer part had a more oblique or longitudinal layer. Other combinations have been described.

This problem of the direction of the muscle fibers of the media probably has been resolved by the methodical studies of von Hayek (10). He sectioned the whole ductus arteriosus in different planes. He found two coats of smooth muscle. The fibers in both of these formed a set of helicoid spirals, but the two spirals went in opposite directions. The spiraling was more acute in the outer layer and, therefore, the fibers appear more nearly circular, but in the inner layer the spirals formed more gradually and appeared to be more longitudinal. The more the ductus is dilated the more circular the muscle fibers become, and the more contracted the ductus becomes the more longitudinally the muscle fibers are oriented. Thus, sections give different appearances in different states of contraction or relaxation and differ according to the plane of the section.

The ligamentum arteriosum may contain a small slitlike lumen which may course throughout the vessel or may be confined to a small area. Degenerative processes increase, and the media becomes dense in collagen and elastic tissue. Fragments of the internal elastic lamina may remain, but the border between intima and media becomes lost. Usually the ligament is represented by a mass of dense elastic tissue, collagen, hyaline material and a small amount of smooth muscle in the outer portion of the wall. The intima of the pulmonary artery and aorta becomes thickened over the ends of the ductus and later atheromatous placques may be found there. Cartilage, calcification or even bone formation may be found in the remains of the ductus arteriosus.

Rarely, in the newborn, peculiar pathological changes may be found. Hemorrhages may appear in the wall with elevation of the intima, and Jager and Wollenman (13) reported mucinous degeneration with cyst formation in the ductus from a full term infant. A dissecting aneurysm has been seen in the wall of the ductus.

It is clear the histological processes of anatomical closure may be slow or rapid, and variation in obliteration of the lumen may occur in different parts of the same vessel.

A brief summary of closure of the ductus may be made: the vessel is relatively muscular and contains less elastic tissue than the aorta or pulmonary artery. The internal layer of the ductus has peculiar properties, and produces protuberances or mounds or pillows which appear to arise from the elastic lamina which fragments beneath them. These mounds are composed of smooth muscle and elastic tissue and make the lumen eccentric by projecting into it. Connective tissue caps may appear at the summit of the mounds, aiding in occlusion of the lumen. Collagen infiltrates the mounds. Meanwhile, the elastic tissue increases in the intima and media. The muscle fibers of the media atrophy and elastic and connective tissue takes over this area, leaving only a remnant of the muscular layer which previously had been a characteristic and differentiating point.

If anatomical closure is determined by variation in the newborn hemodynamics, it is difficult to explain the instances of closure only at the pulmonary artery end of the ductus, sometimes only by a membrane, with the aortic terminus widely patent, as a funnel. Closure by membrane apparently does not occur at the aortic end.

There is, in addition a rich supply of nerves, an accumulation of cells similar to those in the carotid body at the junctions of the ductus with the aorta and the pulmonary artery. These lie in the angle of these junctions in such a way that they should be very susceptible to pressure stimuli. It is possible they are chemo-receptor mechanisms, and there is some evidence they are sensitive to changes in oxygen concentration.

This question of artifact by contraction has been the subject of different kinds of studies. The question has been raised why postmortem contraction should produce contraction and wrinkling of the intima since postmortem blood vessel contraction is not a feature of other vessels. Prellot (15) believed the ridges and folds characteristic of the obliterating ductus were due to proliferation. He immersed a piece of guinea pig aorta in adrenalin and the vessel, contracted evenly and concentrically without showing ridges and mounds of the ductus. A control piece remained smooth and uncontracted without adrenalin.

Bunce (16) made a systematic study of distended and collapsed arteries. Using an instrument which was essentially two pairs of hemostats with a simple handle he removed arteries normally distended with blood from animals in vivo. These were compared with similar collapsed vessels obtained postmortem.

He found that a collapsed vessel removed from living animal contracts more than a postmortem vessel. In distended vessels the intima is compressed but in the collapsed artery the intima may be greatly thickened and the lumen greatly reduced. Subendothelial cushions may be formed in collapsed vessels and appear to protrude into the lumen.

Bakker (17) used fixation of the ductus under pressure for the study of this question and found a smooth lumen without endocardial cushions and a thin wall. The danger of overdistention is recognized. Hornblad (18) used whole body freezing in five species of animals and found at birth a smooth inner surface lined by a single layer of flat endothelial cells.

STUDIES OF COSTA

The study of Costa (9) is considered by some to be the best. This is difficult and highly personalized and rambling but is a detailed study based upon sixty human embryos at the second and third months and fetuses and infants during the first year.

He noted the ductus wall had three layers in all fetal cases studied. These were more or less marked in various stages but were always present.

The intima he said is characterized by (a) great thickness and irregularity, (b) scarcity of elastic fibers, (c) an abundance of muscle cells oriented longitudinally and (d) presence of much mucoid material.

He emphasizes the thickness of the intima in all fetal ages by a table (Table IV).

TABLE IV

THICKNESS OF INTIMA AND MEDIA OF THE
DUCTUS ARTERIOSUS AND AORTA IN FETAL LIFE

Age	Intima of Duct	Intima of Aorta	Media of Duct	Relationship of Media to Intima	Media of Aorta	Relationship of Media and Intima of Aorta
4th-5th mo	(30)-50	10	200	4	150	15
6th-7th mo	70-150	10	500	3	450	45
8th mo	100-150	15	500	3	450	30
9th mo	150	15	500	3	500	30

(From Costa, A. Cuore E Circolazione 14:546, 1930.) Thickness of the intima and media of the ductus and the aorta are shown in micro meters. The relation of these in each vessel are shown.

The intima has layers of longitudinal muscle cells which are prominent early in fetal life and grow throughout this period.

Connective tissue is very rare in the intima and media early, but increases slightly.

The intima and inner two thirds of the media have a very intense impregnation with a substance which reacts metachromatically and makes the area involved appear edematous. This imbibation is characteristic of the ductus in contrast to the walls of the aorta and pulmonary vessels. It is present throughout fetal life.

Elastic tissue is always very sparse in the media, but a rare thin lamella is seen occasionally. The specific differentiation of mucle structures make the vessel a muscular type vessel.

A circular mucle layer is found in the internal two thirds of the media. Outside of this but without a boundary of elastic or connective tissue there is an oblique or longitudinal muscle layer.

The insertion of the ductus into the aorta and pulmonary artery can be seen from the first part of fetal life. The wall of the ductus is lacking in elastic tissue and highly impregnated with a mucoid substance. The ductus intima with all of its characteristics penetrates between the endothelium and the media of the aorta. Sometimes the adventitia of the aorta for a short distance is the external portion of the media.

The wall of the ductus enfolds the aortic wall squeezing the highly elastic media of the aorta between its layers. Normally the ductus tissue doesn't completely encircle the aortic circumference but is limited to the area of attachment of the ductus. This insertion into the aorta lengthens caudally in the aortic wall, but not cranially, as Costa showed in longitudinal sections parallel to the aortic wall. These show the caudal part of the aortic wall under the ductus with a subintimal wedge of tissue rich in mucin in contrast to the elastic tissue of the aorta.

There is no real discussion relating to the junction of the ductus and pulmonary artery. All investigations in all studies, both of the ductus and of coarctation of the aorta, concentrate on the ductus-aorta connection. This connection, however, is said to resemble the insertion at the aorta.

This meticulous long term study of Costa in 1930 probably continues as the best single study of the histology of the ductus. In addition to his own observations, of great interest is his section entitled "Confrontation with the reports and interpretations of other investigations" in which he reviews previous studies and discusses differences.

He makes these points:

1. He believes a typical chronology of events does not exist, but there is striking diversity in the facets of closure. In fetal life the intima is thick and irregular with little elastic tissue, rich in longitudinal muscle cells and in mucoid substance.

2. Proliferative processes of elastic and connective tissue which lead to progressive and irregular thickening of the intima are some of the first morphological modifications the vessel undergoes in extra-uterine life. There is intense hyperplasia of the internal elastic membrane and elastic differentiation of the media.

3. The mucoid impregnation diminishes, but intimal proliferation is not sufficient to complete anatomical closure which is produced by a calcareous cylinder surrounded by fibro-elastic sclerosis.

Involution of the Ductus

Again he emphasizes the variability of the process and that no simple chronology can be ascribed to closure. He notes in some cases the ductus remains perfectly pervious, the intima keeps its fetal thickness, the elastic lamella in the intima and media remain thin and the elastica intima more autonomous. Mucoid impregnation remains intense. There is no atrophy or degeneration of the muscle cells.

In others, the intima is greatly thickened, sometimes double that of the late fetal stages. Elastic lamella become more numerous, the elastica intima appears as a wide fascia, an entanglement of disordered fibrils. Elastic structures of the media are well developed, the circular type predominating. The muscle tissue at this stage does not have an increase of collagen or precollagen connective tissue, but mucoid imbibation disappears in most of the media.

The processes continue, the lumen completely or nearly disappears and has a central and calcareous residue. Extremely active proliferation of precollagen and collagen produces destruction of groups of muscle cells.

This long and detailed study continues to be an important and current document related to study of the ductus arteriosus. The histological events are being studied further with the electron microscope. The study of Silva and Ikeda (19) was primarily concerned with innervation especially the distribution of cholinesterase containing fibers, but a description of ductus tissue was included. However, the paper does not clearly distinguish references to ductus tissue from that of the aorta and pulmonary arteries.

The anatomic ultrastructure of the ductus was studied in the rat fetus and twenty-four hours postdelivery by the technique of electron microscopy by Jones, Barrow and Wheat (20). Postdelivery the ductus was closed and light microscopy showed only a trace of a lumen. The center was fitted with pyknotic nuclei and endothelial cells with remnants of internal elastic membrane layers of rounder smooth muscle cells and spindle-shaped smooth muscle cells.

The prenatal ductus arteriosus studied with the electron microscope was found to have an endothelium projecting into the lumen in many places. These conspicuous projections were thought to be preliminary to necrosis seen in the central endothelial cells of the closed ductus.

Smooth muscle cells extended through and interrupted the internal elastic membrane and lay between the subendothelial space and the media. This cellular arrangement was thought to be preliminary structural change to later obliteration. Elastic lamellae were often broken or split by the intruding smooth muscle cells.

This cellular organization is similar to the changes described by Esterly, Glagov and Ferguson (21) in their study of the changes in small pulmonary arteries following the production of pulmonary hypertension in the dog.

Evidence of protein synthesis was believed indicated by many smooth muscle cells with extremely distended cisternae of rough endoplasmic reticulum. This was especially evident in the ductus prior to delivery.

Further examination of the twenty-four hour specimens indicated the medial smooth muscle cells of the ductus are different than those described in other arteries, they show evidence of active metabolism and protein synthesis as indicated by "abundant endoplastic reticulum and ribosomes with intimately associated mitochondria."

The differences between the ultrastructure of the ductus and the aorta and pulmonary artery which are suggested as preparation for closure, are (a) subendothelial vacuolization, (b) extension of medial smooth muscle cells through the internal elastic membrane into the subendothelial space, (c) interruption of the elastic lamellae and (d) distended endoplastic reticulum.

They consider their observations compatible with closure of the ductus in rats as an active process that is initiated before birth of the fetus.

REFERENCES

1. Rokitansky, C.: Ueber einige der wichtigsten Krankheiten der arterien. *Demkschr Akad Wissensch Wien, 4*:1, 1852.
2. Pfieffer, B.: Zur Kenntniss des histologischen Baues und der Ruckbildung der Nabelgefasse und des Ductus Botalli. *Virchows Arch, 167*:210, 1902.
3. Langer, C.: Zur Anatomie der fotalen Kaeislaufsorgane, Z. Gesell Aertze, *13*:328, 1857.
4. Walkoff, F.: Das gewebe des ductus arteriosus und die obliteration. *Disselben Ztschn Med Leipz Heidele, 3,* R: 109, 1869.

5. Trew, C.J.: Dissertatio epistolica de differentiis quibusdam inter hominem natum et nascendum intercedentibus deque vestigiis divini numinis inde colligendis. Accedunt tabulae aeneae V. in duplo, alterae variis coloribus illustrate. Norimaerge prostat apud Ped. Cone. Monath, 1736.

6. Gerard, G.: Of the obliteration of the canal arterial, the theories and the facts. *J Anat Physiol, 36*:323, 1900.

7. Variot, G. and Cailliau, F.: Research on the process of obliteration of the arterial canal. *Bull Mem Soc Med Hop Paris, 44*:1598, 1920.

8. Melka, J.: Beitrag zur kenntnis der morphologie and obliteration des ductus arteriosus Botalli. *Anat Anz, 61*:348, 1926.

9. Costa, A.: La Minuta Struttura e le transformagioni involutive del botta arteriosus di Botallo vella specie mana. *Cuore Circ, 14*:546, 1930.

10. Von Hayek, H.: Der funktionelle Bau der Naberlarterien und des ductus Botalli. *Z Anat Entwicklungsgesch, 105*:15, 1935.

11. Barnard, W.B.: Pathological changes in wall of the ductus arteriosus. *St. Thomas Hosp Rep, 4*:72, 1939.

12. Swensson, A.: Beitrag zur Kenntnis von dem histologischen Bau und dem postembryonalen Verschluss des ductus arteriosus Botalli. *Z Mikrosk Anat Forsch, 46*:275, 1939.

13. Jager, B.V. and Wollenman, J.Jr.: Anatomic study of closure of the ductus arteriosus. *Am J Pathol, 18*:595, 1942.

14. Reynolds, S.R.M.: The proportion of Wharton's jelly in the umbilical cord. In relation to distension of the umbilical arteries and veins, with observations on the folds of Hoboken. *Anat Rec, 113*:365, 1952.

15. Prellot, G.L.T.H.W.: *Histologischer Bau und Rueck bildong des Ductus Arteriosus Botalli.* Histological structure and involution of ductus arteriosus. Dissertation Heidelberg, 1909, p. 31.

16. Bunce, D.F.M.: Structural differences between distended and collapsed arteries. *Angiology, 16*:53, 1965.

17. Bakker, P.M.: *Morfogenese en Involutie van de Ductus Arteriosus by De Mens.* (Thesis) Mouton and Co., Den Haag, 1962.

18. Hornblad, P.Y.: Experimental studies on closure of the ductus arteriosus utilizing whole-body freezing. *Acta Paediatr Scand,* Suppl. 190, 1969.

19. Silva, D.G. and Ikeda, M.: Ultrastructural and acetylcholinesterase studies of the innervation of the ductus arteriosus, pulmonary trunk and aorta of the fetal lamb. *J Ultrastruct Res, 345*:358, 1971.

20. Jones, M., Barrow, M.V. and Wheat, M.W.: An ultrastructural evaluation of the closure of the ductus arteriosus in rats. *Surgery, 66*:891, 1969.

21. Easterly, J..A., Glagov, S. and Ferguson, D.J.: Morphogenesis of internal obliterative hyperplasia of small arteries in experimental pulmonary hypertension. *Am J, Pathol, 52*:325, 1968.

Six

ANATOMY

THE ANATOMICAL POSITION OF THE DUCTUS ARTERIOSUS was described to some extent by the early anatomists. Most of the descriptions were brief notes relating to the origin and insertion of the vessel and to its dimensions, the length and width. Later, there was more detailed description of the topographical relation to other thoracic organs, and a more detailed analysis of this relationship formed the basis for one of the theories of closure.

The gross anatomy is both simple and complicated. It is simple because its embryology restricts the usual position which it can assume. It must extend from the pulmonary artery at its branching, slightly to the left of the midline and posterior to the surface of the right ventricle, to the aorta lying against the thoracic wall to the left of the vertebral column. Its course must be to the left, slightly upward and posteriorly, but this will vary some with (a) the length of the main pulmonary artery, (b) the position of the aorta and (c) the place of junction with the aorta.

The anatomy of the ductus can be considered in relation to (a) its origin at the aorta and its termination by junction with the pulmonary artery, (b) its size, in terms of length and diameter, (c) its shape and the normal variations of this, (d) its topography in relation to thoracic contents and (e) its relation to the pericardium. In addition, some of these anatomical aspects must be considered in relation to age and especially to the size and course of the artery. There are some studies of ductal size and variations in the fetus. An unusual study of the ductus size in twin fetus was made by Tsuchiya (1). This included monovular and fraternal twins. The percent variation in length was about 3.18 in monovular and 1.73 percent for fraternal, and in circumference 8.91 for mono-vular and 3.78 in fraternal. However, the variation in length was sometimes considerable (Table V).

TABLE V

THE SIZE OF THE DUCTUS ARTERIOSUS IN TWIN FETUS

Age (months)	Number Of Cases	Male length (cm)	Circumference (cm)	Number Of Cases	Female length (cm)	Circumference (cm)
5	0	—	—	2	0.35	0.50
6	2	0.38	0.65	6	0.35	0.61
7	12	0.41	0.92	2	0.48	1.27
8	1	0.40	1.15	3	0.42	1.30
9	5	0.50	1.15	1	0.50	1.30

The circumference of the ductus equaled that of the aorta in 6 of 34 fetus, was greater than in 24 and less than in 7. There was considerable variation in this ratio in the same monovular twins.
(From Tsuchiya, S.: Okahimas Folia Anatomica Japonica, *16*:275, 1938)

The position of the aortic arch which governs the site of the aortic end of the ductus varies considerably during growth. In the newborn the aorta arches nearly directly posteriorly, about 80 degrees to the frontal plane. Consequently, the left border of the arch cannot be identified by a conventional x-ray, even if the thymus did not obscure the area. With growth, the arch gradually assumes an adult position of about 65 degrees to the frontal plane. The presence or absence of a normal left aortic arch, so important in surgical considerations, can usually be identified in the early childhood age group. The size of the aorta plays a role in visibility, and with patency of the ductus arteriosus it tends to be larger, commensurate with increased blood flow. Whether enlargement and dilatation of the left ventricle and some rotation of the heart plays a role in the position of the aorta is not clear.

Noback and Rehman (2) have emphasized that in the newborn the ductus joins the aorta on the anterolateral border and not on its medial aspect. Consequently, it bulges laterally beyond the border of the aorta. This can be seen rarely in the x-ray because of the obscuring thymus. However this junction on the anterolateral border of the aorta was noted by Gerard (3) and has been confirmed by Wilson (4). This can be seen in the newborn when the thymus is dissected free and the lung retracted. Figure 10 shows this quite well. The drawing was made from a full term infant, age one day. The descending aorta has been omitted for clarity. Figure

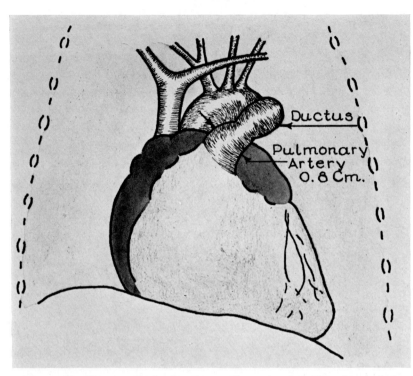

Figure 10. Heart and vessels of a newborn in situ. The ductus bulges laterally to the aorta. The descending aorta has been omitted for clarity.

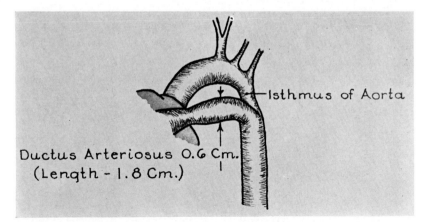

Figure 11. The ductus arteriosus has been displaced downward. The ductus diameter is 0.6 cm, the aorta and pulmonary artery 0.8 cm.

11 and Figure 12 give measurements of the descending aorta, ductus arteriosus and aortic isthmus.

In the fetus and newborn the ductus is usually described as a direct continuation of the pulmonary artery (5, 6) so it may appear that a large vessel extending to the aorta arises off two branches, the right and left pulmonary arteries. Later it is usually noted to arise from the base of the left pulmonary artery 1 to 2 mm distal to the bifurcation of the main pulmonary artery. There are a few reports of what must be an unusual origin from the same site on the right pulmonary artery, or on the posterior surface of the pulmonary trunk. Consideration of the embryology of the pulmonary artery and the left pulmonary arch and the fact that the ductus itself starts as a ventral sprout and meets a dorsal sprout from the primitive aorta makes it clear that the position of the ductus in relation to the pulmonary artery may be variable.

The description of Gerard (3) seems reasonable and accurate:

> Sometimes it arises at the level of the bifurcation of the pulmonary artery and then the ductus seems to give rise to the left pulmonary artery itself. At other times it arises a little to the left of the bifurcation, 1 to 2 mm from the left pulmonary artery itself, from which it can be differentiated by a paler color and a less dense consistency. Rarely it can commence on the posterior surface of the pulmonary artery, a little to the left of the bifurcation, or on the anterior surface in front of the bifurcation.

However, this anatomical bulge of the ductus lateral to the aorta can be seen on x-ray if penetration is appropriate. This was referred to as the *ductus bump* by Berdon, Baker and James (7). This disappears on serial examinations and probably is the correct interpretation of the observation. This is shown in Figure 13 in a one-day old infant. The percent of newborn x-rays in which this can be seen is not known.

The position of the ductus is easily seen in Figure 14, where a catheter retrograde in the aorta enters the ductus and shows its position lateral to the aorta (8).

Perhaps a reasonable thesis would be that the primitive left pulmonary artery carries with it the ventral sprout or the terminus of the ductus in its amalgamation with the main pulmonary trunk. If the taking up of the left pulmonary artery into the main pulmonary trunk is very complete the ductus arises at the bifurcation. If it is less complete it arises from the base of the left pulmonary artery. During this process of shortening the left pulmonary artery may

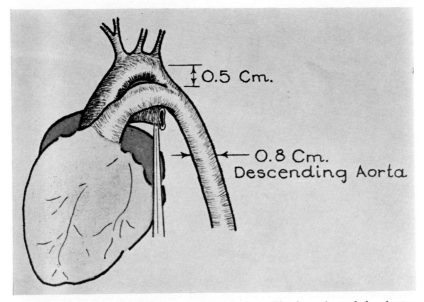

Figure 12. The same dissection, lateral view. The insertion of the ductus on the anterolateral border of the aorta is seen well. The arching of the ductus arteriosus has been disturbed some.

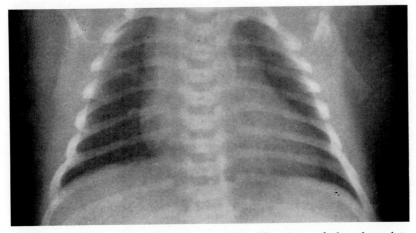

Figure 13. X-ray of a one day old infant. The ductus bulges lateral to the aorta, the ductus *bump* of Berdon, Baker and James (7).

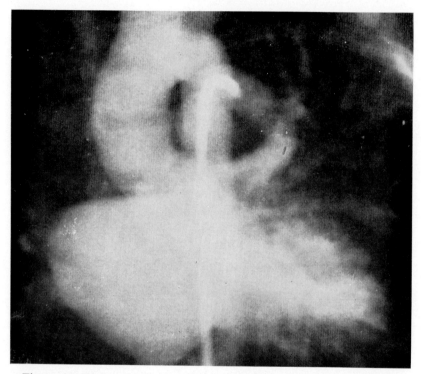

Figure 14. The patent ductus arteriosus fills from a catheter introduced retrograde in the aorta. The large flow outlines the ductus and pulmonary artery.
From Prec, K.J., Cassels, D.E., Rabinowitz, M. and Moulder, P.V.: *J Pediatr, 61*:843, 1962.

carry the ductus well on to the main pulmonary artery, although this should be considered anomalous. Likewise, minor changes in rotation will carry the ductus insertion a little anteriorly or posteriorly.

It seems necessary to assume some differential growth of the left pulmonary artery which carries the ductus insertion to the left, since in the newborn it is rather uniformly a direct continuation of the pulmonary artery, and in the majority of cases of patency of the ductus beyond infancy the ductus arises from the base of the left pulmonary artery.

The termination in the aorta has been called an insertion, a junction or a union. From the standpoint of its embryology this is one origin. In the sense of direction of blood flow the ductus might be considered to originate where flow begins and to insert where flow ends, but the flow reverses after birth to become aorta to pulmonary artery. However, Noback and Rehman (2) point out the course of the vessel is parallel to that of the arch of the aorta and the vessels gradually approach each other to form a junction, and the term union can be used. This is especially true when size is considered since at birth the vessels, the aorta, ductus and pulmonary artery are about equal in diameter. This junction should not be considered as a small vessel inserting into a large one as seen in most clinical situations in older infants and children.

The anatomy of the ductus has been studied in great detail by Noback (9) and Rehman (10) and by Noback and Rehman (2). Their descriptions are followed.

In the newborn the ductus parallels the arch of the aorta. The vessels are separated by loose tissue. They merge or unite about 1 cm below the origin of the left subclavian artery, although the position of this junction can vary upward or downward. It is rare and unusual for the ductus to enter the aorta above the left subclavian.

In the human newborn the ductus enters the descending aorta on its anterolateral aspect at an acute angle of about 30 to 35 degrees (Fig. 15) and it overlaps its aortic entrance. Mancini (11) found an average angle of 31.8 degrees. It is large and bulges beyond the lateral wall of the aorta. In older subjects both the ductus ligament and the patent ductus join the aorta more medially. This medial juncture is probably related to a more lateral position of the aorta and to a more oblique arch which occurs with growth and age. Increase in size of the left ventricle relative to the right may rotate the heart and open the aortic arch and tend to make the course of the ductus more oblique.

The left vagus nerve crosses the ductus arteriosus near its entrance into the descending aorta. The recurrent laryngeal nerve crossed the arch of the aorta proximal to the vagus, and it forms a loop under the ductus near the aortic end. Its position can vary, and it probably lies toward the middle of the ductus in the newborn and closer to the aortic end in older patients.

In the newborn the pulmonary trunk passes upward and slightly to the left and almost parallels the beginning of the arch of the

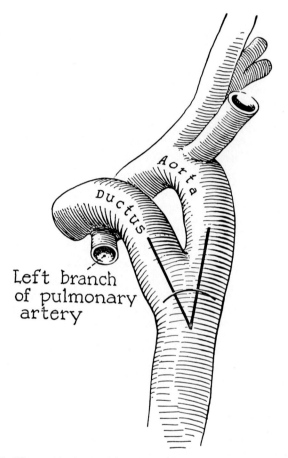

Left branch of pulmonary artery

Figure 15. The angle formed by the ductus and descending aorta in the newborn according to Mancini. This was found to be about 30 to 35 degrees in a study of a newborn.
From Mancini, A.J.: *Anat Rec, 109*:535, 1951.

aorta. It lies anterior and superior to the left atrium and rests on this. The right and left pulmonary arteries leave the pulmonary trunk opposite the origin of the innominate artery. A point of practical importance is that the innominate artery arises from the arch of the aorta to the left of the beginning of the arch and thus is normally to the left of the trachea and not anterior to it as in the adult. It therefore passes to the right across the anterior surface of the trachea and makes a groove upon it. This is no doubt sometimes important clinically, but can be overemphasized as a cause of tracheal obstruction and respiratory distress since this position is normal. This anatomical fact of the newborn and small infants explains the often obvious and readily palpable pulsation in the suprasternal area in those infants, often a normal finding.

Since the pulmonary arteries leave the pulmonary trunk close to the midline, the pulmonary trunk is shorter and the ductus longer than sometimes described. After a variable length of a common wall with the aorta, the vessels become separated just proximal to the bifurcation of the pulmonary artery, and the ductus remains separated from the aorta, although parallel, and it may be close to it. Thus the ductus, like the aortic arch, has an arch which is a little oblique from right to left and has an inferior concavity. If the junction of the aorta is quite high on the arch, the general direction of the ductus forms nearly a right angle with the general directions of the pulmonary artery.

Gerard (3) believed the ductus is always situated in about the same position in relation to external topography and a probe put into the anterior thoracic wall would always pass through it. But its exact location depends upon the volume of the pulmonary artery and the position of the aorta.

In the fetus the origin of the ductus at its pulmonary end is in relation to the left border of the sternum at the upper margin of the second rib. In the stillborn this point is not much different and is still in the first intercostal space but at the angle formed by the left border of the sternum and the second left costal cartilage.

During the first few months of infancy this point moves a little lower, behind the second left costochondral junction and then into the second interspace at the left border of the sternum. Posteriorly, the level is the sixth rib and the sixth intercostal space.

From front to back the inferior surface of the ductus is in relation to (a) the left pulmonary artery, (b) the recurrent laryngeal nerve, (c) the left bronchus and (d) the vagus nerve. The medial part of the inferior surface rests upon the left bronchus and follows the curvature of this to some extent. The ductus can be separated from this by pretracheal-bronchial lymph nodes.

The left bronchus crosses the ductus nearly perpendicularly, or the ductus crosses the left bronchus nearly horizontally.

The ductus is in relation to the thymus anteriorly and superiorly and frequently laterally, and the medial surface of the left lung presses against it and contains an impression formed by the lateral bulge of the ductus. The left lung and the thymus press the ductus against the left bronchus.

Both the size and shape of the ductus are variable. The critical point about the length seems to be that it is determined by the distance between the aorta and pulmonary artery, and it accommodates itself to this. The retraction of the ductus when cut during surgical procedures clearly indicates either it is consistently on a long axis stretch, or it is remarkably contractile longitudinally. There is some indication traction contributes both to pulmonary artery bulge and the conus at the aortic end.

The usual ductus in the newborn varies from 7 to 11 mm in length, but a number will be shorter or longer. Gerard (3) mentions one 18 mm long with a diameter of 9 mm. The normal length is the distance between the pulmonary artery and the point of junction with the aorta and abnormalities of length must be explained by variation in size or position of these vessels. The question whether the ductus grows in length after birth is not settled, but it certainly must be able to stretch or contract to accommodate itself to any variation in the necessary length. There is apparently no good evaluation of the length of the newborn ductus compared to the length of the ligamentum arteriosum through childhood and adult life, although again Gerard (3) believes the length does not vary much. Increase in length of the pulmonary artery and in the diameter of the aorta may be minimized by the increased anterior-posterior diameter of the thorax. It is possible the ductus reaches its maximum size at birth, and it changes little during body growth. The patent ductus which is abnormal in length when found at surgery or at autopsy was probably abnormal in length at birth and this anomaly has merely persisted.

The diameter of the ductus in the newborn is not as variable as the length. During the last month of pregnancy the average diameter is 2.5 to 4 mm and at term this may increase to 4 to 5 mm in the middle and 7 to 8 mm at the ends. A few days after birth the canal is flabby and flattened and there is a difference in color and consistency between the canal and the great vessels. The ductus is engorged with blood in the fetus and cannot be differentiated from the pulmonary artery or aorta.

Thus the diameter of the ductus at birth is about the diameter of some patent ductus at a later date. However, the patent vessel may vary greatly in diameter, and there may be such a discrepancy that postnatal growth must have occurred. Just as unusually large patent ductus may be found clinically in older children this may be present also in early infancy, although this is unusual.

Before birth the diameter of the canal is about the size of the pulmonary arteries and at birth is probably 1 to 3 mm larger. At the end of a week the pulmonary arteries are noticeably larger and increase about 1 mm in diameter a month during most of the first year. While the diameter of the pulmonary artery and the aorta are about the same at birth, the aorta enlarges rapidly and at one month is 1 to 3 mm larger than the pulmonary artery.

After obliteration of the canal the ligamentum is fairly uniform in diameter and varies 2 to 3½ mm in infancy and 4 to 5 mm in adults.

The shape of the ductus can vary considerably. There is little to add to the classification of the patent ductus arteriosus devised by Gerhardt (12) in 1867. It may be (a) cylindrical, and about the same calibre throughout its length, or with an hour glass shape with a slight constriction in the middle point. (b) It may have a funnel shape with the dilated part at the aortic end, although rarely the larger end may be at the pulmonary artery. (c) It can have no length at all, the walls of the pulmonary artery and, aorta being approximated and the communication between the two being an oval or elliptical opening usually referred to as *a window ductus,* and (d) there can be an aneurysmal dilatation of any portion or throughout all its length. To c and d, which must be considered anomalous or unusual, some other forms can be added, such as incomplete patency, with occlusion only at one end, either the aortic or pulmonary artery terminus or in another isolated area. The ductus may open into an aneurysmal dilatation at the point of junction with either the pulmonary artery or aorta.

In general these forms are unusual or pathological, and the great majority of ductus whether normally open in the newborn period or patent into later life are in a or b.

From consideration of the shape of the ductus attempts have been made to draw conclusions regarding the site of the initial impetus to closure. Thus the funnel shape, with the funnel attachment of the aorta, has been cited as evidence of beginning closure at the pulmonary end, and the hour glass shape has suggested beginning closure in the middle portion. In regard to this latter shape, it should be noted Rehman (10) reported examination of the interior of the ductus in the newborn showed a transverse valve or ridge projecting into the lumen and occluding up to one half of the lumen. This was present in 25 percent of the vessels examined microscopically. This was situated almost halfway between the pulmonary and aortic ends where there was an external constriction of the lower border.

It is apparent that the ductus can vary considerably in shape, in length and in diameter. The usual length is 7 to 11 mm, the usual diameter is 4 to 7 mm, its usual shape is slightly funnel, with the dilated portion at the aortic end. But these values must be violated considerably before the ductus can be considered abnormal or pathological in terms of size or shape.

While some consideration has been given to the nerve supply of the ductus itself, the nerve plexus in the region of the ductus is important, since this area is often explored surgically and involves the problem of possible interruption of nerve supply to the heart and great vessels.

The distribution of nerves to the area was studied in detail by Allan (13).

Postmortem contraction of the ductus was studied by Wilson (4). Clinical evidence of delayed closure of the ductus in the premature is not compatible with the anatomical observations of Wilson since in 46 cases of neonatal death where the ductus was contracted, forty were premature and eighteen weighed less than 1250 g. He noted the most striking appearance of ductus contraction was found in the more premature infants. There appeared to be a preponderance of uncontracted ductus in mature infants.

There were three stillbirths with contracted ductus in twenty-five cases, one each over 2500 g. If increase of oxygen to the lung or ductus is indeed required for contraction these few cases are difficult to explain.

He confirmed the observation of Noback and Rehman (2) that the ductus in the newborn enters the aorta on the anterolateral aspect.

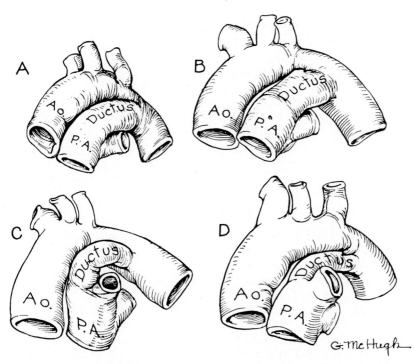

Figure 16. A. Stillborn, 2370 gm, ductus uncontracted. B. Stillborn, 3490 gm, ductus uncontracted. C. Twelve hours old, 2935 gm, ductus contracted. D. Three months of age, 4790 gm, ductus slightly narrower than C. Ductus probably patent.
Redrawn from Wilson, R.R.: *Brit Med J, 1*:810, 1958.

TABLE VI

POSTMORTEM CONTRACTION OF THE DUCTUS ARTERIOSUS IN 100 CASES

State of Ductus	Over 2,500 g.	1,250-2,500 g.	Under 1,250 g.	Total
	Neonatal Deaths			
Contracted	6	22	18	46
Partly Contracted	1	2	2	5
Uncontracted	6	3	2	11
Dilated	—	—	1	1
Total	13	27	23	63
	Stillbirths			
Contracted	1	1	1	3
Partly Contracted	5	3	—	8
Uncontracted	16	8	1	25
Dilated	—	1	—	1
Total	22	13	2	37

(From Wilson, R.R.:Brit Med J, *1*:810, 1958.)

This data is shown in Table VI and the illustration has been redrawn (Fig. 16).

A. Stillborn, 2370 gm, ductus uncontracted.

B. Stillborn, 3490 gm, ductus uncontracted.

C. 2935 g, died age twelve hours, ductus contracted.

D. 4790 g, died age three months, contraction about the same as C.

He notes that all of the contracted ductus would pass a probe and probably blood could pass in either direction. He believes the use of a 2 mm probe in a critical way as done by Mitchell (14) gives results which were, in general, compatible with his study.

REFERENCES

1. Tsuchiya, Satoshi: Uber die Lange und den Umfang des Ductus Arteriosus Botalli bei den Japani-schen Zwillingsfeten. *Okajimas Folia Anat Jap, 16*:275, 1938.

2. Noback, G.J. and Rehman, I.: The ductus arteriosus in the human fetus and newborn infant. *Anat Rec, 81*:505, 1941.

3. Gerard, G.: An anatomical study of the arterial canal. *J Anatomie Physiologie, 36*:1, 1900.

4. Wilson, R.R.: Postmortem observations on contraction of human ductus arteriosus. *Brit Med J, 1*:810, 1958.

5. Walkoff, O.: Das Gwebe des Ductus arteriosus and die Obliteration desselben. *Z ration Med,* 2 Reike, Bd. 36, S. 128-129, 1860.

6. Wrany, A.: Du ductus arteriosus Botalli in seinen physiologischen und pathologischen Verhaaltnissen, Osterr. *Jahrb Padiat,* Bd. 1, S. 1-24, 1871.

7. Berdon, W.E., Baker, D.H. and James, L.S.: The ductus bump. *Am J Roentgenol, 95*:91, 1965.

8. Prec, K.J., Cassels, D.E., Rabinowitz, M. and Moulder, P.V.: Cardiac failure and patency of the ductus arteriosus in early infancy. *J Pediatr, 61*:843, 1962.

9. Noback, G.J.: Changes in relation and form of the ductus arteriosus during early infancy. *Anat Rec, 61*:60, suppl. 2, 1937.

10. Rehman, I.: Topography of the ductus arteriosus in the fetus, newborn and young infant. *Anat Rec, 67*:40, suppl. 3, 1937.

11. Mancini, A.J.: A study of the angle formed by the ductus arteriosus with the descending thoracic aorta. *Anat Rec, 109*:535, 1951.

12. Gerhardt, G.: Persistenz des arteriosus Botalli. *Jenzische Z Med Natur, 3*:105, 1867.

13. Allan, F.D.: The innervation of the human ductus arteriosus. *Anat Rec, 122*:611, 1955.

14. Mitchell, Shiela: The ductus arteriosus in the neonatal period. *J Pediatr, 51*:12, 1957.

Seven

INNERVATION OF THE DUCTUS ARTERIOSUS

THE RELATION OF INNERVATION to early functional constriction or closure of the ductus in the newborn has been a source of concern since the early physiological studies of closure. These studies have been in animal fetus and newborn, and both *in vitro* and *in vivo* studies indicated the smooth muscle of the ductus media contracted with either noradrenalin, adrenalin or acetycholine.

More specifically, the response to noradrenalin could be blocked by dibenamine, a beta adrenergic blocking agent.

There has been considerable literature related to both, and the gross anatomic and microscopic distribution of nerve fibers to and in the wall of the ductus in mammals other than man. In the species studied, however, persistent patency of the ductus arteriosus is rare and no methodical study of intraductal nerve supply is possible in the patent ductus.

In the human, for reasons not clear, the patent ductus occurs in one in 2 to 4,000 live births. The animal population probably does not have this close surveillance, and perhaps the general incidence in lambs or dogs is this high. But lack of a laboratory model of patency has required that most clinical and laboratory studies be applied, when advantageous to the patient, to clinical instances of patent ductus.

Allan (1) outlined the distribution of nerves to the ductus arteriosus in careful dissection, as shown in Figure 17. The innervation as shown in Figure 18 arises chiefly from the thoracic sympa-

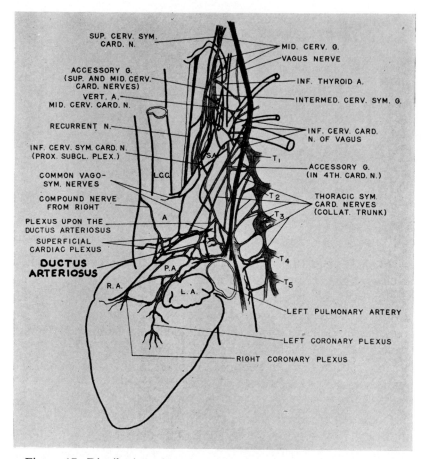

Figure 17. Distribution of nerves to the ductus arteriosus. Redrawn from Allan, F.D.: *Anat Rec, 122*:611, 1955.

thetic trunk and predominantly, in fifteen dissections, from the inferior cervical sympathetic nerve.

However, there was some vagus derivation, as indicated. Further studies by Silva and Ikeda (2) suggest vagus fibers to the ductus as indicated by the presence of cholinesterase granules in the lamb ductus. The problem of vagus distribution to the ductus is confused by the observation of Holmes (3) that cholinesterase was absent in the rabbit ductus although present in the rabbit aorta and pulmonary artery. Indeed, he felt the anatomical limits of ductus insertions could be delineated by negative cholinesterase tissue.

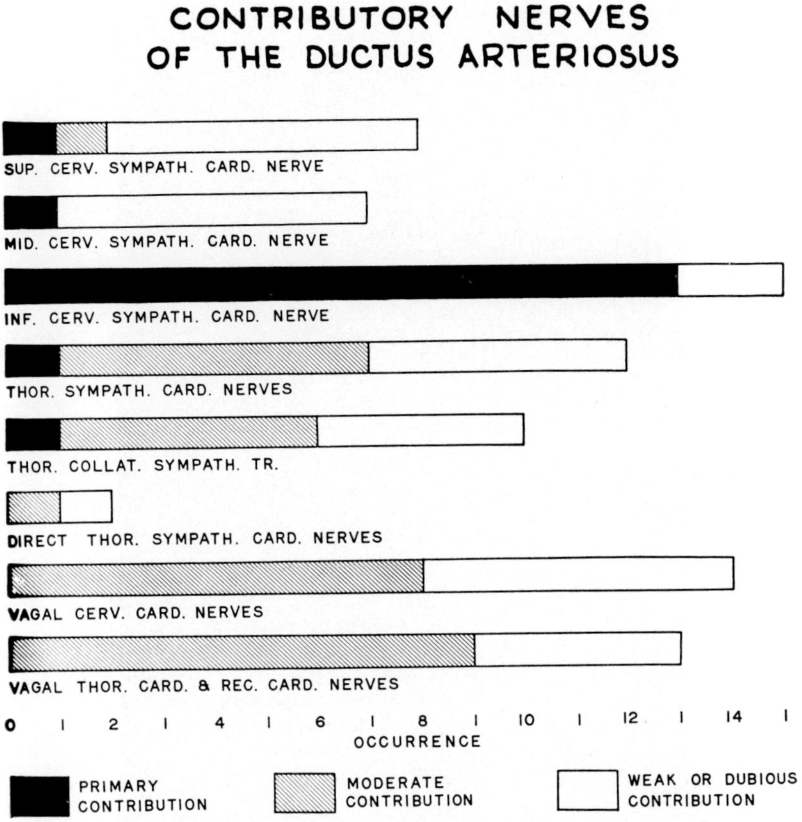

CONTRIBUTORY NERVES
OF THE DUCTUS ARTERIOSUS

Figure 18. Distribution of nerves to the ductus arteriosus in fifteen dissections. The primary contribution in thirteen was from the inferior cervical sympathetic cardiac nerve.

From Allan, F.D.: *Anat Rec, 122*:611, 1955.

Stimulated by the observations of Gregg (4) that patency of the ductus as well as deafness and cataract was related to rubella early in pregnancy, it seemed possible nervous tissue in or to the ductus arteriosus was involved in patency. Efforts to stain patent ductus tissue obtained at surgery with the silver impregnation methods of Cajal (5) gave negative results.

However, when the method of catecholamine fluorescence, which was introduced by Falck et al. (6, 7, 8), became available, tissue from the patent ductus was again examined by Cassels and Moore (9). Boreus et al. (10) showed evenly distributed catecholamine

Figure 19. Photomicrograph of human fetal ductus arteriosus, upper
one-half and aorta, lower one-half as shown by Boreus, et al. (x 120).
Varicose nerve terminals appear as white dots rather evenly distributed in
the media of the ductus. In the aorta, the lower one-half, fluorescent nerve
are absent but ascending elastic lamellae have some autofluorescense.
From Boreus, L.O., Malmfors, T., McMurphy, D.M. and Olson, L.: *Acta
Physiol Scand, 77*:316, 1969.

fluorescence throughout the media of the fetal ductus (Fig. 19).

In contrast, a representative section of a patent ductus obtained
at surgery from an infant age thirteen months (Fig. 20) and from
a patient age six years (Fig. 21) had isolated patency of clinical
significance.

Autofluorescence of connective tissue occurs with this technique

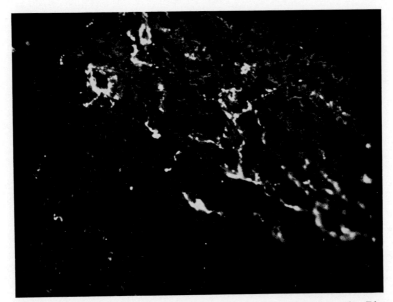

Figure 20. Patient B.S., age thirteen mos., (U of C #108-91-46). Photomicrograph from media of ductus arteriosus showing scattered fluorescent structures arranged largely in rings around apparent vessels. This was the largest accumulation of such structures evident, and the majority of the media was free of specific catecholamine fluorescence. Falck-Hillarp method, x 15.

of examination, but there is absence of specific catecholamine fluorescence in the media and fluorescence is restricted to the walls of vasa vasorum, seen well in Figure 22.

Tissue from patent ductus of fourteen patients age three months to nine years and nine months were examined by the same method. The illustrations shown are representative and in no instance was catecholamine fluorescence seen widely distributed in the media.

This lack of adrenergic activity in the smooth muscle layers and restriction of catecholamine fluorescence to the periphery of the vessel wall was also noted by Brundin, Norberg and Soderlund (11).

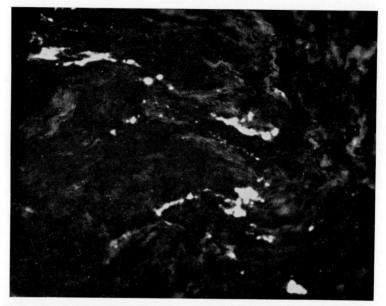

Figure 21. Patient M.G. (U of C #107-18-56). Photomicrograph taken through the media of the ductus arteriosus. The scattered fluorescent structures are large, varicose nerve terminals in close association with the walls of the vasa vasorum of the ductus. Falck-Hillarp method, x 100.

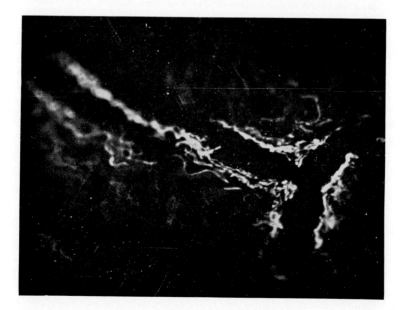

PHARMACOLOGY OF DUCTUS TISSUE

The pharmacology of the ductus tissue has been studied by Kovalcik (12), and his complex and thorough study tabulated in Table VII. Again, the outstanding and constant feature of the study was the rather universal reaction of muscle strips or rings from the ductus arteriosus of sheep and guinea pig fetuses to oxygen. Contraction by oxygen stimulus was not prevented by a concentration of sodium cyanide greater than required for inhibition of cytochrome oxidase. But abolition of response to oxygen was obtained by chloropromazine and promethazine and amytal, and Kovalcik suggests contraction may involve a flavoprotein oxidase not inhibited by cyanide.

The constrictive action of noradrenalin and adrenalin was abolished by dibenamine, but constriction by oxygen was not abolished. It is suggested this drug may be of use in distinguishing between contraction (a) caused by a large rise in arterial oxygen tension or (b) through release of sympathetic amines by asphyxia (12).

Figure 22. Patient M. G. (U of C #107-18-56). Photomicrograph of a branching artery in the adventitia of the ductus arteriosus with a rich catecholamine-containing innervation. The adjacent media was largely free of catecholamine-containing neural structures except about the vasa vasorum. Falck-Hillarp method, x 115.

TABLE VII

I. RESPONSE OF ISOLATED DUCTUS ARTERIOSUS
TO OXYGEN AND ANOXIA (GUINEA PIGS)

Isolated rings of vessels from guinea pig fetuses near term were suspended in Tyrode's solution, or normal Ringers, or potassium-Ringer or calcium free Ringer solution. The constriction of the ductus arteriosus in fetal guinea pigs was also studied by tying right and left pulmonary artery, perfusing the ductus through a cannula in the main pulmonary artery, with warm Tyrode gassed with 5% CO_2 in N_2.

Conditions of Experiment   *Reaction*

Temperature

Cold Tyrode solution .... Contracted

Warm:

with 5% CO_2 in N_2 .... Dilated, at different rates

with 5% CO_2 in O_2 .... Dilated slightly, then contracted over an hour

pH

changing pH of Tyrode .... No change in responsiveness to O_2

solution pH 6 to pH 8 .... No change in responsiveness to O_2

CO_2

increasing content of gas ....

in the solution   .... No effect on tightly constricted ring in presence of O_2 but more rapid relaxation in presence of N_2

Glucose

in Tyrode, with 5% CO_2 in N_2

no glucose .... Abolished response to O_2

add glucose .... Contraction with O_2 in a few minutes

Drug Affecting Autonomic Nervous System
in Tyrode bath with 5% CO_2 and O_2

Hexamethonium 10 to 15 $\mu g/ml$ .... No change in response to O_2

Dibenamine 20 $\mu g/ml$ .... No change in response to O_2

Phentolamine 10 to 50 $\mu g/ml$ .... No change in response to O_2

Atropine 30 $\mu g/ml$ .... No change in response to O_2

Mepyramine 50 $\mu g/ml$ .... No change in response to O_2

Benadryl 20 $\mu g/ml$ .... No change in response to O_2

Dichloro-isoprenaline 20 to 100 $\mu g/ml$ ... No change in response to O_2

Iproniazid 50 $\mu g/ml$ .... No change in response to O_2

Cocaine 1 to 10 $\mu g/ml$ .... No change in response to O_2

TABLE VII

II. RESPONSE OF ISOLATED DUCTUS ARTERIOSUS
TO OXYGEN AND ANOXIA (LAMBS)

In sheep fetus of 75 to 144 days, spiral strips 2 to 4 cm long cut from the ductus and other vessels were suspended in a bath with a writing level and the contractions recorded on a kymograph. Tyrode solution was used with variations.

Conditions of Experiment   *Reaction*

Temperature Effect

Cold Tyrode bath .... Contracted

Warm:

with 5% CO_2 and N_2 .... Relaxed at once, then slowly contracted over 2 hrs.

with 5% CO_2 and O_2 .... Contracted immediately with increasing O_2 concentration; progressive contraction later, with 5% CO_2 in N_2......................Relaxation

38° to 28° to 18° C with O_2 or N_2......Contraction with O_2 slower; maximum contraction not affected; relaxation with N_2 slower

Drugs Affecting Autonomic Nervous System
in Tyrode bath with 5% CO_2 or N_2

Noradrenalin 0.1 to 10 μg/ml......................Contraction

Adrenalin   without O_2......................Contraction much reduced

Acetycholine   0.1 to 10 μg/ml......................Contraction

Bradykinin   0.1 to 1.0 μg/ml......................Contraction
              (low doses)

Isoprenaline   100 μg/ml......................No effect

Hystamine   100 μg/ml......................No effect

Tyromine   100 μg/ml......................No effect

Nicotine   100 μg/ml......................No effect

Dibenamine   100 μg/ml......................No effect

Atropine   100 μg/ml......................No effect

5 Hychoxytryptomine......................No effect or relaxation

Metabolic Inhibitors

Sodium cyanide (1 mM)

   with O_2......................Contraction the same, but slower

   with N_2......................No effect

Sodium cyanide......................Abolished O_2 consumption (measurable within 10%)

Metabolic Inhibitors

Chlorpromazine 0.1 mM......................Abolished response to O_2

Amytal 1 mM......................Abolished response to O_2

Promethazine 1 to 10 mM......................Abolished response to O_2

Dinitrophenol 1 mM......................Abolished response to O_2; reversible by washing

Sodium iodin acetate 1 mM......................Abolished response irreversibly

Sodium fluoride 1 mM......................No change in response

Mersalyl 1 mM......................No change in response

Adenosine triphosphate 0.1 mM......................Reversible inhibition of response to O_2

Adenosine monophosphate 1.0 mM......................Reversible inhibition of response to O_2

Adenosine 1.0 mM......................Reversible inhibition of response to O_2

Creatine phosphate 1 mM......................No similar action

Potassium and Calcium

Calcium-free Ringer's solution......................Relaxation

   with 5% CO_2 and O_2......................No change in length if calcium removed

   with 5% CO_2 and N_2......................Subsequent O_2 did not cause contraction

Calcium added 1 mM......................Contracts with O_2

Ethylenediamine tetra-acetate added 1 mM Abolished response to O_2; this reversible with calcium or washing

REFERENCES

1. Allan, F.D.: The innervation of the human ductus arteriosus. *Anat Rec, 122*:611, 1955.
2. Silva, D.G. and Ikeda, M.: Ultrastructural and acetylcholinesterase studies on the innervation of the ductus arteriosus, pulmonary trunk and aorta of the fetal lamb. *J Ultrastruct Res, 34*:358, 1971.
3. Holmes, R.L.: The rabbid ductus arteriosus. *Nature (Lond), 180/4594*: 1058, 1957.
4. Gregg, N.McA.: Further observations on congenital defects in infants following maternal rubella. *Trans Ophthalmal Soc Aust, 4*:119, 1944.
5. Cajal, S.R.y.: *Degeneration and Regeneration of the Nervous System.* Two volumes, London, 1928.
6. Falck, B., Hillarp, N.A., Thieme, G. and Torp, A.: Fluorescence of catecholamines and related compounds condensed with formaldehyde. *J Histochem Cytochem, 10*:348, 1962.
7. Falck, B.: Observations on the possibilities of cellular localization of monoamines by a fluorescene method. *Acta Physiol Scand, 56*:1, suppl. 197, 1962.
8. Falck, B. and Owman, Chr.: A detailed methodological description of the fluorescence method for the cellular demonstration of biogenic conoamines. *Acta Univ Lund,* sect. 2, no. 7, p. 1, 1965.
9. Cassels, D.E. and Moore, R.Y.: *Absence of Catecholamines in patent Ductus Arteriosus.* Abstract, 81st American Pediatric Society Scientific Session, Atlantic City, N.J., 1971.
10. Boreus, L.O., Malmfors, T., McMurphy, D.M. and Olson, L.: Demonstration of adrenergic receptor function and innervation in the ductus arteriosus of the human fetus. *Acta Physiol Scand, 77*:316, 1969.
11. Brundin, T., Norberg, K.A. and Soderlund, S.: Lack of adrenergic nerves in the circular smooth muscles of ductus arteriosus persistens. *Scand J Thorac Cardiovasc Surg, 5*:16, 1971.
12. Kovalcik, V.: The response of the isolated ductus arteriosus to oxygen and anoxia. *J Physiol, 160*:185, 1963.

Eight

THEORIES OF CLOSURE

G ALEN (1) HAD WRITTEN THE DUCTUS ARTERIOSUS not only
stopped growing but became smaller and *after a time* became shrivelled and solidified. It became the concern of many to identify more
exactly the period *after a time* and to understand the process by
which it became shrivelled and solidified. Observation and especially speculation led to the formulation of several theories of closure and to considerable polemic discussion. Observations on the
time of closure were confusing, and while material for anatomical
dissection of the newborn infant was plentiful and there was great
interest, investigation, was confused by different criteria of closure.
Some considered the ductus closed when the lumen was obliterated
sufficiently that blood flow through it seemed impossible. Others
considered the ductus patent if either grossly or microscopically
there was a slitlike opening present. Closed but probe patent was a
term sometimes used.

Carcano (2) in 1574 had sought to establish the time of closure
by examination of the fetus of man and animals. He found that the
foramen ovale and the ductus did not become closed a few days
after birth. They closed anatomically little by little and even after
three months were not completely obstructed. The walls of the
ductus had become thicker, but a probe could be passed into it.
Harvey (3) was more intent upon the problem of the general circulation and merely stated the channel gradually shrinks after birth
and finally obliterates. During the next century authors suggested
the onset of respiration modified the position of the thoracic organs
so that the canal was drawn laterally and the blood flow became
retrograde.

Senac (4) also suggested a dynamic aspect of closure related to changes in pressure in the pulmonary artery and aorta following birth. He said as soon as air enters the lung the vessels supplying the lung expand and lengthen. The resistance diminishes in the pulmonary vessels, blood enters more easily, and consequently there is less flow through the ductus—that is, more of the pulmonary artery blood flows to the lungs leaving less to enter the aorta. But when the resistance in the pulmonary flow and the flow through the aorta is equal, no blood passes through the canal which has no use and therefore closes. He suggested an analogy. If there was a transverse artery between the two iliac arteries and resistance to flow in the iliac arteries was equal, then there would be no flow in the transverse artery and this vessel would gradually close, as the ductus does.

However ingenious the argument was in 1773, he did not know the pressures in the two vessels connected were very unequal even though the connecting vessel closes. Not secure in his speculations, he could not resist adding arguments related to possible mechanical aspects of closure.

When the infant breathes, he said, the heart action is more powerful and the arch of the aorta is dilated and pushed higher, and consequently the ductus is pulled and lengthened. He noted some believed the duct closed by a change in the angle it forms with the aorta, and agreed it became more transverse and pulled backward by the left branch of the pulmonary artery and the aortic end could bend and become partially obstructed. These mechanical factors contributed to the arrest of flow through it.

However, it was in the next century that detailed observation on the time of closure were made. Billard (5) in 1828 published the results of a systematic study of closure through the first eight days but included observations on a few older infants. He found the time of closure variable and the ductus could be permeable during the first twenty days. Thore (6) studied the problem in 1850 and reported the fetal channels rarely closed before the fourth or fifth day after birth and often were patent to the twelfth or fifteenth day. A narrow opening was found in a six week old infant.

In 1854 Flourens (7) wrote a short review, "Histoire de la deconverte de la circulation du sang," and in this short history he included observations on babies eighteen to twenty-four months of age. Curiously enough, he found the ductus open at this time. As Gerard (8) pointed out, he either encountered an exceptional series of cases or he considered the canal permeable in ductus ligaments which showed on cutting a small central lumen "which one always observes."

DeAlmagro (9) wrote a thesis, "Etude sur la persistance du canal arteriel," in 1862 and concluded closure was complete and the ductus ligament was always present by the end of the first month. Bernutz (10) agreed that closure of the ductus arteriosus occurred in the first fifteen days after birth and it was abnormal to have closure occur at three weeks. He extended the observations on closure which Billard had ended, for practical purposes, at the eighth day. In twenty-one infants age ten to twenty days the ductus was completely closed in fourteen and somewhat permeable in seven. It was found very unusual to have patency after twenty days.

Whether by a fortunate guess or as a result of clinical or pathological observation, he made the shrewd comment that when the foramen ovale or the ductus arteriosus were found at one month or six weeks of age, this did not necessarily mean that if the baby lived he would have had cyanosis.

Alvarenga (11) studied the problem further. He remarked, incidentally and without any description or reference, that the ductus sometimes remained open, even to an advanced age, or it could be completely absent in the fetus.

On the basis of his observation he came to the conclusion that (a) the ductus obliterates after the thirtieth postnatal day, (b) there is no fixed period for obliteration and (c) in general, it is two or three months before the obliteration of the canal is complete. (d) It is rarely persistent beyond three months and if it is still open, it is usually greatly reduced in size and would not transmit blood. Elsasser (12) examined the ductus in nearly 300 autopsies during the first month of life and found obliteration in only 2 percent.

Gerard (8) in 1900 wrote a long and very good exposition on the closure of the ductus. He made the important distinction which clarified some inconsistancies that occlusion referred to physiological function and obliteration to the anatomical and histological process which changed a vessel into a ligament. The ductus is occluded when no blood passes through it, although anatomically it may have a partial or filiform lumen.

He made some carefully considered and reasonable proposals. Physiological obliteration begins with the establishment of respiration. Histological obliteration begins in the first day of life, takes some time for completion and is rarely definitive before the fortieth day. After forty days a patency is rare and later than this the lumen of the canal is so narrow and the walls so thick that passage of blood is impossible. The ductus should be called persistent only if the calibre is intact. Nonobliteration refers to those with incomplete obliteration in part of their length.

He reviewed the literature up to 1900. He found the ductus was completely permeable in stillborn infants, and he then examined the ductus in ninety-six children from one day to twelve years of age. He again emphasized that he had never found the ductus closed at birth or in the first ten days. While it may not be gaping when cut, it is always patent for this period. He agreed with Bernutz (10) that obliteration commenced during the first fifteen days and often was complete by the end of the first month. In addition, he made the observation that anatomical obliteration begins at the pulmonary artery end of the ductus. Condensation of the walls, thickening of the internal layers with diminution of the lumen were observed first at the pulmonary end of the ductus. Obliteration rarely commenced at the aortic end and in older patients it was there that obliteration was incomplete.

This point deserves some emphasis since it has both a clinical application and is of interest in relation to the general argument about closure.

During the same period other authors published observations relating to the time of closure of the ductus. They agreed in general with the findings of Elsasser (12) and Alvarenga (11). The problem was brought up to date in 1918 by Scammon and Norris (13) who summarized the previous studies (Fig. 23) and tabulated their own observations (Fig. 24). During the first postpartum week there is less than 0.3 percent obliteration. There is 2 percent in the second week and about 11 percent in the third and fourth weeks. Obliteration then accelerates with 37 to 47 percent during the second month

TABLE 3

Data on the frequency of post-natal obliteration of the Ductus arteriosus. Numerals enclosed in parentheses indicate number of obliterated cases

OBSERVER AND DATE	0 TO 8 DAYS	8 TO 15 DAYS	15 TO 22 DAYS	22 TO 32 DAYS	32 TO 46 DAYS	46 TO 61 DAYS	61 TO 91 DAYS	3 TO 4 MONTHS	4 TO 12 MONTHS	1 TO 10 YEARS
Alverenga, '69	19	11	15	28 (1)	17	8 (1)	14 (5)	9 (3)	1	7 (7)
Bernutz, '65			* 21 (14)		** 38 (36)					
Billard, '28	118 (16)	20 (11)								
Elsässer, '52	150 (1)	63 (3)	61 (6)	23 (1)	3					
Faber, '12			° 5		3			15 (14)	6 (6)	23 (18)
Gérard, '00	52	2	2 (2)	4	2 (2)	2 (2)	2 (2)		16 (12)	13 (13)
Kucheff, '01						† 40 (18)				
Letourneau, '58	12	1								
Theremin, '87	67	66	61 (6)	56 (8)	50 (26)	43 (23)	68 (55)	53 (48)	54 (54)	
Theremin '95	11	5	4 (2)	6 (3)		4 (1)	8 (8)	1 (1)	12 (12)	4 (4)
Totals	429 (17)	168 (14)	143 (18)	117 (13)	75 (28)	57 (27)	92 (70)	63 (52)	89 (84)	47 (33)

* 10 to 20 days.
** 21 to 60 days.
† 2nd month (data for other periods not available).
° 0 to 30 days.

Figure 23. Observations on obliteration of the ductus arteriosus compiled by Scammon and Norris.

From Scammon, R.E. and Norris, E.H.: *Anat Rec, 15*:165, 1918.

and 76 percent during the third month. During the fourth month 82 percent of the canals are closed and by the end of the first year nerly 100 percent are obliterated.

Christie (14) again reviewed the subject in 1930 and contributed his own observations. For practical purposes the graph of

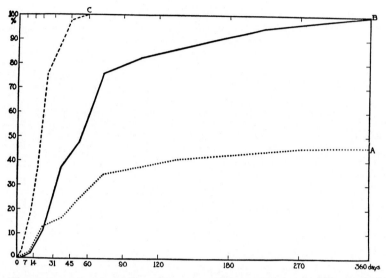

Three curves representing the average percentages of obliterated fetal blood-passages at different periods in the first year of life. *A,* dotted line, foramen ovale, *B,* solid line, ductus arteriosus; *C,* broken line, ductus venosus. These curves are based upon the material summarized in tables 2, 4 and 5.

Figure 24. The solid line represents the closure of the ductus arteriosus as found by Scammon and Norris. The dotted line is the foramen ovale and the broken line the ductus venosus.
From Scammon, R.E. and Norris, E.H.: *Anat Rec, 15*:165, 1918.

Christie seems the most useful (Fig. 25). Mitchell (15) in 1957 examined this problem again and pointed out that the normally closing ductus will admit only a 2 mm probe by the end of the first week. This does not describe possible flow which would be related to the pulmonary vascular resistance and aortic pressure, as well as the resistance of the reduced lumen itself.

All of these studies relate to postmortem material and do not take into consideration the possibility of (a) postmortem constriction or changes in calibre due to methods of fixation or (b) the influence on lumen size of aortic or pulmonary artery pressure or ductus flow.

There is general agreement that the normal ductus is closed by the end of the first year and evidence of patency after one year should be considered as persistent patency with very little likelihood of subsequent closure.

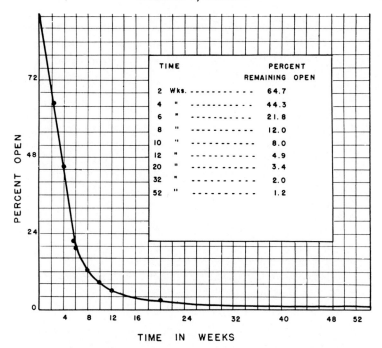

TIME | PERCENT REMAINING OPEN

2 Wks.	64.7
4 "	44.3
6 "	21.8
8 "	12.0
10 "	8.0
12 "	4.9
20 "	3.4
32 "	2.0
52 "	1.2

TIME IN WEEKS

NORMAL CLOSING TIME OF THE DUCTUS ARTERIOSUS IN 558 NORMAL HEARTS OF INFANTS FROM I DAY TO I YEAR OF AGE

AMOS CHRISTIE, AM. JOUR. DIS. CHILD. 40: 323, AUG. 1930

Figure 25. The normal closure of the ductus arteriosus as found by Christie.
From Christie, Amos.: *Am J Dis Child, 40*:323, 1930.

Throughout the whole period of study and discussion regarding the time of closure of the ductus, there was never any debate regarding the fact of anatomical histological closure. This had been observed grossly by those who had first described the vessel, and by all subsequent students of the ductus arteriosus. A considerable literature accumulated regarding the details of the active mechanism. There has been no knowledge or even debate concerning the origin of the embryonic drive toward active tissue proliferation in such a circumscribed area, and this may be analogous to any other proliferative growth mechanism.

But a great discussion arose concerning the question of immediate or early functional occlusion of the ductus arteriosus and the possible mechanism by which this was or could be produced. It was the opinion of most authors that immediate functional closure did occur. The mechanisms proposed may be outlined briefly:

I. Mechanical means
  A. Thrombus formation
  B. Occlusion by change in position of thoracic organs when the lungs inflate with external pressure—by a bronchus, by stretching, by tightening the left recurrent nerve around the vessel.
  C. By a valvelike obstruction at either end, but especially at the aortic juncture.
II. Physiological means
  A. Hemodynamic changes—equalization of pressures, with collapse and closure; diminution of pressure, becoming *useless* and occluding.
  B. Contraction due to nervous mechanisms
  C. Contraction due to local stimulation with the oxygen of oxygenated blod after respiration occurs.
  D. Contraction, cause undetermined.

A great deal of study and investigation was expended by proponents of the various theories, many ingenius experiments were performed and ingenious arguments submitted.

Immediate occlusion of the ductus by some alteration of thoracic mechanics was an attractive and reasonable theory, especially since certainly there was considerable shift in the position of the heart and lungs following the onset of respiration. King (16) suggested the dilatation of the left bronchus at the moment of respiration compressed the ductus posteriorly-anteriorly, since the ductus rests upon the bronchus. Chevers (17) even suggested traction by the left recurrent laryngeal nerve which passes under the ductus at the aortic insertion could lead to closure. Others also noted the larynx became elevated after birth and could thus tighten the loop of the recurrent laryngeal and compress the vessel.

While changes in the topography of the thoracic organs was used by many in different ways in consideration of the mechanical aspects of closure, Walkoff (18) gave a detailed and specific description of these events, and this is of considerable interest:

> The thoracic cavity in the stillborn child is restricted in volume. The lungs, still in a collapsed state, are crowded closely against the vertebral column; the diaphragm is raised high into the cavity and the

heart is placed horizontally. After the onset of respiration, a great change occurs. The lungs assume twice their former volume and exert a pull on the pulmonary branches. These are consequently deflected from their outward and backward course into a lateral direction, whereby the bifurcation of the pulmonary artery and the insertion of the ductus arteriosus are strongly bent and retracted. The bend is further augmented by the increase in pressure in the pulmonary circulation which at the same time results in a tension and development of the walls. The future position of the ductus is furthermore influenced by the change in the position of the heart and by a bending to the right and outward of the aorta ascendent resulting from the intensified muscular activity of the left ventricle. All these factors combine to produce, not only a shunting of the blood into the branches of the pulmonary artery but also a bending of the ductus in such a way, that instead of forming an outward continuation of the artery, it now runs inward at a slight angle and perpendicular to its outer wall, rising steeply towards the aorta and inserting in the latter at an approximately right angle, as I have observed in three day old children on several occasions. As a result the anterior and posterior walls of the ductus are brought so closely together that no injection penetrates after three days. A further factor contributing to this latter phenomenon may be that the enlarged pulmonary branches dilate the posterior wall of the artery at its bifurcation, with the result that the pulmonary ostium of the ductus is forced against the anterior wall with a valvelike effect. In the course of obliteration this initial shifting and bending is gradually counterbalanced by shrinkage, so that no trace of it remains in the ligamentum arteriosum.

This idea that change in position obstructs the ductus occurs many times in different forms, all suggesting that bending of the ductus immediately after birth as a result of change in position of the heart played a role in closure.

Since the pulmonary end of the ductus is free, it is readily subject to changes in direction. The German authors especially were concerned and injected the ductus, inflated the lungs and obtained casts which demonstrated the knuckling of the ductus as previously postulated.

As recently as 1926 mechanical closure was explained by the greatly increased pressure in the aorta after birth which prevented blood flow through the ductus into the aorta and the enlarged pulmonary artery and the aorta compressed the empty ductus between them.

While some were concerned with the pulmonary side of the ductus, others emphasized the importance of the aortic end. Frieux (19) attached a tube of water to the great vessels and noted flow through the ductus stopped when the lungs were inflated. He agreed with others that the increased angle at the pulmonary insertion prevented flow. But the greater issue was the physiological implications of the anatomy of the aortic connection of the ductus, particularly the juncture of the two vessels which occurs at a rather acute angle said to be always 33 degrees. In a more comprehensive study of the angle formed by the ductus arteriosus with the descending aorta, Mancini (20) was more liberal allowing variation from 25 to 37.5 degrees. There was little difference in those who had breathed and infants who had not. This is contrary to speculation that the acquisition of a more acute angle was a factor in obstructing ductus flow at the aortic end. At this junction there would be a common wall for a short distance, where the upper border of the ductus and the lower wall of the aorta came together. Indeed, Barclay and associates (21) coined a name for this ridge, calling it the *crista reuniens*. While the possible importance of this as a mechanical flap to occlude the aortic opening of the ductus had been mentioned previously, Strassman (22) entered the discussion of closure with great energy and ingenuity, asserting with great emphasis the importance of this valvelike action. His conclusion rested upon experiment and injection into carotids, aorta, pulmonary artery and umbilical vein in the mammalian fetus and in newborn infants. He denied the importance of thrombosis, muscular contraction or the topographic changes in the thoracic organs. He believed closure occurred instantaneously and mechanically by this valve. He found that after the fifth fetal month the ductus opening into the aorta at an angle pushed its anterior wall forward to form a roof over the opening of the ductus in humans, sheep, dogs and cats. The separation of the pulmonary and aortic circulation was analogous to the separation of the atrial flows by the foramen ovale. The act of respiration diminished the pressure in the pulmonary artery and raised the pressure in the aorta and the valve was forced closed.

He then found a very curious thing, injection of the ascending aorta with a pressure up to 100 mm of mercury did not fill the ductus in the newborn even if the pulmonary end was open, but retrograde injections from the umbilical artery always filled the ductus. Only under special circumstances could the ductus be injected from the aorta in premature infants with premature respiration, and if the pressure in the aorta was too high, then the aortic end of the ductus could be forced open and the flap inverted. He published striking illustrations of the change of anatomy in the ductus insertion before respiration, after respiration, in the presence of atelectases and after excessive injection of blood.

This was a restatement of previous speculation but with experiment and documentation. His suggestion became the focus of considerable polemic discussion. The criticism of Graper (23) was probably the most complete.

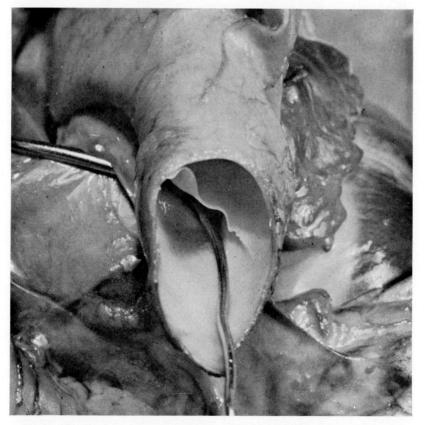

Figure 26. Patent ductus arteriosus with a valvelike flap covering the aortic entrance in a male mongrel dog.

Scharfe (24) was unable to find the valvelike flap and considered it an artifact. He devised another theory of ductus closure, the ductus itself functioned like a tubular valve. He demonstrated this. He made a model of two vessels with tubes leading from them which were connected transversely by a thin walled tube. If the vessel representing the pulmonary flow was raised higher than the *aortic* one, flow occurred through the ductus, but if the aortic flow increased by raising the aortic flow the ductus collapsed. He postulated that if there was increased pressure in the pulmonary artery due to increased resistance in the lungs, aneurysms and other pathological conditions would result. Strassman (22) at once criticized the demonstration.

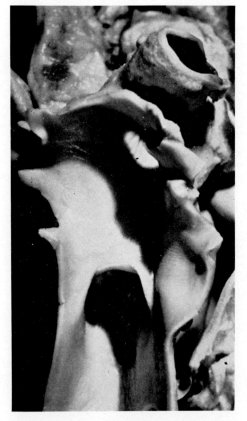

Figure 27. A flap and valve at the entrance of the ductus arteriosus into the aorta in an adult male, human.
Courtesy of Dr. Maurice Lev.

The concept of closure in the human species by a valve has been discarded, but there are subsequent pathological reports which mention a pronounced flap at the junction of the ductus and aorta.

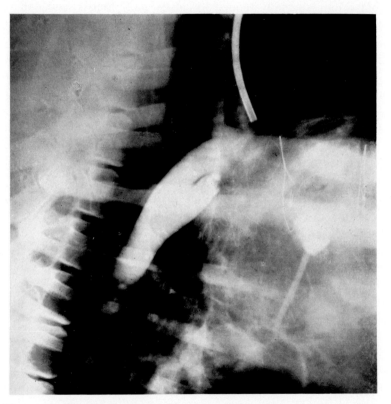

Figure 28. The angle formed by the opacified aorta and ductus is even less than 10 degrees. The ductus arteriosus is nearly as large as the aorta at their juncture.

Since valvelike flaps occur in some animals, but especially in the dog, it is of interest to speculate that Strassman relied on this species in developing and propounding his theory so vociferously. Figure 26 shows this flap and valve associated with a patent ductus arteriosus in a dog and Figure 27 in an adult human. The usual coalescence which covers the aortic orifice had not occurred and the ductus remained patent. The valve in the dog was identified in an aortogram, and retrograde flow occurred (Fig 28).

Before the advent of microscopic examination of differentially stained tissues, it was easy to postulate closure of a vessel by inflammation or thrombosis, and both of these processes had been invoked as explanatory of closure of the ductus arteriosus. This explanation especially tended to satisfy pathologists who had seen instances of ductal thrombosis. Simple thrombosis was considered as the cause of closure by many German authors and by Virchow (25).

Others did not deny its occurrence but considered it rare and pathological. Rauchfuss (26) for instance found the ductus thrombosed four times in 1,400 infants, and Variot and Cailliau (27) discovered one ductus thrombosis in seventy-four infants. While a thrombus could be found occluding a canal that otherwise would be patent this was certainly not the usual method of closure, and tended to be associated with infection and sepsis.

Many were impressed with the analogy of the healing of aneurysms and the resemblance of the obliteration of the ductus and venous thrombosis. Dumontpallier (28) carefully considered the process of inflammation as applicable to the closure of the canal and as analogous to the process which occurs in the obliteration of other vessels, especially of aneurysms. It seemed logical that when the blood flow became more sluggish the calibre of the vessel would become smaller and leucocytes would infiltrate and organize, forming connective tissue. Also proposed was obliteration by fibrinous clots and many argued for this idea or some modification of it. Even Walkoff (18) following his exhaustive histological study of obliteration in 1869, noted fibrin deposits on the longitudinal wrinkles of the inner surface. The ductus, said Bernutz (10) is the site of complex changes which are similar to those observed in inflammation of arteries, and there is deposited on the inner surface of the internal membrane a fibrinous layer which doubles the thickness of the vessel walls.

While students of the ductus problem considered the possibility of relatively early closure by mechanical events and by obstruction, there was continued interest in immediate closure by physiological means. There are references to a possible suction action of the pulmonary artery in diverting blood from the ductus, a situation favorable for collapse and closure. Perhaps the sucking action could be exerted by the flow through the aorta, as the ingenious experiment of Scharfe (24) had suggested. In addition to this immediate reduction of blood flow through the ductus resulting from diversion of blood into newly opened channels in the vascular bed of the lungs, Haberda (29) suggested the ductus closes temporarily at birth by contraction of its muscular walls.

Schultze (30) thought of occlusion in terms of thrombosis or by contraction of the vessel walls following a great fall in blood pressure. When the fall in pressure was associated with stagnation, the situation encouraged obliteration without thrombosis when there was no current in the canal. Some agreed the ductus closed temporarily at birth by contraction of its muscular walls, and the contraction caused diminution of flow through it. Virchow (25) had accepted the concept of closure by contraction of the walls, but he believed obliteration included the formation of a thrombus.

Subsequently, most authors have accepted muscular contraction as an element in early functional closure although not agreeing on its relative importance. As recently as 1939 Swensson (31) in an extensive review of the subject of closure includes muscular contraction as only one factor involved, the others being the acute angle of insertion into the aorta and the change in position of the heart, causing a bend in the ductus wall.

As early as 1851 Kiwisch (32) described some of the peculiar anatomical attributes of the ductus arteriosus. He stated its walls were thicker than those of other arteries and its internal layer was *ponctiforme* and its middle layers cavernous and loose. He found that the muscle bundles in the muscular layer were easily separated and that there were *abundant* vessels and nerves. All of these circumstances combined to favor closure. He suggested a nervous mechanism which both made the canal contract spontaneously and the pulmonary arteries relax. Complete obliteration was then produced by progressive loosening of the internal membrane so that the sides of these opposed each other and became adherent.

FUNCTIONAL CLOSURE

Suggestive and intriguing as the nervous anatomy of the ductus and neighboring aortic and pulmonary artery areas are, another type of study reveals other possibilities in the variety of mechanisms

suggested as the stimulus for the functional closure of the ductus
arteriosus. This was the extraordinarily comprehensive physiological
study of Kennedy and Clark (33). Extensive quotation is necessary
and summary inadequate:

> When guinea pig fetuses were delivered into saline baths at body
> temperature, the ductus remained open for several hours if the pla-
> centa and cord were kept intact and respiration prevented. Closure of
> the vessel, which was under direct observation, could be caused by
> a variety of stimuli and reopening followed removal of the stimulus.
> For instance, even rhythmic inflation of the lungs through a tracheal
> cannula, mechanical stimulation or weak electrical stimulation of the
> wall caused closure.
>
> Pursuing the observation that respiration caused closure, experiments
> were designed to test the effect of interruption of the reflex path-
> ways. (1) Both vagi were sectioned, (2) both stellate ganglia were
> removed, (3) stellate ganglia removed with section of both vagi,
> (4) the carotids were ligated below their bifurcation, (5) both caro-
> tids and their bifurcations were removed, (6) the carotids and bifur-
> cations were removed and both vagi sections, (7) all vessels, nerves,
> other structures above the arch were ligated tightly, (8) the spinal
> cord on each side of the section destroyed, (9) the spinal cord was
> destroyed from the second cervical to the second thoracic, the third
> cervical to the caudal end, and from the first thoracic to the eleventh
> thoracic segment, (10) all of the cord was destroyed from the
> second cervical segment to the caudal end, the vagi sectioned and
> the mediastinal structures above the aortic arch ligated, and finally
> (11) the whole medulla and spinal cord was destroyed, the vagi
> sectioned and the stellate ganglia removed.

The procedures interrupted all known pathways between the
central nervous system and the region of the ductus. There was no
evidence of a local reflex mechanism. Electrical stimulation of the
left vagus, right vagus, left cervical sympathetic, left phrenic, left
stellate ganglion and left splanchnic nerve did not affect the ductus.
They concluded that a nervous pathway or a neuromuscular reflex
was not essential for the closure of the ductus. The utility of the
demonstrable nervous paths to the ductus are, therefore, not known,
although it is possible that in a different species the findings may
be different, and still different in the human. No report of stimulation of the ductus area, other than mechanical, is known.

Supplementary findings are of great interest, and a variety of
stimuli caused closure under direct observations. Inflation of the

lungs with oxygen, or with oxygen and nitrogen caused closure. But inflation with nitrogen alone did not. Mechanical or electrical stimulation caused rapid closure as did mechanical stimulation of the carotid sinus on either side. Hemmorhage, or injection of adrenalin or the intravenous injection of oxygen also caused closure.

It, therefore, appeared that (a) the ductus arteriosus is capable of marked muscular contraction as a response to a variety of stimuli and (b) it was not possible to discover the specific principle which governs this contraction, except respiration with gases containing oxygen.

Kennedy and Clark (34) as a result of a thorough study of this problem conclude that respiration is the most important stimulus, providing that respired gases contain oxygen. Kennedy (35) entitled a paper "A New Concept of the Cause of Patency of the Ductus Arteriosus." Born and colleagues (36) also demonstrated that in lambs under a variety of conditions, the ductus constricts when arterial oxygen is increased and dilates when this is lowered. But also deliberate under-ventilation and consequent asphyxia could cause constriction. Infusion of adrenalin and noradrenalin into the lambs also cause constriction of the ductus.

The fetal and newborn ductus is a muscular vessel with a demonstrable innervation, and is delicately balanced between muscular contraction and muscular relaxation. All of the biochemical factors involved in muscle contraction in other areas are not yet completely resolved, and the factors involved in early ductus contraction are not fully known.

It is presumed that the persistent patent ductus arteriosus in the human is not balanced in this way between contraction and relaxation, and indeed it must be supposed that this kind of contraction is not possible. Its goal is nonclosure.

The stimulus of oxygen in contributing to the temporary occlusion of the ductus arteriosus in lambs (36), guinea pigs (37), colts (38), chicks (39), piglets (40) and dogs (41) has been amply confirmed in many laboratories since the original report of Kennedy and Clark (33).

The complex study of Fay (42) shows that double perfusion of the ductus arteriosus of the guinea pig, a situation more normal, shows a greater sensitivity to oxygen than reported for isolated preparations. The data indicates an increase of PO_2 from 30 to 80 mm Hg would be sufficient to initiate closure against arterial pressures up to 110 mm Hg.

Further studies suggested oxygen causes contraction of ductus smooth muscle because of an increase in the rate of oxidative phosphorylation from increased supply to the terminal cytochrome component presumed to be cytochrome a 3.

Intermittent occlusion has been shown by angiography by Lind and associates (43) and the unstable physiological status of the ductus has been studied by dye dilution curves, and changing shunts demonstrated. It was noted by Prec and Cassels (44) in 1955 and studied by others in more detail (45, 46) that the ductus did not close by contraction as early and possibly not as completely in the human as in the lamb. As Mitchell (15) has pointed out, the relation of a 2 mm lumen at seven days to flow through it is not established.

However, the problem remains whether physiological occlusion is related in any way to anatomical closure. Is this transient occlusive phenomenon required in the orderly process of histological closure. The question can be posed succinctly: has the ductus in which patency will persist had an episode of functional closure and was it capable of contraction. The histology of the patent ductus suggests fibrosis, loss of muscle fiber and the accumulation of collagen makes contraction impossible in the ages in which the vessel was examined. It is not known whether the patent ductus is this abnormal in early infancy and whether both functional and histological closure was impossible from an inherent anatomic defect which originated in early fetal life. There are no hemodynamic studies through this critical period which can answer these questions. There is no animal model in which functional closure or nonclosure can be compared with appropriately traced histology.

In the absence of more or less continuous hemodynamic data through a period of functional closure the relation of this closure to distending pressure within the vessel is not clear. McIntyre (47) made tension-radius studies on the guinea pig ductus and by analysis of its physical properties determined this vessel would undergo critical closing at low intravascular pressure. The term critical closing pressure was devised by Burton (48) to describe forces in a blood vessel which tend to produce cessation of flow in the presence of active tension and a driving pressure.

REFERENCES

1. Galen: Opera Omnia IV:243. Kuhn Edition. Translation from Dalton, J.C.: *Doctrines of the Circulation.* Philadelphia, Lea's Son & Co., p. 68, 1884.
2. Carcano, Leone Grambattista: *Anatomici Libri II,* 1574.
3. Harvey, William: *Exercitatio Anatomica de Motu Cordis et Sanguinis in Animalibus.* Francofurti, Sumptibus Gulielmi Fitzeri, 1628.
4. Senac, J.B.: *Traite de la Steut, du Coeur I.* p. 369, 1773.
5. Billard, C.M.: *Traite des maladies des enfants nouveau-nes et a la mamelle, fonde sur de nouvelled observations cliniques et d'anatomie pathologique, faites a' i' hospital des enfants trouves de Paris.* Paris, 1828.
6. Thore, M.: De l'aneurysme, du canal arteriel. *Arch Gen Med Par, II*:30, 1850.
7. Flourens, P.P.: *Historie de la Deconverte de la circulation Du Sang Chez.* J.B. Vailliere, 1854.
8. Gerard, G.J.: Of the obliteration of the canal arterial, the theories and the facts. *J Anat Physiol, 36*:323, 1900.
9. De'Almagro, M.: *Etude Clinique et Anatomo-Pathologique sur Persistence du Canal Arteriel.* Paris, Theses, 1862.
10. Bernutz, G.: De la persistence du canal arteriel. *Arch Gen Med Par, XX*:415, 4th serie, 1849.
11. Alvarenga, P.F. DaC: *Considerations et Observations sur L'epoque de L'occlusion du Trou Ovale et Canal Arteriel.* Lisbon 1869.
12. Elsasser: Uber den Zustand der Fotuskreislaufwege bei neugeborenen Kinder, *Z Staafsarzneik, Bd LXIV,* 1852.
13. Scammon, R.E. and Norris, E.H.: On the time of the postnatal obliteration of the fetal blood passages (foramen ovale, ductus arteriosus, ductus venous). *Anat Rec, 15*:165, 1918.
14. Christie, A.: Normal closing time of the foramen ovale and the ductus arteriosus. *Am J Dis Child, 40*:323, 1930.
15. Mitchell, Shiela: The ductus arteriosus in the neonatal period. *J Pediatr, 51*:12, 1957.
16. King, T.W.: On the open state of the ductus arteriosus after birth, with illustrative cases. *Lond Edinbur Month J Med Sci, 11*:83, 1842.
17. Chevers, Norman: Observations on the permanence of the ductus arteriosus and constriction of the thoracic aorta, and on the means by which the duct becomes naturally closed. *Lond Med Gaz, 36*:187, 1845.
18. Walkoff, F.: Das Gewebe des ductus arteriosus und die obliteration disselben. *Z Med Leipz Heidelb 3,* R 36, 109, 1869.

19. Frieux: De L' obliteration du canal arteriel. *Bull Soc Anat Physiol Bordeaux, XV*:36, 1894.
20. Mancini, A.J.: A study of the angle formed by the ductus arteriosus with the descending thoracic aorta. *Anat Rec, 109*:535, 1951.
21. Barclay, A.E., Franklin, K.J., Prichard, M.L.: *The Foetal Circulation.* Oxford, Blackwell Scientific Publications, Ltd., p. 187, 1944.
22. Strassman, P.: Anatomische und physiologische untersuchungen uber den Blutkreislauf bei Neugeborenen. *Arch Gynzkol, 45*:393 1894.
23. Graper, Ludwig: Die anatomischen veranderungen kurz nach der Beburt. III. Ductus Botalli. *Z Anat Entwicklungsgesch, 61*:312, 1921.
24. Scharfe, H.: Der ductus Botalli, Beitrage zur physiologie und pathologie de verschlusses. *Beitr Geburtsch Gynak, 3*:368, 1900.
25. Virchow, R.: Die thrombosen der neugebornen. Gesammelte Abhandlungen zur Wissenschaftlichen Medicin Frankfurt, Meidinger, p. 591, 1856.
26. Rauchfuss, C.: Verber thrombose des ductus arteriosus Botalli. *Arch Pathol Anat, etc Berl, xvii*:376, 1859.
27. Variot, G. and Cailliau;: Research on the process of obliteration of the arteriel canal. *Bull Mem Soc Med Hop Paris, 44*:1598, 1920.
28. Dumontpallier, M.: Ru Retezsseiment Aortigue Auniveau de ll Abouchement du canal arteriel. *Mem Soc Biol III*:273, 1856.
29. Haberda, A.: *Die Fotalen Kreislaufswege des Neugebornen und Ihre Veranderungen nach der Geburt.* Wien, 1896.
30. Schultze, B.: *Der Scheintod Neugeborener.* Jena, Mauke, 1871.
31. Swensson, A.: Histologic structure and postembryonic closure. *Z Mikrosk Anat Forsch, 46*:275, 1939.
32. Kiwisch: Quoted by Gerard, G.: De L' obliteration du canal arteriel, les theories et les facts. *J Anat Physiol, 36*:323, 1851.
33. Kennedy, J.A. and Clark, S.L.: Observations on the ductus arteriosus of the guinea pig in relation to its method of closure. *Anat Rec, 79*:349, 1941.
34. Kennedy, J.A. and Clark, S.L.: Observations of the physiological reactions of the ductus arteriosus. *Am J Physiol, 136*:140, 1942.
35. Kennedy, J.A.: A new concept of the cause of patency of the ductus arteriosus. *Am J Med Sci, 204*:570, 1942.
36. Born, G.V.R., Dawes, G.S., Mott, J.C. and Rennick, B.R.: The constriction of the ductus arteriosus caused by oxygen and by asphyxia in newborn lambs. *J Physiol (Lond), 132*:304, 1956.
37. Record, R.G. and McKeown, T.: The effect of reduced atmospheric pressure on closure of the ductus arteriosus in the guinea pig. *Clin Sci, 14*:225, 1955.
38. Amoroso, E.C., Dawes, G.S., and Mott, J.C.: Patency of the ductus arteriosus in the newborn colt and foal. *Br Heart J 20*:92, 1958.
39. Rowe, R.D., Sinclair, J.D., Kerr, A.R. and Gage, P.W.: Duct flow and

mitral regurgitation during changes in oxygenation in newborn swine. *J Appl Physiol, 19*:1157, 1964.

40. Coughlin, F.E. and Husson, G.S.: Effect of hypoxia on the closure of the ductus arteriosus in the chick. *Am J Dis Child, 100*:531, 1960.

41. Everett, N.B. and Johnson, R.J.: A physiological and anatomical study of the closure of the ductus arteriosus in the dog. *Anat Rec, 110*:103, 1951.

42. Fay, F.S.: Guinea pig ductus arteriosus. I. Cellular and metabolic basis for oxygen sensitivity. *Am J Physiol, 221*:470, 1971.

43. Lind, J., Stern, L. and Wegelius, C.: *Human Foetal and Neonatal Circulation.* Springfield, Thomas, p. 22, 1964.

44. Prec, K.J. and Cassels, D.E.: Dye dilution curves and cardiac output in newborn infants. *Circulation, XI*:789, 1955.

45. Adams, F.H. and Lind, J.: Physiologic studies on the cardiovascular status of normal newborn infants (with special reference to the ductus arteriosus). *Pediatrics, 19*:431, 1957.

46. Moss, A.J., Emmanouilides, G.C. and Duffie, E.R.: Closure of the ductus arteriosus in the newborn infant. *Pediatrics, 32*:25, 1963.

47. McIntyre, T.W.: An analysis of critical closure in the isolated ductus arteriosus. *Biophys J, 9*:685, 1969.

48. Burton, A.C.: On the physical equilibrium of small blood vessels. *Am J Physiol, 164*:319, 1951.

Nine

THE FETAL DUCTUS —
PULMONARY ARTERY SYSTEM

I. Conventional concepts of the fetal circulation
INDICATE:

1. there is medial hypertrophy, contraction and perhaps tortuous
distal pulmonary artery vessels. Some of this may be related to complete atelectasis or at least no air expansion of alveoli. These observations indicate there is a high resistance to blood flow through the
lungs with a consequent small pulmonary flow up to the time of
birth, perhaps 10 percent of the pulmonary artery flow. However,
there remains some controversy regarding this, some maintaining that
toward term there is a much larger flow to the lungs. There is no
explanation why medial hypertrophy with small lumen to wall-ratios
exists in the neonate in the absence of increased pressure/flow in
this system unless vasoconstriction produces hypertrophy.

2. At birth, concomitant with lung expansion, there is a marked
drop in resistance, the alveoli oxygenate blood and increase of oxygen
affects constriction of the ductus which is sensitive to oxygen, and
an independent functioning oxygenation-circulation system is acquired.

II. On closer inspection of the voluminous literature, chiefly related
to newborn animals especially lambs, this conventional concept
has many exceptions. Sciacca and Condorelli (1) have reviewed
critically the early data both in relation to the pioneer work of
Barclay et al. (2) demonstrating the fetal circulation angiograph-
ically in the lamb and that of Kennedy and Clark (3) relating to
vasoconstriction of the ductus by the influence of oxygen. The
stimulus of oxygen in vasomotion of the ductus, although the
mechanism is unknown, seems well substantiated by many subse-

quent reports. But the ductus responds to other stimuli, as they pointed out, and more than one receptor may be present. Response to mechanical stimulation, norepinephrine, acetylcholine and sometimes spontaneous constriction without a known stimulus have all been documented.

1. Naeye and Blanc (4) find the muscle mass in small pulmonary arteries is increased in premature closure of the foramen ovale. This means that when blood flow/volume/pressure is increased in the main pulmonary artery-ductus-descending aorta complex there is an effect on the distal small vessels, presumably due to increased flow, pressure or both. These vessel changes are present before birth. Whether the medial muscle is a response to increased pulmonary pressure-flow exerted by hemodynamic oriented constriction of the ductus is not known but is a reasonable speculation.

2. Naeye (5) also points out increased muscle mass was present in instances of coarctation of the aorta with a distal open ductus both before and after birth. This increase was found in all arteries and arterioles observed. The left ventricle is hypertrophied also. The pulmonary vascular bed is therefore caught between an overactive left heart, with pressure overload from aortic obstruction, and increased pulmonary artery flow from diminished left atrium, left ventricle filling through the foramen ovale. Again, it is a reasonable assumption that the pulmonary arterial system has increased flow and pressure, and again, pressure/flow hemodynamic stimulus in the ductus may cause contraction in this area. The effect of transfusion and increased ductus flow/pressure as a stimulus to ductus contraction are not known.

3. It has been shown (6) in the recipient twin in the monovular twin-placental syndrome, where the recipient twin has an increased volume but low pressure return from the placenta, the pulmonary artery muscle mass is increased at birth, while the donor has normal or lowered pulmonary artery mass. These facets must be a reflection of (a) increased flow/pressure, or (b) left heart distress. Frank heart distress or frank heart failure may occur and it is believed fibroelastosis may occur as a consequence of these hemodynamic events.

4. When right ventricle-pulmonary artery and ductus-aorta flow is increased due to left heart malformations, medial muscle mass in the pulmonary vascular bed is increased. Again, prenatal increase of flow seems to be the underlying factor.

This presumes increased flow through the pulmonary artery and ductus has as a side effect increased flow through the right and left branches of the pulmonary artery.

It should be noted this increased flow must contain a greater percent of oxygenated blood than normal, and vasoconstriction of the
ductus with proximal elevation of pulmonary artery pressure may
occur.

5. The possibility of the readiness of the lung for the assumption
of full pulmonary flow has been indicated in fetal or newborn animals, for the ductus has shown unmistakable evidence of preparation
for closure prenatally.

GUINEA PIG[1]. (a) There was histological evidence of early
events of closure during late fetal life. The media was invaded by
mucoid substance and cells which later bacame connective tissue.
The muscle fibers in the media atrophied. There was no acceleration
of events in the first few postnatal days. (b) There was an arrest of
growth of the ductus, but the pulmonary artery increased in size.
(c) The walls of the ductus became narrower. (d) Ligation of the
ductus near term did not result in right ventricle dilatation or serious
circulatory disturbance. Angiographic studies indicated no appreciable change in the appearance of the pulmonary vessels before or
after ligation of the ductus. Earlier ligation produced dilatation of
the right ventricle and distress occurred.

PUPPY. Occlusion of the ductus in the fetal dog near term is compatible with life in utero, but not with live birth. Cineangioghaphic
studies, however, showed no evidence of increased flow in the pulmonary vessels after ligation. Increased flow through the foramen
ovale with immediate opacification of the ascending aorta was
noted (8).

However, in the ductus ligated puppies, there was marked increase in pulmonary flow following inflation of the lungs.

LAMB. Live birth after fetal occlusion of the ductus occurred three
times in twenty. Pulmonary artery pressure increased 25 to 35 percent following ligation, but reverted to normal within ten minutes.
The increased blood flow was accommodated presumably by diminution of resistance. It would then appear that considerable species
variation occurs in the fetal lung (9).

RAT. In the rat prenatal ultrastructural studies show changes
thought to represent preparation for closure since the ductus is
closed anatomically twenty-four hours after birth. There is: (a) subendothelial vacuolization, (b) extension of medial smooth muscle
cells through the internal elastic membrane into the subendothelial
area, (c) interruption of elastic lamellae and (d) distended endoplasmic reticulum. Late hemodynamic changes or the relation of
anatomical change to pulmonary blood flow are not known (10).

HUMAN. Potter and Adair (11), in a study of the cause of death
of the fetus and death in the neonatal period, did not find evidence
for sudden augentation of pulmonary blood flow after birth. For in-

stance, weight of the lung was not increased enough to determine whether death occurred before or after birth. They concluded that in the human late prenatal pulmonary blood flow was not changed considerably after birth.

The prenatal embryology of the lung indicates that at seven to seven and one-half months, 1400 to 1500 gm, there is a sudden change in the anatomy. Arteries assume some mature characteristics and capillaries are widely open (12).

Since direct and indirect radiological observation in animals indicate the postnatal constriction of the ductus, the problem of (a) the presence of fetal ductus tone and changing diameter and (b) the possibility of a hypoplastic ductus media in prenatal life can be considered.

Uterine contraction changes the oxygenation of fetal blood as a basis for constriction of the ductus. Vascular tone in the ductus arteriosus has been demonstrated (13).

Apparent reduced muscle in the ductus was suggested in an instance of severe heart failure in a neonate (14). While the histological features of the patent ductus have been studied in the older infant and child, the critical information would be in early infancy before vascular degenerative disease has appeared in the vessel.

Certainly surgeons report considerable variability in wall thickness and in systolic distensibility of the ductus in infants. Postoperative quantitation of biopsy specimens or autopsy material becomes difficult due to contraction, or to overdistension of the pressure fixed ductus.

CLINICAL ASPECTS

Ziegler (15) was among the first to emphasize the importance of the patent ductus in the severe heart failure in early infancy. Following the analysis of the fetal pulmonary vessels by Civin and Edwards (16) instances of early failure were explained by accelerated involution of high resistance fetal vessels due to increased lumen to wall ratio in small vessels.

Variation with increased muscle mass in special situations has been studied. Less emphasis has been placed on the absence of such medial hypertrophy. The consequent low resistance, high flow pulmonary circulation in early infancy may be associated with heart failure.

Heath, et al. (17), as well as Keith, Rowe and Vlad (14) have reported such infants with hypoplastic pulmonary vessels and heart failure.

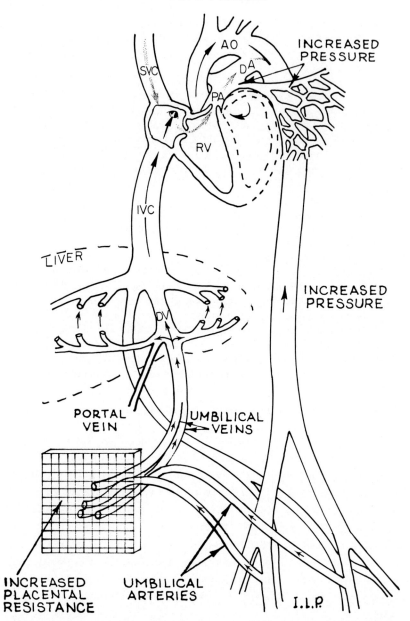

Figure 29. A schematic diagram of the possible role of the placenta in the fetal pulmonary vascular system. If increased resistance is produced by infarction and vascular obstruction increased pressure occurs in the aorta, the open ductus arteriosus and the pulmonary artery. Whether this affects the smaller pulmonary vessels is not known.

The two infants with patent ductus arteriosus studied by Heath et al. (17) were two days of age and neither survived intractable heart failure. The lumen to wall ratios in all vessels were 3.6:1 in one infant and 4.5:1 in the second patient in contrast to the normal control of 1.4:1 during the first day and 2.3:1 the subsequent month.

This involution did not occur in two days. The status of intra-uterine pulmonary blood flow is not known.

In the patient referred to by Rowe and Mehrizi (18) it was thought there was less than usual muscle mass both in the ductus and in the small pulmonary arteries.

The hemodynamic or metabolic control of small vessel medial hypertrophy is not clear, but exceptions to the usual fetal physiology are exceptionally important. For instance, Dawes (19) produced evidence that high resistance in the unexpanded lung was due almost entirely to vasoconstriction and could be changed remarkably by vasodilating substances as acetylcholine.

The Placenta and The Ductus

Inadequate attention has been given to the possible role of the placenta in relation to pulmonary vascular hemodynamics and medial wall hypertrophy.

In Figure 29, a schematic portrayal of the fetal circulation, increased placental resistance must raise the pressure in the aorta to ductus to pulmonary artery and branches. The role of placental dysfunction in the circulation of the postmature infant is not clear, although neonatal systemic hypertension tends to be present in the postmaturity syndrome. It is believed in case 2 of the report of Prec, et al. (20) who had pulmonary hypertension and thick walled pulmonary arterioles and heart failure at age two weeks, postmaturity played a role.

While it seems reasonable that this scheme plays a role in determining the status of the pulmonary vascular bed, the necessary studies are incomplete. It is not known, for instance, if increased aortic pressure is transmitted to the pulmonary artery, or if this stimulus causes constriction of the ductus and prevention of transmission of pressure to the pulmonary system.

REFERENCES

1. Sciacca, A. and Condorelli, M.: Involution of the ductus arteriosus. *Bibl Cardiol,* suppl. to Cardiologica Fasc. *10,* S. Karger, Basel, Switzerland, 1960.
2. Barclay, A.E., Barcroft, J., Barron, D.H. and Franklin, K.J.: A radiographic demonstration of the circulation through the heart in the adult and in the foetus and the identification of the ductus arteriosus. *Br J Radiol, 12*:505, 1939.
3. Kennedy, A.J. and Clark, S.L.: Observations on the physiological reactions of the ductus arteriosus. *Am J Physiol, 136*:140, 1942.
4. Naeye, R.L. and Blanc, W.A.: Prenatal narrowing or closure of the foramen ovale. *Circulation, 30*:736, 1964.
5. Naeye, R.L.: Perinatal vascular changes in coarctation of the aorta with distal patent ductus arteriosus. *Circulation, 24*:754, 1961.
6. Naeye, R.L.: Human intrauterine parabiotic syndrome and its complications. *N Engl J Med, 268*:804, 1963.
7. Naeye, R.L.: Perinatal vascular changes asociated with under development of the left heart. *Am J Pathol, 41*:287, 1962.
8. Haller, J., Morgan, W., Rodgers, B. Gengos, D. and Margulies, S.: Chronic hemodynamic effects of occluding the fetal ductus arteriosus. *J Cardiovasc Surg, 54*:770, 1967.
9. Almond, C.: In discussion of Haller's Paper: Chronic hemodynamic effects of occluding the fetal ductus arteriosus. *J Cardiovasc Surg, 54*:770, 1967.
10. Jones, M., Barrow, M. and Wheat, M.: An ultrastructure evaluation of the closure of the ductus arteriosus in rats. *Surgery, 66*:891, 1969.
11. Potter, E. and Adair, F.: *Fetal and Neonatal Death.* Chicago, U of Chicago Pr, 1949.
12. Engel, S.: *The Prenatal Lung.* Oxford, Pergamon, 1966.
13. Bromberger-Barnes, B., Rowe, R.D. and Bor, I.: Vascular tone in the ductus arteriosus. *Circulation, 32*:259, 1965.
14. Keith, J.D., Rowe, R.D. and Vlad, P.: *Heart Disease in Infancy and Childhood,* 2nd 5d. New York, MacMillan, p. 178.
15. Ziegler, R.: The importance of patent ductus arteriosus in infants. *Am Heart J, 43*:553, 1952.
16. Civin, W.H. and Edwards, J.E.: Postnatal structural changes in intrapulmonary arteries and arterioles. *Arch Pathol, 51*:192, 1951.
17. Heath, D., Swan, H.J.C., DuShane, J.W. and Edwards, J.E.: The relation of medial thickness of small muscular pulmonary arteries to immediate postnatal survival in patients with ventricular septal defect and patent ductus arteriosus. *Thorax, 13*:267, 1958.
18. Rowe, R. and Mehrizi, A.: *The Neonate With Congenital Herat Disease.* Philadelphia, Saunders, 1958, p. 183.
19. Dawes, G.S.: Vasodilation in the unexpanded foetal lung. *Med Thorac, 19*:345, 1962.

20. Prec, K.J., Cassels, D.E., Rabinowitz, M. and Moulder, P.V.: Cardiac failure and patency of the ductus arteriosus in early infancy. *J Pediatr, 61*:843, 1962.

Ten

THE PATENT DUCTUS ARTERIOSUS

I. HISTORICAL ASPECTS OF CLINICAL RECOGNITION OF PATENCY

D R. BABINGTON (1), IN 1847, PUBLISHED IN THE LONDON MEDICAL GAZETTE details of a patient he had seen:

> The patient was a female of 34 years of age who had palpitation, precordial pain, dyspnea and cough. The heart impulse was forceful. Both the heart sounds were prolonged, especially the second, and both wre accompanied by loud sawing murmurs, which are heard over the whole precordium but loudest over the third and fourth sternocostal articulations, right as well as left. Immediately after the flap of the valves, which is loud, there follows a sharp click which is the commencement of the second murmur. This is distinctly heard over the second sternocostal articulation. Both sounds were heard over the back and down the spine to the sacrum. Ecchymotic spots appeared on each cheek, and could be felt. She was seen by Dr. Wilkinson King, who made the diagnosis of patescence of the ductus arteriosus.
>
> Autopsy showed fluid in the abdomen, patchy areas in the lungs looking as if they had never been expanded. The whole heart was enlarged, both ventricles dilated, their walls thickened. The aortic orifice was diminished in calibre, from a large vegetation the size of a filbert nut which occupied two thirds of the ventricular surface of the anterior leaflet. There was a perforation on the aortic surface of the valve, leading into the vegetation, forming a small aneurysm. There was abnormality of the other valves, one bound down by a band from the ventricular surface. The aorta was narrowed through-out, and above the left subclavian a narrow band over one third the

circumference of the vessel further narrowed it at this point. There was a circular opening the size of a goose quill at the position of the ductus, between the aorta and pulmonary artery, which were in perfect opposition at this point.

Dr. Williams (2), unidentified, in further commenting on this case stated:

a sure ground for diagnosis of the patent ductus arteriosus when there is no other serious lesion to obscure it, that the murmur accompanying the first sound of the heart is prolonged into the second, so that there is no cessation of this murmur before the second has already commenced. From this sign, of course, with other symptoms, he was able in two cases which lately fell under his notice to diagnosticate this lesion, and postmortem examination proved the accuracy of this diagnosis.

This is a concise description of the clinical diagnosis of the patent ductus, although unfortunately the protocols of Williams's cases have not been published. The case of Babington is complicateed by subacute bacterial endocarditis and coarctation of the aorta, but is probably acceptable as one of the first recorded instnces of clinical diagnosis. The ductus was of the unusual *window* type.

In 1873 Fagge (3) described:
a female, aged 42 years, who was reported never to have had rheumatic fever, and who gave birth to four children without any difficulty. He entitled his paper "A case of patent ductus arteriosus attended with a peculiar diastolic murmur". She became ill six months before her first admission to Guy's Hospital in 1869. She had been confined, and afterwards her abdomen began to swell, she was breathless, and was not able to lie down. The pulse was slow, thirty-four to forty-three per minute. There was a systolic murmur, loudest between the fourth and fifth costal cartilage, near the sternum, with the intensity diminishing toward the axilla. There was a "wavy bruit" loudest at the second left costal cartilage, close to the sternum. It had a musical quality, and there was no interval between the second sound and the bruit, although lower there was such an interval, and here the murmur was separated from the next first sound by a considerable interval. A diagram of the murmur was given, which showed separate systolic and diastolic murmurs. Autopsy showed great enlargement of the heart, the foramen ovale was closed, the tricuspid valve greatly enlarged, the base of the aorta was of less size than the base of the pulmonary artery, whose branches were greatly dilated. The ductus was patent and a size six to seven catheter could

be passed through a short canal. He refers to the case of Wade where there was an aneurysmal communication between the aorta and the pulmonary artery, where the murmurs were of a loud bellows quality, and Bennet (4) had also recorded a case of a communication with the pulmonary artery, with two murmurs at the base of the heart, with the second sound clear and healthy.

Soon after this, others reported cases of patent ductus, with greater attention to the auscultatory findings. During the period from 1850 to 1900 the art of auscultation improved and became routine in the examination of the heart. These descriptions did not crystallize into criteria generally accepted for clinical diagnosis of the patent ductus arteriosus, but several of these have the familiarity of current literature. Thus Gerhardt (5) spoke of prolongation of the murmur during diastole, and Durosiez (6) found a double thrill and a double murmur at the level of the pulmonary artery in a female aged 28 years. Autopsy showed a patent ductus and a dilated pulmonary artery, but the two sigmoid valves were fenestrated and insufficient. Gilbert (7) showed a patient with a continuous thrill, with reinforcement after the *systolic shock,* diminishing progressively to the end of diastole. And Hochhaus (8) in 1893 observed a young man with an accentuated pulmonary second sound in the second left interspace, followed by a diastolic murmur. Autopsy showed an open ductus, shaped like a funnel, a distended pulmonary artery and altered pulmonary valves. And there are other isolated cases reported, where the murmurs described resemble the current literature.

Descriptions of the auscultatory findings in the presence of a communication between the aorta and the pulmonary artery gradually accumulated. These observations were confused by the papers of Francois-Franck (9) which were quoted widely. In 1878 he published a paper on the diagnosis of the persistence of the arterial canal. He discussed two points of diagnosis, (a) the location and the type of murmur present, and (b) the effect of the persistent ductus on the peripheral pulse. In regard to the first he said the typical murmur was a systolic murmur posteriorly, to the left of the vertebral column, at the level of the third and fourth dorsal vertebra. This description was republished in other places, and became quite popular, both in the subsequent literature and as an aid to clinical diagnosis. In regard to the second point he wrote the radial pulse diminishes in amplitude during inspiration, and increases on expiration, and he showed this by sphygmography. He explained this phenomenon by saying there was greatly increased blood flow into the lungs on inspiration, by dilatation of the intra-pulmonary vessels, and the opposite effect occurred during expiration. Again, he wrote of this in more than one place (10) and was quoted avidly. This shrewd observation was correct, if the ductus is of any size, but his auscultatory criteria retarded understanding of the murmur produced by an arteriovenous fistula. He summarized his diagnostic criteria as (a) a systolic murmur posteriorly, to the left of the vertebral column, (b) inspiratory reinforcement of the murmur, (c) a change in the pulse with respiration and (d) the absence of any cyanosis.

In the same year he published a further consideration of the change in the peripheral pulse in the presence of a patent ductus. He noted the influence of respiration on the pulse is considered an abnormal phenomenon, called in Germany pulsus parodoxicus. He said with the patent ductus, during inspiration the blood flows more freely into the pulmonary bed, and the pulse is less, while on expiration the blood passes less freely from the aorta to lungs, and pulse is fuller. Therefore, he concluded, the paradoxical pulse is only an exaggeration of the normal influences of respiration.

Description of the cardiac murmurs diagnostic of patency of the ductus arteriosus were published with increasing frequency. It remained for Gibson (11) to evaluate these suggestions and to propose diagnostic criteria for the diagnosis of the average instance of patency of the ductus which have not been improved upon. He stated these simply, and without reservation. It is of interest that he did so in a clinical demonstration for third year medical students, which was then published in the Edinburgh Medical Journal.

Gibson wrote (11):
congenital affections of the heart do not lend themselves in general to ordinary clinical teaching. Most of the lesions as so complicated in their nature that the resulting symptoms are difficult of explanation. They are without doubt of the deepest interest to a speculative mind, but for you in your arly student days they are but a waste of time, which may be much more usefully employed otherwise. There is, nevertheless, amongst the many different congenital lesions of the

heart one particular variety of malformation so easy of detection as to
be instructive even for the junior student of clinical medicine. This
is persistence of the arterial duct, which will form the subject of lecture today, in order to give me the opportunity of formulating its
diagnosis, as well as provide me with an occasion of replying to
certain strictures recently passed on me . . . This malformation is
easily recognized during life by the physical examination.

In consequence of the higher pressure of the blood in the aorta, as
compared with the pulmonary artery, there must be a current from
the former to the latter, and this stream will be almost, if not quite,
continuous. It will of necessity flow with its greatest velocity during,
and immediately after, the ventricular systole, when the aortic blood
pressure is at its highest; from that phase it will gradually become
less swift, as the pressures in the two great vessels approximate more
nearly to each other during the period of repose. It must therefore be
expected that, as evidence of patent ductus arteriosus, there will be a

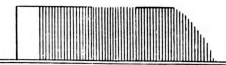
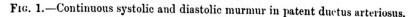

Fɪɢ. 1.—Continuous systolic and diastolic murmur in patent ductus arteriosus.

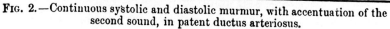
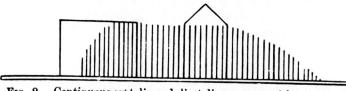

Fɪɢ. 2.—Continuous systolic and diastolic murmur, with accentuation of the
second sound, in patent ductus arteriosus.

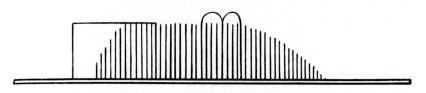

Fɪɢ. 3.—Continuous systolic and diastolic murmur, with doubling of the
second sound, in patent ductus arteriosus.

Figure 30. Reproduction of the diagram of Gibson showing the pathognomic murmur of patent ductus arteriosus. He noted it began distinctly
after the first sound, occupies systole, accompanies the second sound which
may be accentuated or doubled and dies away during diastole.
From Gibson, G.A.: *Edinb Med J, 8:*1, 1900.

long murmur, filling up the short pause (systole) and continuing beyond the second sound. The murmur may be, in fact it almost invariably is, accompanied by a well-marked thrill. The localization of murmur was well as of vibration will naturally be in the second or third left intercostal space, just outside of or inferior to the conventional pulmonary area . . . From a careful study of these cases, the diagnosis has come to seem in my eyes almost as exact as the solution of a mathematical problem. The rhythm of the murmur is laid down definitely, and figured diagrammatically in my work on the Heart.[12] (Fig. 30)

. . . Let me, in conclusion, gather up briefly the essential facts upon which the diagnosis of persistent ductus arteriosus may be founded with perfect confidence. There may be no dyspnea, cyanosis, oedema, or other evidence of disturbance of the general circulation, and the recognition of the lesion may depend entirely on the presence of a few physical signs. Inspection may fail to yield any facts of diagnostic importance; palpatoin usually reveals the long thrill following the apical impulse, and enduring beyond the recoil of the blood on the semilunar cusps, which may be felt during the thrill; percussion may not show any enlargement of the cardiac dullness; while auscultation gives convincing evidence of the lesion in a murmur which may be regarded as almost pathogonomic. Beginning distinctly after the first sound, it accompanies the latter part of that sound, occupies the short pause (systole) accompanies the second sound, which may be accentuated in the pulmonary area, or may be, and often is, doubled, and finally dies away during the long pause (diastole.)

II. THE SYNDROME OF PATENCY

The clinical syndrome of patency of the ductus varies from (a) remarkably complex and changeable status in the newborn and early infancy, through (b) the more typical and identifiable manifestations of a free blood flow from the aorta to pulmonary artery due to a positive pressure gradient, to (c) the complicated pathological, hemodynamic and clinical aspects of the patent ductus associated with pulmonary hypertension.

The typical and usual syndrome is defined as (a) persistent patency of the ductus arteriosus which has junction below the left subclavian artery with a normal aorta, (b) it usually has length, often to 8 to 10 mm. (c) It is often described as a continuation of the main pulmonary artery in the newborn or usually arises at or joins the base of the left branch of the pulmonary artery and rarely the right in older patients, and (d) is associated with a systolic and diastolic pressure gradient from aorta to pulmonary artery and consequently blood flow and murmur in both phases of the cardiac cycle.

The position of the ductus arteriosus in relation to the heart and great vessels in shown in Figure 31. A venous catheter (a) from the right arm passes through the superior vena cava, the right ventricle and pulmonary artery. It traverses the ductus arteriosus into the descending aorta. A second catheter (b) ascends the aorta and passes through the ductus into the left pulmonary artery. The ductus arteriosus lies medial and posterior to the point where the catheters cross.

The large ductus and the window type, a side to side direct communication with the aorta at the ductus side, are usually

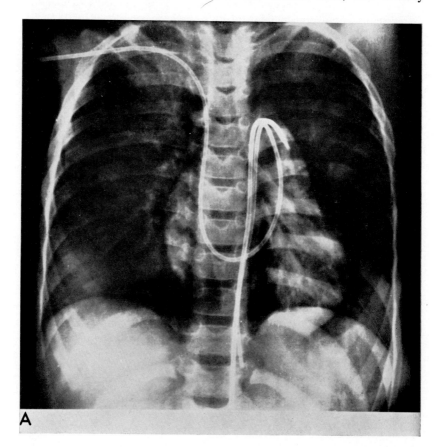

A

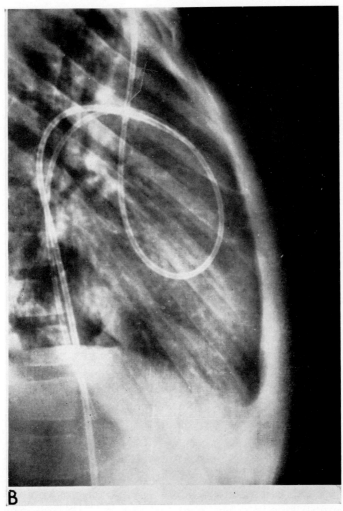

B

Figure 31. Patent ductus arteriosus with moderate increase of pulmonary flow, two times systemic. Catheters placed to indicate some anatomical facets. Catheter 1, right arm, passes through superior vena cava, right atrium, right ventricle, pulmonary artery, ductus arteriosus and down the descending aorta. Catheter 2 ascends the aorta, passes through the ductus arteriosus and into the left pulmonary artery. The ductus lies at the point where catheters cross in the A-P view and in the lateral view about at this same landmark.

associated with pulmonary hypertension and represent a special complex problem. The ductus is termed giant at 15 mm but in the younger child is very large at 10 mm.

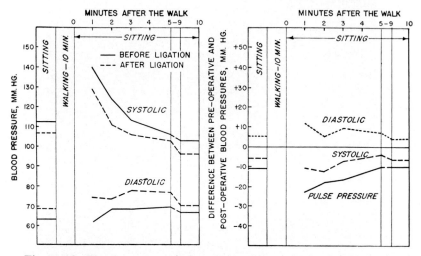

Figure 32. Blood pressure before and after closure of patent ductus arteriosus. Average of seven patients.
From Cassels, D.E., Morse, M. and Adams, W.: *Pediatrics,* 6:557, 1950.

The systemic blood pressure as determined clinically has an increased pulse pressure usually due to diminished diastolic pressure. The fall in systolic pressure found by Rudolph et al. (13) within a few beats after opening an aortic pulmonary artery shunt is not sustained, as the left heart return from the lung becomes augmented by the large shunt from the aorta with consequent increase of aortic flow. The typical response after exercise is shown in Figure 32 (14). In the infant and in the young child who objects to a blood pressure cuff this increased pulse pressure can be appreciated by palpation in the brachial or femoral artery by a typical bounding or collapsing character. However, this characteristic depends upon aortic run off and can occur in aortic valvular regurgitation. But simple dilatation of the peripheral arteriolar bed can produce increased diastolic flow which imitates these lesions and the visible capillary pulse in the subungual region is visible in the absence of heart disease in some children.

A low diastolic pressure becomes especially important in the presence of a slow heart rate, when low pressure and perfusion may affect the sensorium. This is illustrated by congenital heart block in association with a patent ductus in addition.

The peripheral pulse and blood flow has been studied by finger plethysmography (15). The essential observation again was the widened pulse pressure with a low diastolic component.

The pathognomic murmur of patency of the ductus was described by Gibson (11). Some details may be added and additional murmurs related to augmented blood flow are shown schematically in Figures 33 and 34.

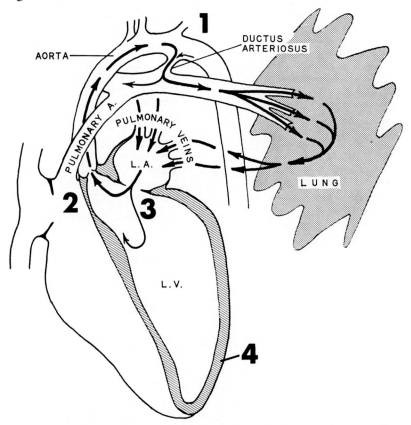

Figure 33. Representation of the site of origin of murmurs associated with a patent ductus arteriosus. 1 - murmurs at the ductus and pulmonary artery, 2 - systolic ejection murmur at the aortic valve due to increased stroke volume and 3 - mid-diastolic murmur arising from augmented flow at the mitral valve, sometimes called the flow murmur of relative mitral stenosis. 4 - Indicates a dilated left ventricle with a typical V6.

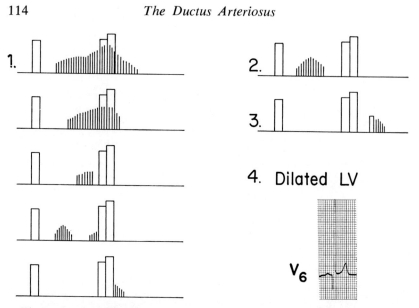

Figure 34. Diagram of murmurs which may occur with a patent ductus arteriosus. 1. With increasing pulmonary artery pressure the systolic component becomes a shorter, the diastolic disappears. With bidirectional shunting the systolic element disappears. There is a diastolic murmur of pulmonary valve insufficiency. An ejection murmur may appear related to pulmonary artery dilatation and this may persist after closure (see Fig. 45). 2. An ejection murmur occurs at the aortic valve with a large left ventricular stroke volume. 3. A mid-diastolic murmur may be present due to a large volume blood flow across the mitral valve often referred to a murmur of relative mitral stenosis. 4. V6 of a typical dilated left ventricle is shown to complement the hemodynamics.

1. The murmur of Gibson, filling most of systole, continuing through S_2 and into diastole for a variable period never starts with the closure of the atrioventricular valves, or with S_1. Time is required for systolic ejection of a pulse wave through the aortic arch, the ductus and into the turbulence of the pulmonary artery blood flow where major components of the murmur arise in most instances.

2. A mid-systolic or ejection murmur may occur at the aortic valve, with the same explanation: a large flow gives a murmur arising at the inflow valve of the left ventricle during left ventricular diastole. The same large flow produces a murmur at the aortic valve, during systolic outflow from the left ventricle. This murmur may be lost in the loud continuous murmur, but sometimes is loud and an associated defect is suspected. The loudness of these functional murmurs will depend upon (a) the size of the blood flow involved and (b) anatomical features of the valves. For instance Rudolph et al.

(13) found an actual pressure gradient across the aortic valve when an aortic pulmonary artery prosthetic shunt was opened.

3. Augmented pulmonary flow from the aorta-ductus communication increases flow into the left atrium by the amount shunted. As this augmented flow crosses the mitral valve, a mid-diastolic murmur is produced, sometimes referred to as the murmur relative mitral stenosis. A normal valve may have twice the normal flow and produces an obstruction type murmur during this flow resembling that of mitral stenosis. This is heard only if the pulmonary flow is large, nearly twice systemic flow. In general, the greater this flow the louder the murmur. This murmur indicates a large flow regardless of other data, if there is only an uncomplicated patent ductus arteriosus and no associated mitral valve disease.

A correlation of the murmur and mean pulmonary artery pressure was found by Krovetz and Warden (16). They noted patients with continuous murmurs tend to have a lower pressure, but a systolic murmur alone and pulmonary artery pressure under 40 mm Hg can occur in the infant group. This is seen especially in early infancy. The reason is not clear although ventricular asynchromy can be invoked with right to left shunting in the face of a mean pressure gradient from aorta to pulmonary artery.

However, a complex study of the cardiac murmur from the ductus was undertaken by Dawes et al. (17), and probably many facets of this murmur in lambs are applicable to the clinical problem.

The hemodynamic conditions which cause a murmur in the patent ductus arteriosus was studied by observation of physical variables related to production of the murmur. A preparation was devised in which velocity and volume of blood flow and the diameter of the ductus and pressure gradient across it could be varied.

The data of a typical example is shown in the diagram of the authors (Fig. 35). This is read conveniently from right to left since this begins with the ductus widely patent with little pressure gradient and a large flow at low velocity through it. There was no murmur. The diameter of the lumen could be changed by a tape around the vessel and when progressively constricted the flow was reduced but the pressure gradient and velocity of flow increased. A murmur appeared, but when the flow was reduced to less than 10 percent it disappeared.

Since the murmur was not related to flow, velocity or pressure gradient, it was thought it was due to turbulence within the pulmonary trunk. The murmur did not appear until the internal diameter was greatly reduced, even when the gradient was increased by 10 mm Hg.

The Reynolds number is a dimensionless quantity which de-

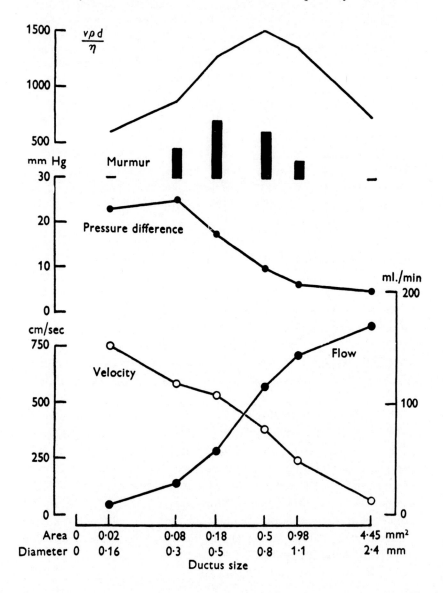

scribes the conditions under which laminar flow changed to turbulent flow.

Turbulence in flow in a pipe, assuming the analogy is suitable, is related to the Reynolds number for the fluid, in this instance blood, and Re $=$ ^{vdp} , where v is the mean linear velocity, p the density of the liquid, d the diameter and n the viscosity. This fraction was plotted against ductus diameter, and the values obtained were thought to be reasonbale for the conditions.

The clinical implication, especially in the newborn period, would be that (a) no murmur is heard early when the ductus is widely patent, (b) a murmur appears when the ductus begins to contract and (c) the continuous murmur, often present for a few days, represents the closing phase of the ductus. The pulmonary artery pressure is reduced, the aortic pressure elevated and the pressure gradient and the narrowed ductus contribute to the continuous murmur.

The changing murmurs of the patent ductus arteriosus shown in Figure 34 resemble those produced by narrowing of the aorta by a clamp in the closed chest of a dog (18). The murmur was recorded by a phonocatheter in the aorta below the constriction. As narrowing began a murmur occurred in late systole with a gradient of 10 to 15 mm Hg. With increasing gradient the murmur extended retrograde into systole and across S_2 and gradually became a continuous murmur. This is analogous to the late systolic murmur with pulmonary hypertension and a small gradient, a longer systolic murmur with less hypertension and a continuous murmur across S_2 with a more modest hypertension.

The x-ray in the typical patent ductus with 20 to 50 percent of

Figure 35. Study of Dawes, Mott and Widdicombe of the ductus murmur. Lamb, chest open, positive pressure ventilation. The pressure difference between the two ends of the ductus arteriosus and the volume and velocity of blood flow through the ductus arteriosus are plotted against its calculated internal diameter and cross-sectional area. The comparative intensity of the murmur in the pulmonary trunk is shown as estimated from phonocardiograph records. The Reynolds number has been calculated from the equation Re $=$ vd/0.02, assuming the density of blood $=$ 1.0 and viscosity $=$ 0.02. From Dawes, G.S., Mott, J.C. and Widdicombe, J.G.: *J Physiol, 128*:344, 1955.

aortic flow directed through the ductus is not diagnostic of this lesion. The findings are those of (a) increased pulmonary flow, (b) increased pulmonary venous return to the left atrium, (c) increased flow and volume in the left ventricle and (d) sometimes evidence of increased flow in the ascending aorta, dilatation.

X-rays of the typical patent ductus arteriosus may be diagnostic of increased pulmonary flow, depending on whether this flow is large or small. Since the pulmonary artery silhouette is accentuated in normal children, the normal prominence of the pulmonary artery in children may be over read in the presence of known heart disease.

Increased flow entering the pulmonary vessels returns to the left atrium, the left atrium does not distend as readily as the atrium on the right and increased blood flow and distention is not obvious at once. However, the shadow of the left atrium when seen in an A-P or lateral view is almost always abnormal and suggestive of (a) increased pulmonary venous return or (b) obstruction at the mitral valve. Figure 36 illustrates this, perhaps in an exaggerated way, in a child with a large flow patent ductus.

Enlargement or dilatation of the left ventricle is difficult to identify unless at least of moderate degree. The average patent ductus flow does not enlarge the left ventricle definitely by x-ray, but often this question can be raised. Enlargement of specific chambers in the presence of left-to-right shunts increase with age, a left ventricle doubtfully enlarged at five years may be diagnostically dilated at age ten or fifteen years.

The ascending aorta may appear visible or even prominent in the presence of a large left ventricular output. This never resembles the gross poststenotic dilatation observed in the presence of valvular aortic stenosis. But it may be sufficiently distinct to be confused with a visible border of the left atrium.

Figure 36. K.T., age three months, PA pressure 75/35, Qp/Qs 4.3. X-ray shows dilated left atrium and some left ventricular overfilling. V1-V6 double standardization, paper speed 100 cm. The left atrial enlargement is indicated as the negative component of P in V1 and the prominent terminal segment of P in V6. T in V6 is biphasic but prominent and upright after surgery. P, V1, shows right atrium with diminution of left atrial forces.

The relation of age to pulmonary artery pressure has been uncertain since there are few documented instances of acquisition of

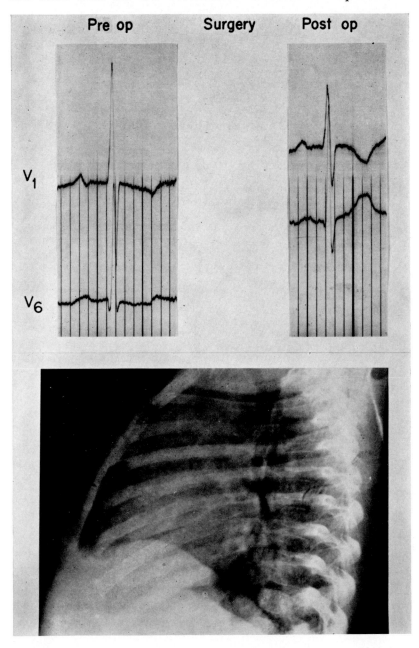

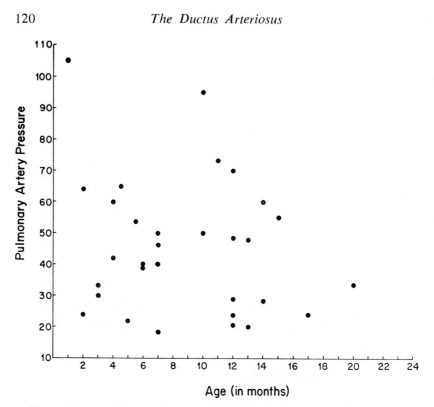

Figure 37. Pulmonary artery peak systolic pressure plotted against age for the first twenty-four months. Pressure is used since it is not possible to calculate flow or resistance with any degree of accuracy in the patent ductus and especially in this age group. No pattern is discernible.

hypertension. The size and hemodynamic status of the patent ductus are so variable it is difficult to compare individual patients or to study a group with serial hemodynamic studies. Nevertheless pulmonary artery pressure plotted against age gives an impression that such a trend exists.

Figure 37 shows a wide scatter in the first twelve or twenty-four months. However, Figure 38 with ages from two years to fifteen years is suggestive.

Shepard (19) examined the pulmonary artery pressure with reference to age in older patients. In Figure 39 he has calculated pulmonary arteriolar resistance and showed this against age. While such a calculation involves some uncertainty in the determination of pulmonary flow, again there is a trend toward increasing resistance

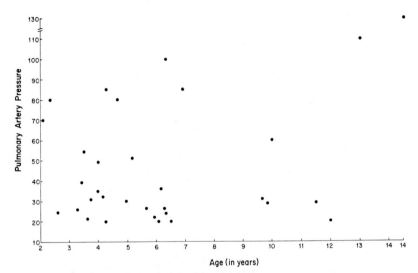

Figure 38. There is a tendency for increasing pulmonary artery pressure with age above two years.

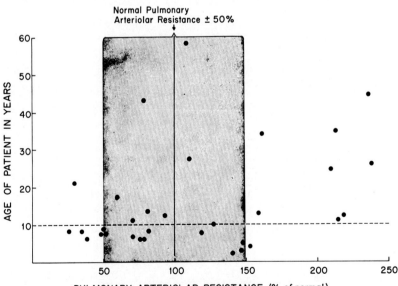

Figure 39. Age of patient and pulmonary arteriolar resistance expressed as percent of normal. No patient under ten years has a value more than 150 percent of normal. Eight older patients had resistances 150 to 250 percent of normal.

From Shepard, R.J.: *Guy's Hosp Rep, 104*:46, 1955.

with increasing age. Below ten years the calculated resistance, the basis of elevation of pressure, is in the area of the normal, and abnormal values are in older patients.

III. DIFFERENTIAL DIAGNOSIS

The differential diagnosis includes lesions which (a) produce continuous murmurs and are therefore confused with the more or less pathognomic murmurs of the patent ductus arteriosus, or (b) gives deceptive data on cardiac catheterization. (c) In the newborn a systolic murmur only associated with a bounding peripheral pulse always raises the question of a patent ductus. Angiocardiograms and especially retrograde aortograms are seldom confusing and cineangiography which gives quantitative estimate of hemodynamics as well as visualization, are usually diagnostic.

Continuous murmurs are seldom produced by a venovenous communication, since a significant pressure gradient and flow sufficient to produce a murmur are seldom persent. An exception to this is complete anomalous pulmonary venous return with some stenosis at the site of the connection to a systemic vein or to the right atrium producing a pressure gradient.

A more common cause of confusion is the loud venous hum originating in the neck thought to be at the jugular bulb. This murmur is usually loudest on the right probably related to increased intracranial venous return, about two fluids being on the right side. This murmur, either right or left side, transmits downward and is readily heard in the infraclavicular aera and may either imitate a ductus murmur or even obscure a ductus murmur.

But the classic murmur of the patent ductus arteriosus is produced by an aorta-pulmonary artery communication, and arteriovenous connections anywhere produce (a) a pressure gradient in systole and diastole and (b) a continuous murmur. In addition, some aspects of aortic or pulmonary valve regurgitation must be included.

Starting with intracardiac lesions the differential diagnosis can be listed and are self evident in Figure 40.

The differential diagnosis includes lesions producing atypical murmurs, since atypical ductus murmurs occur. In general, these are systolic-diastolic murmurs, not continuous, and the diastolic

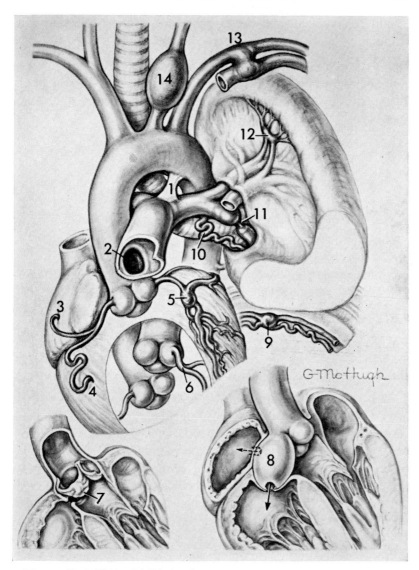

Figure 40. Differential Diagnosis.

element may be rudimentary or decrescendo and prolonged. An atypical murmur or an absent murmur in the presence of pulmonary hypertension and reversal of flow through the ductus are usually self evident, and the diagnosis made or suspected by differential cyanosis between fingers and toes.

DIFFERENTIAL DIAGNOSIS—fourteen instances of the origin of a continuous murmur or a systolic-diastolic murmur in which the diagnosis of patent ductus arteriosus has been considered.

1. Patent ductus arteriosus
2. Aortic-pulmonary artery window (aortic septal defect)
3. Coronary artery—right atrial fistula
4. Coronary artery—right ventricular fistula
5. Coronary artery—coronary vein communication
6. Anomalous origin of left coronary artery from pulmonary artery
7. Ventricular septal defect with aortic valve cup prolapse and aortic regurgitation
8. Communication from right sinus of Valvalva into right atrium or right ventricle.
9. Intercostal artery—vein fistula
10. Dilated bronchial arteries
11. Partial obstruction to a pulmonary artery branch
12. Pulmonary artery—vein arteriovenous fistula
13. Subclavian artery—vein fistula
14. Aneurysm of an artery—carotid artery shown

IV. THE ELECTROCARDIOGRAM

The electrical events of the heart usually reflect the hemodynamic-anatomical status of the heart. The correlation is often very good, usually quite good but sometimes the electrocardiogram bears little relation to known anatomical or physiological measurement. Systemic pressure in the right ventricle may be present with normal voltage and complexes for the age. Severe left ventricular hypertrophy associated with severe aortic stenosis may give slight indication in the electrocardiogram of left ventricular status.

But these recordings are obtained easily, are a reasonabley faithful reflection of cardiac events especially if serial tracings become available and with care are fairly quantitative and reproducible.

A variety of hemodynamic events related to the patent ductus arteriosus may be studied.

1. The late fetal circulatory physiology includes full patency of the ductus with a large flow of blood from the right ventricle to

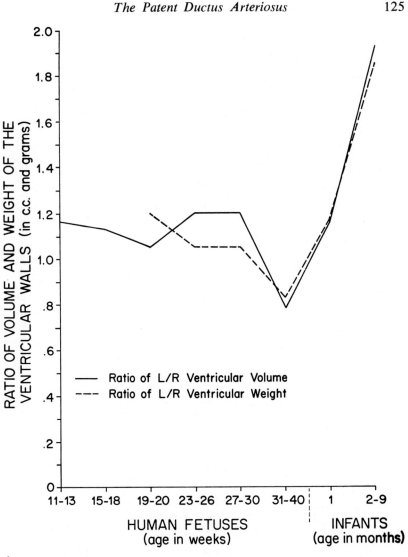

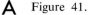 Figure 41.

the aorta. This is due to (a) pressure asynchromy which allows right to left flow in the presence of equal pressure, (b) the large low pressure, low resistance reservoir of the placenta and (c) a modest obstruction in the aorta between the left subclavian and the ductus, the fetal isthmus of the aorta. This probably is both due to and contributes to the low volume flow across it thought to be about 25 percent.

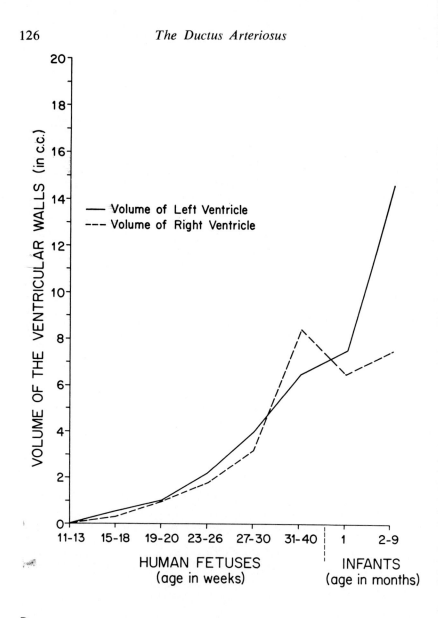

B   Figure 41.

The systemic right ventricle with hypertrophy is seen in all fetal animal studies, human premature and in the full term infant.

Figure 41 shows the weight and volume study in the human fetus of Sciacca (20). He concluded the ratio of weight of the LV/RV dropped late in fetal life, and the right ventricle had func-

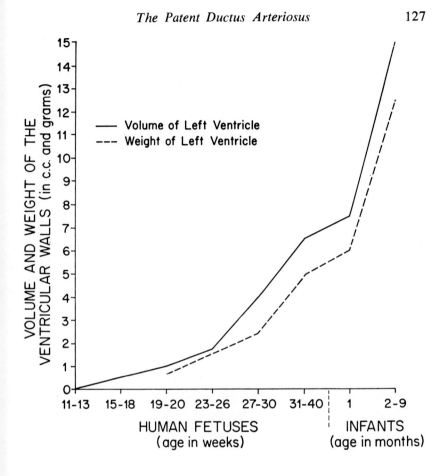

C   Figure 41.

tional hypertrophy which regressed after birth. His suggestion relating to the cause of his observations are of interest and not entirely dependent on changes in vascular resistance. He thought that right to left foramen ovale shunting was reduced by diminution of its functional size, resulting in increased filling of the right ventricle. The flow through the ductus was reduced due to beginning involution and there was more blood flow into high pressure pulmonary arteries.

Naeye (21) has shown the relatively rapid drop in muscle mass

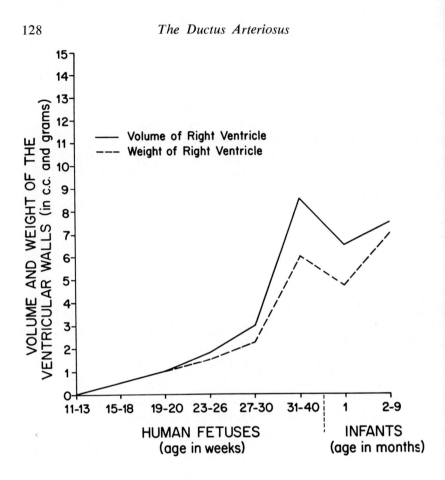

D

Figure 41A-D. Redrawn from Sciacca. *A* shows the ratio of the volume and the weight of the left and right ventricle in fetal and infant age groups. *B* indicates the volume of the right and left ventricle in the fetal and infant ages shown. *C,* volume and weight of the left ventricle. *D,* volume and weight of the right ventricle. From Sciacca, A.: *Monitore Zool Ital, 61:*356, 1953.

of arteries 5 to 30 microns after birth occuring at about the time of drop in right ventricle or pulmonary artery pressure in lamb and man.

The blood flow changes occurring with and subsequent to

(a) obliteration of placental flow and ductus flow, (b) filling of the lungs and the left heart and (c) independent ventilation-oxygenation with PaO_2 and $PaCO_2$ changes which are reflected in the electrocardiogram.

Walsh (22) states changes occur throughout the first week although all intervals and deflections are affected at different rates. She found the most striking changes in the first 30 to 60 minutes of extrauterine life, with prolongation of P wave, P-R, QRS and Q-T intervals, few Q waves on the left and good amplitude positive T waves in all chest leads. After a few hours these change toward normal, Q waves appear in V6, T in left chest leads are isoelectric or negative but positive in the right precordial leads. These change to negative on the right about the third day and positive on the left in the second day.

The T waves were studied in detail in the newborn period by Haight and Gasul (23) and are pertinent since they may reflect ductus closure and increased loading of the left ventricle by full pulmonary flow and an increase in systemic resistance with withdrawal of the low resistance placental flow.

They suggested three phases, (a) 0 to 5 minutes after birth; (b) a transient phase 1 to 16 hours of age, when T's reach maximum position anterior and right; and (c) restitution up to 7 days.

In the horizontal plane in (a) the T's are upright in all leads, in (b) they become isoelectric or negative in the left chest leads and in (c) the T axis returned to the left and at 7 days T's were all positive in the left precordium.

These changes have been confirmed in the vectorcardiogram (24) the T vcetor being anterior then anterior and to the right and finally toward the left and posterior.

These changes in the newborn are related to the circulatory changes at birth, probably chiefly functional closure of the ductus and filling of the left heart with the full circulatory blood volume instead of about 40 to 50 percent of this volume through the left ventricle during late fetal life. While hypoplasia is too strong a word to describe the left atrium and ventricle during this period physiological disuse perhaps describes their status.

The early changes to normal were summarized by Almiurung et al. (25) who noted isolated R waves in V1 were rare and qR is not seen in this lead. Adult R/S progression seldom occurs in the first month, and reversal of adult R/S progression V1 to V6 was present in 50 percent of cases. During this period the related anatomical facet is the reversal of R/L ventricular weight and soon left ventricular dominance by weight increases to 2:1.

The contribution to anatomical and in consequence electrocardiographic changes made by increased filling of the left ventricle through a left to right shunt with the pulmonary artery via a patent ductus is usually not discernable. The normal shift of forces to the left ventricle is so variable that the additional overfill of this flow shows only sometimes as a facet of changing hemodynamics. The diagnosis of patent ductus arteriosus is not made by the ventricular QRS patterns in infants and younger children.

The left atrium is more responsive to the overfill in the average patent ductus arteriosus. Because compliance is less, strain patterns show more easily. Some technical changes are necessary for proper study of the left atrial forces. These include recording of (a) V1 and V6 simultaneously, (b) at twice normal standardization and (c) at least double paper speed and 100 mm/sec is advantageous, as suggested by Ziegler (26) and Green (27). While normal values of amplitude and area for right and left atrial components of the P wave are not yet available qualitative changes are readily discernible.

The left atrium is hemodynamically and electrographically responsive to increased flow imposed by augmented return from the pulmonary circulation.

This device for identification of prior or current left to right shunts is also extremely useful in older infants. Figure 42 shows the electrical events following closure of a large ductus in a male infant age eight months. Since there is considerable mediastinal shift and some change in atrial patterns, more than one complex is shown. The left atrium is hypertrophied and changes following surgery. In addition, there is transient elevation of T in V1 thought to represent augmentation of right heart following closure of the ductus and acquisition of a normal postductal aortic flow. This flow had been reduced both by the large shunt of preductal blood into the lung via the ductus, and retrograde flow from the postductal arterial system into the ductus in diastole.

There are four types of flow associated with the patent ductus arteriosus. The categories are rather loosely defined with over-

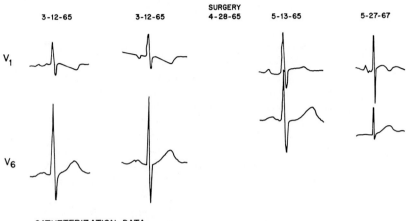

SURGERY

CATHETERIZATION DATA:
PULMONARY ARTERY PRESSURE 46/20 MM HG
PBF:SBF (QP:QS) 4.6:1

G.M. 87-94-17
B.D.: 8/10/64

Figure 42. Simultaneous V1-V6, standardization x2, paper speed 100 cm. Male, age seven months. Preoperatively the prominent left atrial forces are seen in the negative component of P in V1 and in the broad notched P in V6. These nearly disappear postoperatively. Increased flow to the periphery following closure of the ductus is seen as increased return to the right heart, and T in V1 becomes positive for some time.

lapping and changing boundaries. The electrical events do not follow precisely or rigidly but do have relevance.

1. The electrocardiogram is normal. The ductus is small, less than 8 mm or less. The flow is not large with a Qp/Qs of about 1.3. The diagnosis is made by the typical continuous murmur. If there is no thrill, the ductus is small. The x-ray is normal, the blood pressure is normal and there are no symptoms.

2. The electrocardiogram shows real or suggestive changes in the left ventricle. In the left precordial leads, there is increased amplitude of initial forces in QRS and in the T waves. Ziegler (28) makes the point that increased T wave positivity is porportionate to the QRS amplitude when increased volume-flow work is present, in contrast to the disproportionate relation in increased pressure work.

The typical murmur is present and diagnostic, and there is a thrill. The flow is moderately large, with Qp/Qs 1.5 or over. The x-ray shows increased pulmonary flow. There is a brisk S_2 with nearly normal splitting.

The electrocardiogram shows left ventricular overload, there may be early evidence of left bundle branch block. There is some involvement of the right ventricle, with evidence of right ventricular hypertrophy. The T wave may be positive in VI, and the R wave is increased, and RsR[1], or rSR prime may be present, although this is uncommon.

There is a large flow, left to right, with Qp/Qs 2 or over. There is pulmonary hypertension. This phase of the patent ductus arteriosis is likely in infancy. The elevated pulmonary pressure is related to the large flow and vasoconstriction since after surgery it falls to normal. However easy it is to explain hyperkinetic hypertension, the origin of this is not clear since in the adult pulmonary flow it must reach several times normal before elevation of pressure occurs. The vascular facets involved in infants are unknown but presumably different. This pulmonary hypertension associated with patent ductus arteriosus presumably has a component of vasoconstriction since oxygen, acetylchloine and priscoline reduce pressure.

3. Type three may be increased to any degree of mixture of increased flow and resistance. The electrocardiogram shows evidence of biventricular hypertrophy, the left ventricle from prior or present aorta to lung shunting and right ventricular hypertrophy from high pressure persisting and increasing over a period of time. In general, ventricular hypertrophy represents increased work times duration, or age.

The electrocardiographic facets are (a) and R/S ratio resembling the newborn, about one or less, (b) T wave is positive in VI, (c) deep Q waves in the precordial leads, (d) large amplitude R waves in V5 and 6, with a rather deep S and (e) the T waves may be biphasic or inverted as an indication of evidence of prior large shunt.

4. There is almost exclusively right to left shunt. The toes are cyanotic. The electrocardiogram is that of systemic right ventricular hypertension, but not above this as in severe pulmonary valve stenosis. However, on close inspection there is almost always some evidence of a previous left to right shunt under ten years of age. This will problably show most in the left atrium with the technique of increased amplification. This is because there are so few cases of *blue since birth* or a fixed anatomical pulmonary resistance from birth. If the patient is under six years, the question of trial closure deserves serious consideration.

General Considerations

Krovetz et al. (16) noted the presence of an upward concavity in the R-ST segment such as described by Sodi-Palleres et al. This finding of left ventricular diastolic overload was present in one or more leads in 63 percent of cases over one year of age, 26 percent of infants and only 18 percent of those with additional lesions.

McCoughan, Primaeu and Littman (29) studied the character-istics of the precordial T wave with the Frank horizontal plane and precordial V leads, and noted that in this frame V6 is directed more posteriorly electrically than anatomically. The direction of the maximal horizontal T vector varies greatly.

In children the T axis may be in the left posterior quadrant with a greater axis, up to 210.

The angle between the initial efferent and the terminal afferent segment of the T loop was found to be less than 30 percent with the initial vector slow and the terminal vector rapid. In both adults and children the direction is counter clockwise. If the axis was leftward over 150 degrees the T may be inverted in V1, the initial segment on the negative side, resulting in a biphasic T. The further to the right the axis is T waves in V6 may be flatter but not inverted.

In children the T axis may be greater than 180 degrees and T inverted in V2. If the angle of the vector segments is less than that between leads, 30 degrees, and the loop lies between two lead axes, a biphasic T will not be seen.

In the presence of patent ductus hemodynamics with left ven-tricular overload the T axis shifts progressively to the right. When the overload is mild, T becomes flat in V6, then biphasic and in-creasingly upright in the right precordial leads. As overload in-creases, the T axis moves toward zero. The T loop becomes clock-wise as there is more severe overload, with an upright T in lead V1 and negative T over the left precordium with S-T depression. Clockwise T loops are stated to be a function of pulmonary artery mean pressure and occur in 94 percent of patients when this is over 40 mm Hg.

In the usual aorta to pulmonary artery flow a prominent Q in V5 and V6, tall and peaked T waves and an upward displacement of S-T, the overload pattern of the left ventricle, are commonly seen. A problem of interpretation arises, however, since a tall peaked T complex and an elevated S-T are seen in normal chil-dren. Therefore, the left to right shunt ductus cannot be diagnosed by the scalar electrocardiograms alone. The prominent Q probably represents some rotation of the heart clockwise from a dilated left ventricle, making the septum more anterior-posterior. The septum may also be hypertrophied.

With pulmonary hypertension, especially when this is marked, the electrocardiogram pattern is that of right ventricular hypertrophy. However, there are residual elements of left atial and left ventricular hypertrophy which distinguish this electrocardiogram. P may be biphasic in V1, a residual of past left to right shunt. In addition to evidence of high or systemic right ventricular pressure, there are significant R waves in V5 and V6, again a residual of previous left ventricular overload.

The status of ventricular voltage criteria as a facet of analysis in the ductus problem may be seen in Figures 43 and 44.

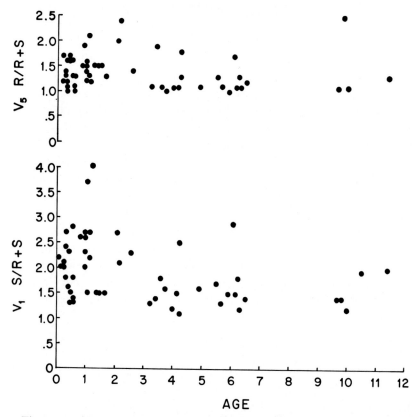

Figure 43. The relation of age to voltage in V1 and V5. In V1 the ratio S/R+S has been calculated to show the contribution of posterior or left ventricular forces to the total QRS voltage, the same ratio is shown for V5 R/R+S. It is noted that only in the one to two year group is there much variation in these ratios.

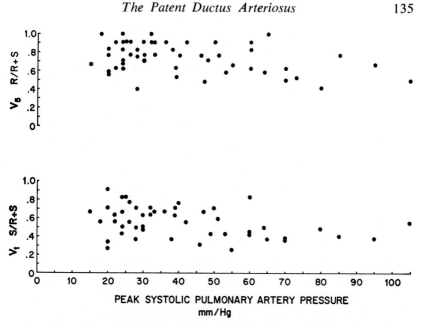

Figure 44. The ratio S/R+S in V1 and R/R+S in V5 is plotted against peak systolic pulmonary artery pressure. There is remarkably little change in the ratio of left ventricular voltage to total QRS voltage with increasing pulmonary artery pressure.

In these figures, the percent of voltage contribution by the left ventricle to the ventricular complexes is shown by the ratio S/R + S in V1 and R/R + S in V5 plotted against age in Figure 43 and pulmonary artery peak systolic pressure in Figure 44. The data was obtained from fifty-six cases of isolated patent ductus arteriosus confirmed by hemodynamic study and by subsequent surgical repair.

The voltage contribution of the left ventricle is scarcely discernible. In this series RsR′ pattern occurred three times and disappeared following surgery. These were not included. In the infant left ventricular influence is apparently masked by high pulmonary artery pressure.

Conduction Disturbances

Disturbance of normal conduction, other than tachycardia, may be seen. In general, these are abnormalities which might be expected with large flow and dilatation of the left atrium and left ventricle. In addition to atrial premature contractions, in rare instances atrial fibrillation or flutter may occur. These are usually easily controlled and disappear after surgery.

Of more concern are premature ventricular contractions when associated with pulmonay hypertension. These may be difficult to control and sometimes ominous.

Mirowski et al. (30) studied first degree A-V block sometimes seen in patent ductus arteriosus patients. In a series of 200 cases first degree A-V block was present in over 10 percent. This disappeared after surgery in 79 percent of those who had this delay. In those who did not have this degree of block there was usually improvement in the mean P-R index.

The hemodynamic origin of the conduction defect is not clear although presumably related to distension of the left atrium.

Congenital heart block in association with isolated patent ductus arteriosus does not appear to have a discernable etiological factor and does not seem to be common in the rubella syndrome. One hundred and ninety-two patients with congenital heart block were analyzed by twelve pediatric cardiology centers in a cooperative study (31). The most frequent single associated anomaly was patent ductus arteriosus which was present in fifteen patients. There are other isolated reports (32).

This association is of considerable hemodynamic interest and importance since when diastole is prolonged there is (a) an accentuation of the aortic runoff into the ductus with a low pressure and increased frequency of syncope and (b) since there continues to be forward flow from the aortic arch in diastole, the problem of coronary steal and T wave inversion becomes important.

These considerations are accentuated during the compensatory pause in premature ventricular contractions which are very undesirable.

V. REVERSIBLE PULMONARY HYPERTENSION

The patent ductus with pulmonary hypertension is a facet of the clinical syndrome and probably has a better prognosis in the younger age. This is illustrated by the very few patients in the blue since birth or in the disappearance of a continuous murmur group. Fixed resistance due to anatomical change at the arteriolar level is not yet the predominant cause of the elevated pressure. Whether complete regression of severe hypertension such as seen in this patient will occur is not known. But in the preschool age group cautious optimism is proper.

> Patient A.C. was age two years. Preoperative hemodynamic data included RV pressure 80/10, PA pressure 85/40, PA wedge mean 13, femoral artery pressure 95/35, all in mm Hg. Qp/Qs was 1.4, although determination of flow values in patency of the ductus are uncertain and consequetly resistance calculations not quantitative. Two weeks postoperative both the RV and pulmonary artery pressure were 48/6 in mm Hg.

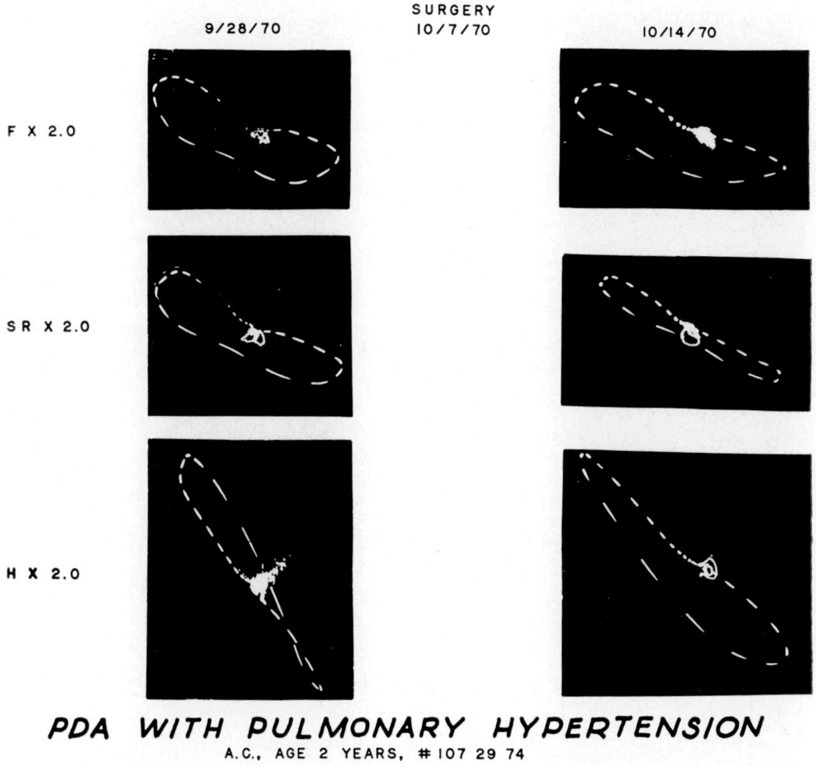

PDA WITH PULMONARY HYPERTENSION
A.C., AGE 2 YEARS, # 107 29 74

Figure 47. The vectorcardiogram, Frank, in the two year old with pulmonary hypertension which was 40 mm Hg postoperatively is of interest. The frontal and right saggital loops showed little change. In the horizontal loop the initial and terminal forces are similar. However, the loop has changed from left of the E point to the right. This would suggest closure of the ductus has increased strain on the right ventricle by obstruction of the communication with the aorta even though the right ventricular pressure was 40 mm Hg fourteen days after surgery.

Figures 45, 46 and 47 show the pre and postoperative phonocardiogram, simultaneous V1-V6 recordings and Frank vectorcardiogram.

In the vectorcardiogram (Fig. 47) there is little change in the frontal and right saggital loops two weeks after surgery, and it shows right ventricular hypertrophy. In the horizontal plane, however, while the initial and terminal forces have not changed the central loop has moved to the right of the E point and is clockwise. This suggests that with closure of the ductus there is at least a temporary increase of right ventricular stress due to withdrawal of the escape valve. The systolic pulmonary pressure remains mildly elevated but the low diastolic value is encouraging.

P and T loop studies were unsatisfactory.

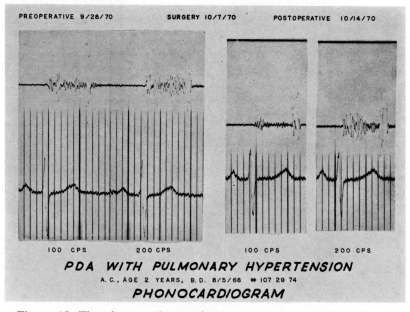

Figure 45. The phonocardiogram before and after surgical closure. The chief features are a systolic ejection click preoperative followed by a systolic murmur filling systole, with no discernible diastolic murmur. Splitting of S2 is obvious only after closure of the ductus. The systolic murmur shortens and is an ejection murmur. This part of the murmur was not changed much from the preoperative appearance and with the click represent the finding associated with a dilated pulmonary artery. This will probably lessen but not completely disappear.

Figure 45 is the pre and postoperative phonocardiogram at the second left intercostal space. There is some difference between the 100 and 200 CPS recordings. There is a prominent pulmonary ejection sound, less evident after surgery. The systolic murmur which continued through systole is shorter postoperatively. S_2 was very narrowly split or single, and splitting became evident although there was not much variation in this. No real diastolic murmur was seen or heard either before or after surgery.

Sutton, Haris and Leatham (33) noted in hyperkinetic pulmonary hypertension with left to right shunt, A_2 continued to be greater than P_2 in the pulmonary area. Splitting could be reversed, S_2 could be single or there could be up to 0.04 second interval.

With greater pulmonary resistance and bidirectional shunting P_2 became louder than A_2 and there was no paradoxical splitting.

In both groups $Q-T_2$ remained constant throughout respiration.

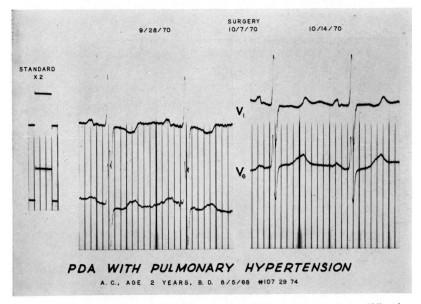

Figure 46. Simultaneous V1-V6 recording of twice normal amplification and four times normal paper speed. The positive element of the P is less broad in V1 and the negative element, thought to represent the left atrium, has not been affected discernibly. P in V6 is less broad and smaller. The P-R interval has shortened. QRS has not changed appreciably. T in V1 has acquired a relatively large positive component.

In Figure 46 the pre and postoperative V1-V6 show little change in the relative voltage RA to LA although LA is less in V6. T in V1 has developed a marked late upright component which is consistent throughout a long tracing, and T in V6 is taller and more peaked.

The immediate results of closure of the ductus in an intermediate type were very good. The pulmonary artery pressure diminished to nearly one half of systemic value. But with a residual of peak systolic pressure of 48 mm Hg the prognosis cannot be predicted. The pulmonary vasculature can (1) remain the same, with moderate elevation of pulmonary artery pressure indefinitely, (2) diminish any arteriolar changes and eventually have normal heart and lungs or (3) the pulmonary pathology responsible for elevated pressure may be progressive even in the absence of an initiating stimulus of greatly increased pulmonary flow and result in extreme pulmonary hypertension and associated risks. Many would label this primary pulmonary hypertension with an associated patent ductus arteriosus.

But another opinion suggests circulatory insult initiates the pulmonary vascular pathology, and after some unknown point this perpetuates itself. Now normal flow but at an increased pressure is sufficient stimulus for progressive pulmonary vascular disease.

REFERENCES

1. Babington, Dr.: *Lond Med Gaz, 39*:882, 1847.
2. Williams, Dr.: In discussion of the paper of Babington.
3. Fagge, C.: A case of patent ductus arteriosus attended with a peculiar diastolic murmur. *Guys Hosp Rep, 18*:23, 1873.
4. Bennet, Hughes: *Principles and Practice of Medicine,* 3rd Ed. p. 595.
5. Gerhardt, C.: Persistenz des ductus arteriosus Botalli. *Jena Z Med Naturwiss, 3*:105, 1867.
6. Duroziez, P.: Memoire sur la persistance du arteriel sans autre cumminucation. *C R Mem Soc Biol, Tom, 4*:279, 1862.
7. Gilbert, A.: Un cas de persistance simple du canal arteriel. *France Med Par, ii*:1062, 1886.
8. Hochhaus, H.: Persistenz des ductus arteriosus Botalli. *Deutsch Arch Klin Med Bd,* 51, S 1, 1893.
9. Francois-Franck, M.: De l' exageration des influences normales de la respiration sur le pouls, dans les cas d' aneurysme intrathoracigne et de la persistance de canal arteriel. *Gaz Hosp, 51*:1115, 1878.

10. Francois-Franck, M.: Sur le diagnostic de la persistance du canal arteriel. *Gaz Hebd Med Chir, Tom, 15*:588, 1878.
11. Gibson, G.A.: A clinical lecture on persistent ductus arteriosus. *Med Press Circ Lond, 21*:572, 1906.
12. Gibson, G.A.: Persistance of the arterial duct and its diagnosis. *Edinb Med, 8*:1, 1900.
13. Rudolph, A., Scarpelli, E.M., Golinko, R.J. and Gootman, N.L.: Hemodynamic basis for clinical manifestations of patent ductus arteriosus. *Am Heart J, 68*:447, 1964.
14. Cassels, D.E., Morse, M. and Adams, W.: Effect of the patent ductus arteriosus on the pulmonary blood flow, blood volume, heart rate, blood pressure, arterial blood gases and pH. *Pediatrics, 6*:557, 1950.
15. Megibow, R.S. and Feitelberg S.: Application of microplethysmography to the diagnosis of patent ductus arteriosus and coarctation of the aorta. *Am J Med, 4*:798, 1948.
16. Krovetz, L.G. and Warden, H.E.: An analysis of 515 surgically proven cases. *Dis Chest, 42*:46, 1962.
17. Dawes, G.S., Mott, J.C. and Widdicombe, J.G.: The cardiac murmur from patent ductus arteriosus in newborn lambs. *J Physiol, 128*:344, 1955.
18. Cassels, D.E. and Tatooles, C.J.: *Auscultatory Features of Coarctation of the Aorta. The Theory and Practice of Auscultation.* Philadelphia, Davis Co., 1963, p. 272.
19. Shepard, R.J.: Pulmonary artery pressures in persistent ductus arteriosus with particular reference to older patients. *Guys Hosp Rep, 104*:46, 1955.
20. Sciacca, A.: La veriazione della massa muscolare dei ventricoli del cuore nella vita fetale e postnatale: suo significato morfo-funzionale. *Monitore Zool Ital, 61*:356, 1953.
21. Naeye, R.L.: Arterial changes in greater or lesser circulation during perinatal period. *AMA Arch Pathol, 71*:121, 1961.
22. Walsh, S. Zoe: The Electrocardiogram in the Neonate and Infant. In Cassels, D.E. (ed.): *The Heart and Circulation in the Newborn and Infant.* New York, Grune, 1966.
23. Haight, G. and Gasul, B.M.: The evaluation and significance of T wave changes in the normal newborn during the first seven days of life. *Am J Cardiol, 12*:494, 1963.
24. Castellanos, A., Jr., Lemberg, L. and Castellanos, A.: The vectorcardiographic significance of upright T waves in V1 and V2 during the first month of life. *J Pediatr, 62*:827, 1963.
25. Almiurung, M.N., Joseph, L.G., Nadas, A.S. and Massell, B.F.: The unique precordial and extremity electrocardiogram in normal infants and children. *Circulation, 4*:420, 1951.
26. Ziegler, R.: Importance of amplification techniques in routine clinical electrocardiography. *Circulation, 24*:1076, 1961.

27. Green, E.W. :Electrocardiographic Pattern of Atrial Enlargement and Abnormal Impulse Formation and Conduction. In Cassels, D.E. and Ziegler, R.F.: *Electrocardiography in Infants and Children.* New York, Grune, 1966.

28. Ziegler, R.F.: The clinical contribution of electrocardiography in mechanical malformations of the cardiovascular system. *Am Heart J, 58*:504, 1959.

Eleven

HEMODYNAMICS

THE MAJORITY OF THE CLINICAL AND PATHOLOGICAL MANI-
FESTATIONS OF THE PATENT DUCTUS ARTERIOSUS are related to
changes in the circulatory patterns of the central circulation introduced by an aortic-pulmonary artery communication. Holman (1)
considered most forms of congenital heart disease as aspects of
either intracardiac or extracardiac arteriovenous fistula. In the
case of the patent ductus arteriosus the communication is extracardiac and much of the hemodynamic events of an arteriovenous
fistula are present except that the right heart is excluded and only
the lungs and left heart are affected.

The three general aspects of aortic-pulmonary communication
through a patent ductus arteriosus are well known, (a) left to
right flow to pulmonary artery, (b) increased flow through the
lungs and (c) increased flow through the left atrium, left ventricle
and aorta. However, newer information concerning these are not
so well known, especially that related to the aorta to pulmonary
artery blood flow of a typical patent ductus arteriosus.

Pulmonary artery and aorta pressures are readily measured and
left atrial or at least pulmonary artery wedge pressures and left
ventricular systolic and end-diastolic pressures are recorded. Blood
flow and especially quantitative aorta to lung flow in relation to
systemic flow, Qp/Qs ratios, have been considered as total pulmo-
nary/total systemic flow and not in relation to the possibility of
difference in aortic flow above and below the origin of the ductus.
While pressure through a column of fluid should be transmitted
equally, there may be differential flow in the aorta above and below
the ductus and in the right in contrast to the left pulmonary artery.

A difference in forearm blood flow pre and postoperatively was observed using a venous occlusion plethysmograph. It was not possible to do leg flow, but table VIII shows a fall in the forearm flow postoperatively, a reflection of diminution of the flow in the aortic arch.

The exceptions were C.M., a six year old with systemic pressure in the pulmonary artery, who later died, and S.M. who also had pulmonary hypertension but who survived and improved. Diminished pulmonary perfusion and subsequent left ventricular output would seem to be the explanation of no change in forearm blood flow.

TABLE VIII

FOREARM BLOOD FLOW IN ISOLATED PATENT DUCTUS ARTERIOSUS
PRE AND POSTOPERATIVE DETERMINATIONS
BY VENOUS OCCLUSION PLETHYSMOGRAPH

ml/100 gm forearm tissue/min

Patient	Age	Pre-op	Post-op	Months Post-op
R.H.	10 4/12	9.06	4.34	5
S.G.	12 9/12	3.08	3.55	4 1/2
S.P.	5 6/12	2.9	1.62	3
N.P.	7 11/12	4.59	4.45	2
T.M.	10 6/12	3.95	2.98	12
M.S.	10 8/12	7.05	2.57	10
S.M.	8 10/12	1.77	4.04	1 1/2
S.H.	7 10/12	3.42	3.04	24
C.H.	5 1/12	4.29	2.44	9
S.K.	10 10/12	4.85	2.5	18
H.F.	9	4.26	3.88	16
J.P.	18 11/12	2.57	1.7	2 1/2
J.G.	10 8/12	4.27	3.1	7
J.V.	14 4/12	3.04	2.27	1/2
R.T.	6 4/12	8.61	5.73	1/2
C.M.	6 6/12	2.2	—	—

Figure 48 illustrates a more precise quantitative study. During thoracotomy for division and suture of isolated patent ductus arteriosus, blood flow was measured in the aorta above and below the ductus using a suitable probe of a Carolina electromagnetic flow meter. The ductus was then clamped and unclamped at least twice. The figure shows the technique and the flow ml/min for a large ductus with a Qp/Qs ratio of 2.1, realizing that representative mixed samples are difficult to obtain in the pulmonary artery and quantitative pulmonary flows are not exact in patent ductus arteriosus.

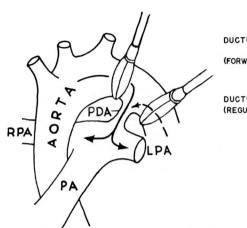

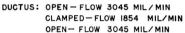

DUCTUS: OPEN—FLOW 3045 MIL/MIN
CLAMPED—FLOW 1854 MIL/MIN
OPEN— FLOW 3045 MIL/MIN

DUCTUS: OPEN—1523 MIL/MIN
CLAMPED — 1720 MIL/MIN
(FORWARD FLOW) OPEN —1457 MIL/MIN
CLAMPED— 1722 MIL/MIN

DUCTUS OPEN—
(REGURGITATED FLOW DURING DIASTOLE)
1986 MIL/MIN
1820 MIL/MIN

Figure 48. Blood flow in the aortic arch above the ductus and in the aorta below the ductus, with the ductus open and then clamped as shown for E.M., age six years, a study done during surgery. She had Qp/Qs of 2.4 and a peak pulmonary artery pressure of 35. There was (a) a much larger flow in the aorta above the ductus when the ductus was open than when clamped and (b) forward flow in the descending aorta was greater when the ductus was clamped. But there is a large regurgitant flow from the descending aorta into the ductus in diastole. There was also forward flow in diastole from the aortic arch through the ductus and into the lung.

With the probe above the ductus and the aorta clamped immediately below, the probe flow, in case 1, was 2649 ml/m. This should be the flow through the duct, augmented by increased pressure in the aortic arch. Using the same technique in a small ductus, the probe flow was 1021 ml/m.

Of great interest in case 1, E.M., was the large regurgitant flow from the descending aorta into the ductus. This is seen only in the presence of a large ductus with a large flow. A recording of such flows in a male, age fifteen months, is shown in Figure 49.

Information obtained with this technique can be summarized:

1. When there is a large ductal flow, this blood flow arises chiefly from the aortic segment above the ductus exit from the aorta. But there is also a regurgitant retrograde flow into the ductus from the aorta below the ductus. The aortic segment below has greatly reduced flow due to (a) diminished forward flow which increases when the ductus is clamped and (b) to regurgitant retrograde flow into

PROBE ABOVE DUCTUS

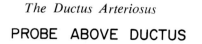

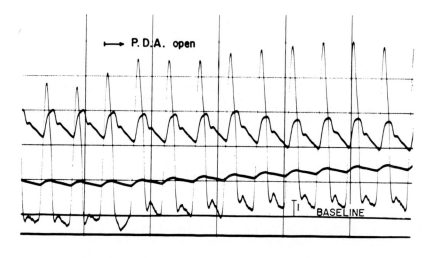

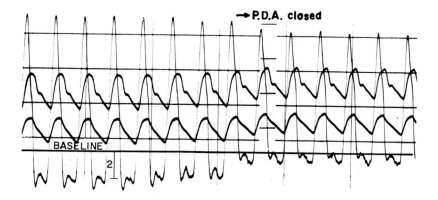

PROBE BELOW DUCTUS

Figure 49. E.C. #1126075, age one yr. PA pressure 25/16, Ao 100/60 mm Hg, Qp/Qs 1.7. Flow probe above ductus arteriosus and below with ductus open and closed. Upper tracing shows *1* that forward flow continues in diastole after the ductus is opened and the flow tracing does not return to the baseline. Lower—when the probe is below the ductus there is regurgitant flow in diastole as shown at *2*, the tracing continues below the baseline until the ductus is closed. The mean flow proximal increases with the ductus open, the mean flow distal increases when the ductus is closed.

the ductus. There is also forward flow from the arch in diastole. Since coronary flow occurs chiefly in diastole, this aortic arch runoff through the ductus and into the lung may be the source of a *coronary steal* and contribute to negative T waves and diminished ventricular function.

2. In smaller or medium sized ductus flow the values are less with modest reduction of a supraductal flow and some reduction of infraductal flow and no regurgitant flow.

3. In the small ductus there is very little change in blood flow in either the supraductal or infraductal segments of the aorta.

In the average patent ductus with normal or slight to moderate increased pulmonary resistance the pulmonary blood flow increased 1.5 to 2.5 times the systemic flow. The segmental nature of the aortic-pulmonary shunt is apparent only in large blood flows. Regurgitant flow can be seen in most large flow ductus if opacification is made into the descending aorta. In Figure 50 this injection has been made through the ductus. Studies of five patients are shown in Table IX.

TABLE IX

AORTIC FLOW DATA

PRE AND POST DUCTUS INSERTION

		Ductus Open	Ductus Clamped	Regurgitant Flow	Clinical Status
1. E.M. #109-04-41	Pre ductal flow	3045	1854	1986	Large ductus
F. 6 yrs.	Post ductal flow	1523	1722	1820	
2. M.G. #105-60-84	Pre ductal flow	1680	1400	—	Moderate ductus
F. 15 mos.	Post ductal flow	1456	1344	—	
3. J.S. #107-64-49	Pre ductal flow	1638	1596	—	Small ductus
M. 4 years	Post ductal flow	1676	1516	—	
4. L.P. #109-01-93	Pre ductal flow	1729	1972	—	Small ductus
F. 6 yrs.	Post ductal flow	1729	1729	—	
5. E.C. #112-60-75	Pre ductal flow	1132	658	435	Moderate ductus
M. 15 mos.	Post ductal flow	922	620	420	

When the ductus is closed the postductal aortic flow increases. This can be reflected in increased venous return to the right heart. Electrocardiographically there may be (a) augmented voltage in the right atrial component of P in V_1, (6) T in V_1 may become positive for a short time, suggesting increased right ventricular load and (c) increased height of R in V_1 and increased R/S ratio.

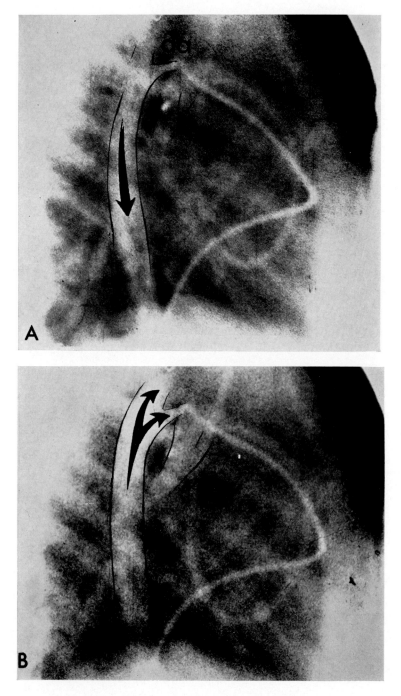

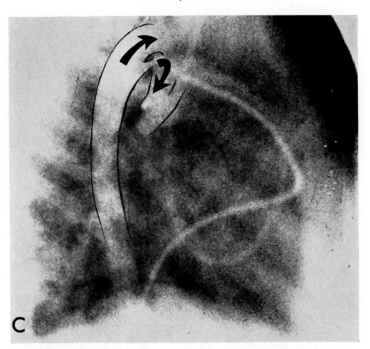

Figure 50. Regurgitant flow from the descending aorta can be seen in most large flow ductus if opacification is done with the descending aorta. In this case this was done through the ductus. The aortic arch is sometimes seen. It had been noted previously that the neonatal ductus visualized if contrast was injected distal to the aortic-ductus junction but not if injected proximally. Hirvonen, L. and Peltonan, T.: *Mem IV Mundial Cardiol,* 5:82, 1962.

These findings are best seen in simultaneous V_1 and V_6 recordings with double standardization and paper speed of 100 mm per minute.

THE PULMONARY CIRCULATION AND THE LUNG

Just as the lung lies between the venous pulmonary circulation and the left atrium-ventricle and the systemic circulation, the lung also lies between the aorta-ductus and the left atrium-ventricle. When large blood flow into the lung occurs from the ductus, the pulmonary circulation and left atrium and left ventricle are overloaded. These segments of the ductus circulation may respond to overfilling in a discernable way. The lung, for instance, responds with diminished pulmonary compliance, and the increased respiratory effort needed for ventilation is observed clinically (2). Compliance improves after closure of the ductus (Fig. 51).

It might be supposed that recirculation of already oxygenated arterial blood through the lungs would affect pulmonary function and some aspects of diffusion and arterial gases.

It was shown in 1950 (3) that PaO_2 resembled normal values very closely in patency of the ductus, but this value was significantly lower two to three weeks post closure. There was no real change in the $PaCO_2$ values. $PaCO_2$, however, tended to be lower

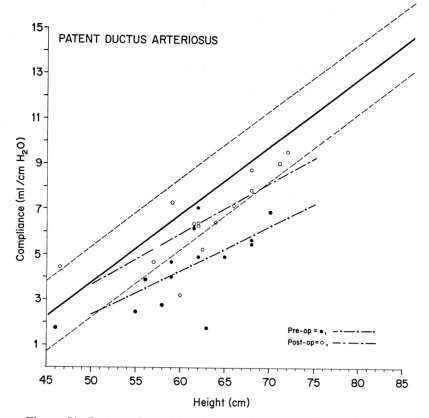

Figure 51. Preoperative and postoperative pulmonary compliance in fourteen infants with patent ductus arteriosus. Following surgical closure there is improvement in compliance which becomes normal in most infants. From Griffin, A.J., Ferrara, J.D., Lax, J.O. and Cassels, D.E.: *Am J Dis Child, 123*:89, 1972.

than the normal values for children. The reason for this is not clear, but it suggests hyperventilation.

Lees, Way and Ross (4) studied ventilation and respiratory gas transfer in infants with increased pulmonary blood flow. This hemodynamic category includes the patent ductus and indicates that in the absence of heart failure there is not much variation from the normal controls except for an alveolar-arterial difference in O_2 tension. This was believed to represent intrapulmonary venous admixture rather than unevenness of ventilation/perfusion.

This intrapulmonary venous shunt was not especially related to either pulmonary hypertension, elevated left atrial pressure or the largest pulmonary blood flow. This finding is of great interest, and suggests shunts in the infant differ from the older child. There is a reciprocal effect in relation to pulmonary flow, and if pulmonary arterial flow is increased, collateral flows diminish.

However, Ehara (5) studied pre and postoperative pulmonary function in great detail. Some important aspects of his study with determinations done preoperatively, two to three months and six to twenty months postoperatively, are summarized.

   1. *Vital capacity,* which averaged 78.6 percent of normal preoperatively, approached normal in six months, especially in those patients with markedly decreased values and left to right shunt over 45 percent of systemic flow.
   2. *Maximum breathing capacity, minute ventilation and one second timed vital capacity* showed a similar trend toward normal values.
   3. *Increased pulmonary capillary blood volume and alveolar diffusing capacity* were increased before surgery and were near normal postoperatively. It is believed increased capillary volume leads to increased diffusing area and thus increased alveolar diffusing capacity.
   4. *In the presence of pulmonary hypertension* with increase in the pulmonary/systemic vascular resistance to 0.8 the ductus is operable and hypertension reversible, providing there is no decrease in alveolar diffusing capacity or capillary blood volume. In these there is a mildly thickened basement membrane.

Patients with greatly increased pulmonary-systemic vascular resistance ratio, markedly thickened basement membrane and decreased diffusing capacity are inoperable.

Ramkin and Callies (6) had previously shown in patients with atrial septal defect or ventricular septal defect, whose pulmonary blood flow varied from 2.6 to 24.2 L/min, the diffusing capacity for CO_2 varied significantly with variation in blood flow and capillary blood volume. In the absence of pulmonary hypertension diffusion increased 11 to 92 percent. With pulmonary hypertension and with significant increase in arteriolar resistance DL was decreased.

In these large left to right shunts reduction of pulmonary diffusing capacity probably indicates pulmonary hypertension or incipient cardiac failure.

CARDIAC HEMODYNAMICS

Ventricular hemodynamics have been studied in detail by Jarmakani et al. (7) and especially in relation to similar parameters in ventricular septal defects. Appropriate data and indices included: Left Ventricular Stroke Volume; Left Ventricular Ejection Fraction (ratio of stroke volume/end-diastolic volume); Left Ventricular Systolic Index (stroke volume x heart rate, normalized for surface area in patent ductus arteriosus = pulmonary blood flow), and Left Atrial Maximal Volume, measured at end of ventricular systole. In addition Left Ventricular Wall Thickness and Left Ventricular Wall Mass were estimated.

There were many similarities in the hemodynamics of ventricular septal defects and patent ductus arteriosus, although one left to right shunt is intracardiac and one supravalvular and extracardiac. Both, in the usual situation, (a) increase pulmonary blood flow, (b) increase return to the left atrium and left ventricle, and the patent ductus arteriosus increases flow in the supraductal aortic arch segment.

1. Thus, LVEDV was greater than normal in all patients with PDA or VSD if the left to right shunt was over 35 percent, up to 2.5 times in infants and less in older children.

2. LVEF, the ejection fraction, was similar and less than normal in all patients, both VSD and PDA.

3. LVSI, the left ventricular volume x heart rate/BSA increased in both if the shunt was over 35 percent.

4. Left ventricular wall thickness was greater than normal in all patients.

5. Left ventricular wall mass was increased in all patients, VSD

and PDA with a linear increase with increasing left to right shunt. The wall mass had a linear increase with LVSI.

6. Left Atrium Maximal Volume elevated in both VSD and PDA when the shunt was over 35 percent, increasing with increasing shunt and LV systolic index. LV end-diastolic volume and Left Atrial Maximal Volume were both elevated in all patients with PDA and VSD and a shunt over 35 percent, suggesting a close relation between the two.

7. Increase in LV muscle mass with increasing shunt and LV systolic index may indicate volume overload of the left ventricle stimulates muscle hypertrophy. In infants with VSD or PDA the LV mass was almost twice normal and the volume to mass ratio was above normal, indicating a greater volume than mass response. Perhaps slowness in developing hypertrophy may explain why failure seems to occur more easily in infancy.

Muscle mass per BSA normalized for degree of shunt over 35 percent was significantly increased in patients with PDA over that in VSD patients. As they pointed out, this is probably related to continued left to right shunting during diastole in the isovolumic contraction period as well as during the systolic ejection period in VSD patients.

This gives a loss of LV volume in VSD and a stable volume in PDA, and a higher peak LV systolic pressure in PDA when the shunt is large. The result is greater stroke work in PDA than VSD for patients with equal shunts.

Regardless of similarities in these two left to right shunting lesions very real differences were found in the patent ductus arteriosus. They were:

1. higher left ventricular end-diastolic pressure
2. elevated left ventricular end-diastolic stress in PDA vs. VSD if shunts were large
3. greater left ventricular mass/BSA and left ventricular wall thickness/BSA, normalized for shunt, in the patent ductus arteriosus patients.

Other studies (8) also indicated that in acute, controlled VSD and PDA lesions of equal left to right shunting, Qp/Qs 2:7, there were real differences in hemodynamics. In PDA, LV end-diastolic pressure and volume increased much more than in VSD. Some parameters of myocardial mechanics varied between the two lesions, mostly related to ejection of all the systolic volume into a high pressure aorta in PDA, but in VSD a portion ejects into a low pressure right ventricle. The distinction is made that LV performance is compromised more in PDA than VSD.

Presumably surgical correction would cause improvement of LV performance and regression of left ventricular muscle mass

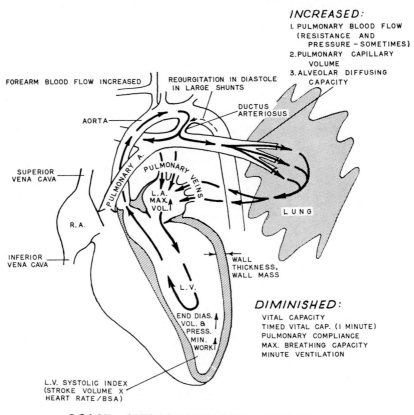

SOME HEMODYNAMIC EVENTS

Figure 52. The major hemodynamic events related to a large flow into the lung through a patent ductus arteriosus are illustrated. It should be noted forward flow from the aortic arch into the ductus also occurs in diastole as well as diastolic regurgitant flow from the descending aorta, if the ductus is clinically significant. There is probably a *coronary steal* during the diastolic flow from the aortic arch, since negative T waves in V5 and V6 become upright after surgical closure of the ductus.

and wall thickness if done before fibrosis or irreversible structural changes occurred.

The major hemodynamic events associated with a patent ductus arteriosus of some size are summarized in Figure 52. This does not include any aspects of pulmonary hypertension. Of special interest is the blood flow into the ductus and lung during diastole from both the aortic arch and the descending aorta. Sometimes this flow is large. The forward flow from the arch during diastole may be important as interference with coronary blood flow which occurs predominantly in diastole.

Further data regarding E.M., case 1 in Table IX, was obtained by obtaining quantitative measurement of cardiac output by angiography (9). This is especially applicable in a study of the ductus arteriosus where there is difficulty in obtaining an adequately mixed blood sample in the pulmonary artery. With cardiac output unreliable, calculation of pulmonary vascular resistance is subject to error.

Chamber size is seen easily during cineprojection, although single frames do not reproduce well. Representative frames showing maximum left atrial filling in diastole and the left ventricle at end diastole are shown in Figure 53 and Figure 54. Volume can be determined by planimeter in anterior-posterior and lateral view for systole and diastole of each chamber in sequence following injection into the right atrium and cardiac output calculated.

Such determinations in E.M. are compared with cardiac output calculated by Fick technique and are shown in Table X. The similarity of Qp/Qs is reassuring, although the Fick value is slightly larger.

The shunt through the ductus may be balanced between the right and left pulmonary artery or may be predominately to either right or left lung. The opinion that ductus flow is chiefly to the left pulmonary artery is not always correct. The predominant flow is presumably directed by the angle of insertion of the ductus into the bifurcation of the pulmonary artery. This is observed to vary considerably and in cases where the flows have been determined, correlates with what inspection of this angle would suggest.

In the presence of a patent ductus arteriosus with left to right shunt Cardio-Green® injection into the left ventricle will result in

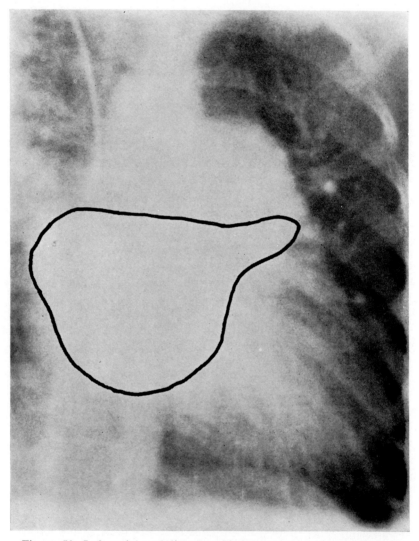

Figure 53. Left atrial end-diastole with left atrial maximum distension. This is seen best during the cine. The large left atrial appendage is a feature of patent shunts. This frontal and the simultaneous lateral projection are used for calculation of volume. Determinations courtesy Dr. Otto Thilenius.

an early appearance of dye in the right and left pulmonary artery. The area under these shunt curves is dependent (a) on the amount of dye being shunted (i.e. the extent of the left to right shunt) and (b) on the amount of undyed blood with which the shunt flow is

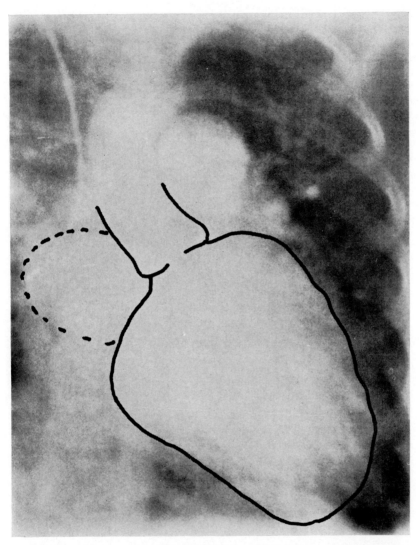

Figure 54. Left ventricular end-diastole. The left ventricle occupies most of the frontal cardiac silhouette. Left atrial systole is indicated. Again, heart chambers are outlined satisfactorily only when the cineangiogram is projected.

mixed (i.e. the distribution of right ventricular output to the right and left pulmonary artery.) If one assumes (a) an equal distribution of right ventricular output to the right and left pulmonary

TABLE X

CARDIAC OUTPUT: FICK METHOD AND CINEANGIOGRAPHY

Cardiac Output, Fick Determination, Vo_2 Estimated

Qp 10.7 1/min   = LV stroke volume 134 ml

heart rate 80/min

Qs. 4.3 1/min   = RV stroke volume 54 ml

Qp/Qs 2:1

Aortic pressure   120/55 mm Hg

(Pullout through
the ductus)

Pulmonary artery pressure   35/20 mm Hg

Cardiac Output, Cineangiography

Right Ventricle

end diastole	82 ml
end systole	23 ml
stroke volume	59 ml

Heart rate 100/min

RV output   5.9 1/min

Left Ventricle

end diastole	149 ml
end systole	31 ml
stroke volume	118 ml

Heart rate 100/min

LV output   11.8 1/min

Qp/Qs 2:1

artery, (b) complete mixing of the shunt flow with the undyed right ventricular component and (c) the use of the forward triangle method for estimation of the blood flow is a reliable one, then and only then, will the area under the time-concentration curves obtained from the peripheral right and left pulmonary artery be proportional to the amount of ductal shunt flow to each pulmonary artery.

Of two patients studied (left ventricular dye injection; withdrawal of blood from the right and left pulmonary artery) one patient showed predominant shunting into the right pulmonary artery by a factor of 3:1, while the second patient showed predominant shunting into the left pulmonary artery by a factor of 1.2:1.

Bisferiens pulse was recorded in the right carotid artery before and after surgery in a ten year old male (Fig. 55). This type of pressure tracing is seen in aortic regurgitation or instances where there is a lowered diastolic pressure (10). This type of collapsing carotid pulse is seen in the patent ductus arteriosus when the flow is large. The electrocardiogram and phonocardiogram were recorded simultaneously.

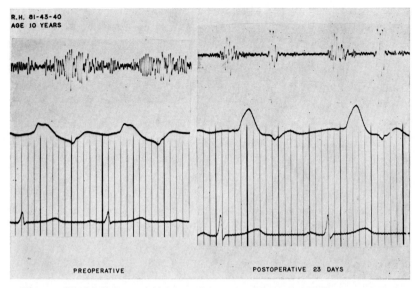

Figure 55. Bisferiens pulse seen in a carotid tracing before surgery has disappeared after closure of a large flow patent ductus arteriosus. The continuous murmur has disappeared. The bisferiens pulse occurs in children, and when there is a large stroke volume and a low diastolic pressure as in any form of aortic regurgitation such as the aortic diastolic runoff in a large flow patent ductus arteriosus.

REFERENCES

1. Holman, Emile: Certain types of congenital heart disease interpreted as intracardiac arteriovenous and venoarterial fistulae. *Bull John Hopkins Hosp, 36*:61, 1925.
2. Griffin, A.J., Ferrara, J., Lax, J. and Cassels, D.E.: Pulmonary compliance. An index of cardiovascular status in infancy. *Am J Dis Child, 123*:89, 1972.
3. Cassels, D.E., Morse, M. and Adams, W.E.: Effect of the patent ductus arteriosus on the pulmonary blood flow, blood volume, heart rate, blood pressure, arterial blood gases and pH. *Pediatrics, 6*:557, 1950.
4. Lees, M.H., Way, R.C. and Ross, B.B.: Ventilation and respiratory gas transfer of infants with increased pulmonary blood flow. *Pediatrics, 40*:259, 1967.
5. Ehara, H.: Pre and postoperative assessment of cardiopulmonary function in patent ductus arteriosus. *J Jap Assn Thor Surg, 14*:30, 1966.
6. Ramkin, J. and Callies, Q.C.: The influence of atrial and ventricular septal defects on the capilliary bed of the lung and on the diffusion

characteristics of the pulmonary membrane. *J Lab Clin Med, 6*:937, 1958.

7. Jarmakani, J.M. Graham, T.P., Canent, R.V. and Capp, M.P.: The effect of corrective surgery on left heart volume and mass in children with ventricular septal defect. *Am J Cardiol, 27*:254, 1971.

8. Spann, J.F., Jr., Mason, D.T., Zelis, R. and Braunwald, E.: Differences in left ventricular performance and myocardial mechanics in patent ductus arteriosus and ventricular septal defect. (Abstract) *Circulation, 37* (suppl VI):184, 1968.

9. Arcilla, R., Tsai, P., Thilenius, O. and Ranniger, K.: Angiographic method for volume estimation of right and left ventricles. *Chest, 60*:446, 1971.

10. Ikram, H., Nixon, P.G. and Fox, J.A.: The haemodynamic implications of the bisferiens pulse. *Br Heart J, 26*:452, 1964.

Twelve

THE DUCTUS ARTERIOSUS & COARCTATION OF THE AORTA

A DISCUSSION OF AORTIC CONSTRICTION at the ductus level becomes necessary because of (a) the anatomical and (b) hemodynamic aspects of the ductus arteriosus and coarctation of the aorta.

The anatomical relation of the aortic end of the ductus and the constriction of the aorta is such that the open ductus or the involuted ligamentum often ends in the aorta at the position of the coarctation. This association gave rise to speculation concerning the possible effect of one upon the other. David Craigie (1) in 1841 noted that in a seven year old girl:

> the region of obstruction corresponds exactly to that of the ductus arteriosus with the aorta and that these circumstances, taken along with the depressed and ligamentous appearance in the outside of the aorta, rendered almost certain that this oblitration had taken place at the part at which the ductus arteriosus joins the aorta. It seems therefore, that the obliterating action which had taken place in the ductus arteriosus, had been from some peculiar cause prolonged into the aorta, and had there given rise first to contraction, and then to obliteration of the coats of that vessel.

He published this case report and quotes from other published reports, and his illustration is shown in Figure 56.

But he included an alternative opinion:

> to me, indeed, it appears that the lesion is the result rather of an arrest of development than of a positive and active disease.

161

These two theories, so nicely formulated by Craigie, have been repeated and debated since then, although sometimes as new and original ideas. Skoda (2), 1855, speculated upon the constriction

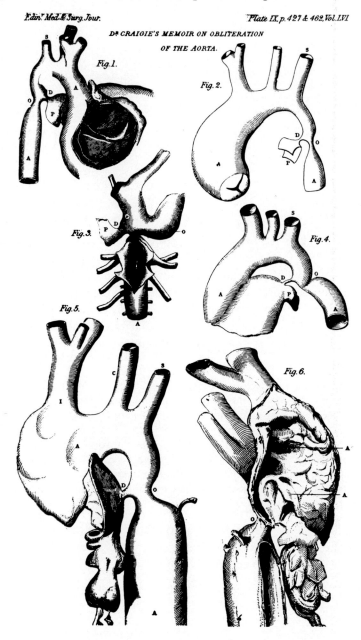

of the aorta as related to closure of the ductus arteriosus extending into the walls of the aorta, and indeed this proposal has been referred to as the Skodiac hypothesis. J. Jordan (3) in 1830 had noted a remarkable similarity between (a) the obliterated part of the aorta and (b) the obliterated ductus arteriosus, and since he thought the closing process of the ductus began in the aortic end, he concluded:

> it seems not unnatural to infer, that, were the closure from any cause to be attended with much contraction, or to be a little extended, it would produce partial, if not total, constriction of the aorta.

He noted Reynaud (4) remarked almost all adult aortas show some degree of constriction at the place at which the ligamentous arterial duct joins the aorta. He has an excellent illustration.

Rokitansky (5) believed the primary fact was nondilatation of the isthmus. An essential corollary, however, was that when the ductus obliterates and regresses there is traction on the aortic ithmus which is too feeble to resist the pull.

The patent ductus arteriosus in association with constriction of the aorta is of special interest since this implies (a) either the ductus is unrelated to constriction or (b) ductus tissue in the aorta had undergone involution, but the ductus itself was not involved in the same process.

There were numerous clinical and pathological reports in the literature during the middle half of the nineteenth century illustrating this association. Many of them are notable for their excellent engravings.

Nixon (6) in 1834 presented a case of coarctation at the insertion of the ductus, with the ductus open, and reviewed the literature prior to that time. An excellent illustration accompanies the case report of Muriel (7). Rees (8) in 1847 reported an open ductus below a contracted aorta in a baby of ten weeks who had a very large heart and hypertrophy of both ventricles, especially the left.

Figure 56. Reproduction of the engraving shown by Dr. Craigie to illustrate the relation of the ductus ligament to narrowing or "obliteration of the aorta beyond the arch."
From Craigie, D.: *Edinb Med Surg J, LVI*:427, 1841.

Chevers in commenting on this case, made the interesting and perhaps astute suggestion that contraction of the aorta distal to the left subclavian might be the lesion determining nonclosure of the ductus.

Dumontpallier (9) collected cases and analyzed them, and he also sought the origin in the closure of the ductus. Peacock (10) wrote prolifically concerning various aspects of congenital heart disease and reported in 1861 a widely open ductus entering the aorta below a constricted area. He considered this as an example of *permanent pervious condition* of the ductus due to congenital contraction of part of the aorta distal to the left subclavian.

There has been some effort to substantiate the early suggestions that the closing ductus was related to coarctation of the aorta, such as the report of Pezzi and Agostini (11). Bremer (12) reemphasized the main types of Bonnet, the fetal type I and adult type II, and noted variations of both types, type IV, depended on the extent of the normal cranial migration of the left subclavian artery or less commonly that of the vertebral artery. The adult type "is due to a fault of development in which the processes of closure of the ductus arteriosus normally occurring at birth extend abnormally to the aorta."

There are many facets of the discussion which persist to the present day. Certainly if a functioning ductus inserting below a coarctation and representing the fetal type should close, the hemodynamics would change markedly and a preductal or infantile coarctation would be transformed into a simple adult coarctation. There are many instances of this closure, and in sections of the ductus-coarctation area in the aorta, it is not always possibe to identify clearly the direction of the ductus flow (13).

The reconstruction of the ductus-aorta junction from serial sections show some similairty to the hypothetical situations illustrated by Bonnet (14). Wielenga (15, 16) especially has pursued this study and showed a clear line of demarcation between collagen rich ductus tissue and elastic vascular tissue of the aorta. In the normal junction with no coarctation the ductus extension into the aortic wall is minimal. When coarctation is present there is variable but greatly increased amount of ductus tissue in the aorta, sometimes as *reins* nearly surrounding the vessel. The diaphragm of the coarctation is directed toward the point of attachment of the ductus or ligament. Schematic representation of the attachment with the normal aorta and the greatly extended extension of the ductus when coarctation is present are shown in Figures 57 and 58.

Brom (17) published histological material from Bakker which showed muscular ductus tissue in the aorta wall in coarctation of the aorta and a closing ductus in an infant of seven days. However, coarctation, degree not specified, was already present and the interpretation of this is not clear.

Coarctation as unusual sites were seen and Figure 59 shows ligamentous ductus tissue preading from the attachment to circle the lumen and form a tube (16).

One of the deterrant to the acceptance of the Craigie-Skoda hypothesis has been the universal observation that coarctation of the aorta may occur with the ductus still patent. However, Wielenga and colleagues (15, 16, 17) have demonstrated that fibrosis of extensive ductus tissue in the aorta considered typical of coarctation occurs independently of closure of the ductus and apparently unrelated to this.

It was found that at the area of attachment at the pulmonary artery ductus tissue extends into the wall for some distance but

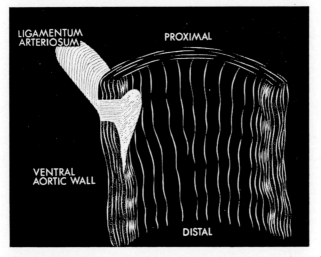

Figure 57. Normal aorta with more or less normal extension of ductus tissue into the aortic wall, schematic illustration. From Wielenga, G. and Dankmeijer, J.: *J Pathol Bacteriol, 95*:256, 1968.

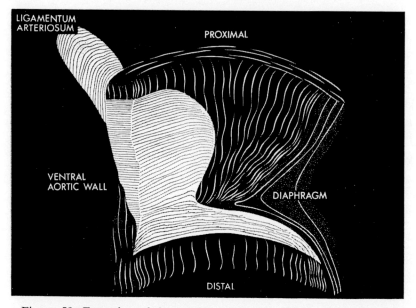

Figure 58. Extension of ductus tissue into the aortic wall in coarctation of the aorta. The diaphragm partially occluding the lumen protrudes from the dorsal wall. The diaphragm is always directed toward the point of attachment of the ductus or ligament.
From Wielenga, G. and Dankmeijer, J. *J Pathol Bacteriol,* *95*:256, 1968.

never involves more than one third of the total circumference. This is considered normal by standards of usual insertion into the aorta. It is suggested that anatomical considerations may be related to abence of coarctation in the pulmonary artery at the insertion of the ductus ligament since the pulmonary trunk is near the insertion and extension of tissue would also involve both right and left pulmonary arteries.

While the Craigie theory is simple and attractive, there are real objections. Costa (18), in his thorough and probably the best study of the histology of the ductus, showed a rather abrupt termination of ductus tissue in the aorta. And Wielenga has fibrous tissue of the ductus in the aortic wall even though the ductus is patent. Bakker (19) concludes in relation to this that the fibrosing process in the wall is independent of closure of the ductus causing involution of ductus tissue in the aorta but not in the ductus. Then there is the occurrence of circumscribed aortic narrowing found in prenatal specimens with the ductus still patent. In the clinical situation typical narrow areas of the constriction with or without an open ductus can be seen on aortography or cineangiography in the first few days after birth, an anatomical status impossible to achieve in so short a time by fibrosis.

The Mayo Clinic group (20) were not able to substantiate the growth of ductus tissue into the aortic wall after histologic examination of a large number of cases. These studies included some reconstructions and serial sections.

Edward and colleagues (21) note as the most striking change an infolding of the media involving the superior, anterior and posterior aspects of the aortic wall, with an overlay of intimal thickening. There is an absence of involvement of the wall into which the ductus inserts. The infolding of the media produces a diaphragm like obstruction as in Figure 60. The ductus part of the wall may evert toward the ductus.

The site of the junction of the right aortic arch with the dorsal aorta was tentatively identified by Kromer (22). The ductus is patent in many instances of coarctation and even in patients over

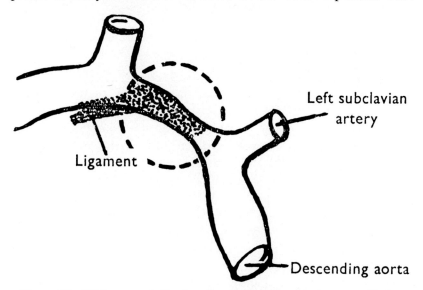

Figure 59. Wielenga and Dankmeijer showed ductus tissue could form a tube narrowing the aorta, resembling tubular hypoplasia.
From Wielenga, G. and Dankmeijer, J. *J Pathol Bacteriol,* *95*:256, 1968.

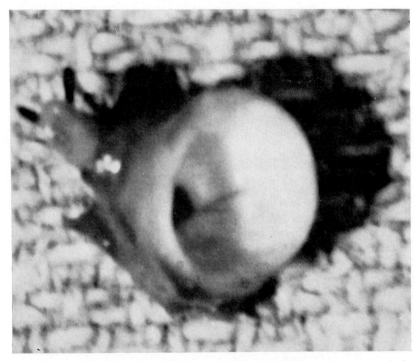

Figure 60. The diaphragm like obstruction due to an infolding of the media. There is no ductus tissue in this diaphragm.

two years of age the association is nearly 10 percent. All surgical series of coarctation include some instances of ductus patency. The ductus may arise from the aorta above or below the site of constriction or appear to be precisely at the coarctation, as in Figure 61, or it may be some distance from it. Figure 62 shows the ductus ligament above the constriction and a poststenotic dilatation below. Figure 63 shows the infantile type *in situ* with a dilated pulmonary artery and a large ductus disappearing into the descending aorta. Figure 64 shows the narrow aortic isthmus and a postcoarctation dilatation in a male infant age six weeks. While the aortic end of the ductus appears patent a ligament was present over two thirds of the vessel. A severe coarctation with similar anatomy is seen by aortogram in a three month old male infant (Fig. 65). There are many reports of isolated areas of aortic constriction far removed from the ductus aorta junction.

In Figure 66 the ductus inserts directly at the site of coarctation.

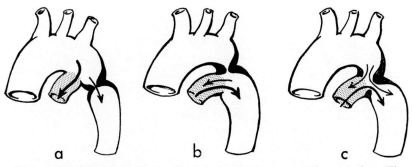

a   b   c

Figure 61. Schematic illustration of the ductus-coarctation relation. The ductus may be above (a) or below (b) the constriction. When it is patent and appears to be exactly at the level of the coarctation (c) it is difficult to determine the direction of blood flow—from the aortic arch into the ductus, or from the ductus into the descending aorta.

There may be complete separation of the aorta with only a hypoplastic cord connecting the segments or no connection at all. The left subclavian may be the terminus of the ascending aorta or it may arise from the descending aorta distal to the interruption.

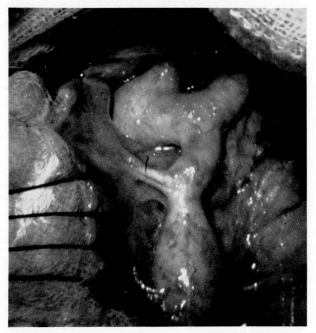

Figure 62. The ductus ligament is just above the coarctation. There is a prominent poststenotic dilatation of the aorta. The isthmus is narrow and the subclavian artery large.

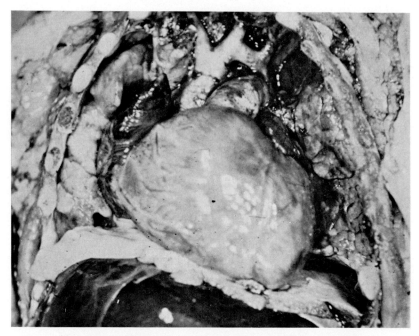

Figure 63. The infantile type coarctation or preductal constriction of the aorta *in situ* in a day old full term infant. The right ventricle and pulmonary artery are grossly dilated. The widely patent ductus continues as the descending aorta. The aortic constriction is very marked. The left subclavian is in its normal position.

Some have made the point that constriction of the pulmonary artery at the site of the ductus-pulmonary artery junction has not been reported, the inference being that if ductus tissue is involved in great vessel constriction it is remarkable that this histological event occurs at one end of the ductus only. Coarctation of right or left pulmonary arteries at or near the bifurcation are commonly seen, but apparently these have not yet been studied for the appearance of ductus tissue at this site.

The typical coarctation at the ductus-aortic junction is not frequently seen or recognized in the fetus and newborn, yet this has been reported by Ingham (23). While in his summary he uses the term infantile type, protocols in 3, 4, 7 and 8, infants at four days of age and one of thirty-eight weeks gestation and two fetus of six months and five and one-half months had coarctation at the junc-

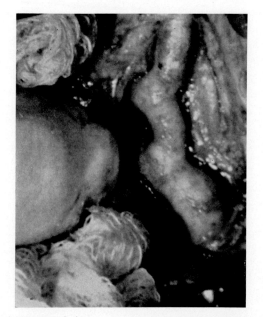

Figure 64. A narrow isthmus coarctation and poststenotic dilatation in an infant age six weeks. Where the aortic terminus of the ductus seems patent actually there was a ductus ligamentum with the aortic end patent, as shown.

tion of the aorta and ductus. Case 2 had narrowing distal to the great vessels, with no statement concerning the site of the ductus junction. As noted, the adult type may be seen in the aortogram in newborn and infants a few weeks of age. It is of interest that Bonnet (14) listed in his classification 3, cases in which there is inversion of the two types. These were his cases 32, 73, 74 and 75. He notes case 32 was absolutely characteristic. But there are not many such reports. However, Kesson (24) reported the clinical diagnosis of coarctation at four days of age, with absent blood pressure in the femoral arteries, and a pressure of 125/90-0 mm Hg in the arms. At four months of age after death from bronchopneumonia, the ductus was seen closed and the aorta constricted just distal to the left subclavian.

Several surgical series include infants with postductus coarctation and usually an open ductus just before and after one month of age. It is difficult to conclude the constriction always occurs

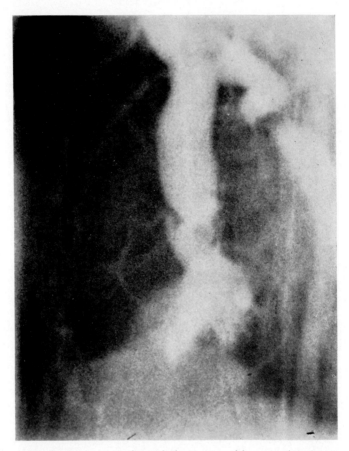

Figure 65. Severe coarctation of the aorta with a partial ductus above it seen in an aortogram in a male infant age three months. There is also aortic valvular stenosis.

postnatally. Morgan (25) concludes that severe coarctation is well developed at birth. In contrast to the presence of a patent ductus in monozygotic twins, he notes coarctation has never been reported in both twins.

The mosaic pattern of the ductus-coarctation anatomy was illustrated by the diagrams of twenty-one cases of coarctation of the aorta in early infancy shown by Calodney and Carson (26) (Fig. 67). Gross believes there is no point in classifying coarctation into types since such a wide variety occur.

The categories Bonnet (14) applied to this defect and his

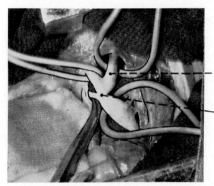

L. Subclavian A.

Coartation of Aorta
at Insertion of Patent
Ductus Arteriosus

Figure 66. The ductus or ligament may insert at the exact level of the coarctation. The identation of the aortic wall opposite is well seen and usually points toward the ductus-aorta junction.

classification, published in 1903, remains the classic reference. However, it is a formidable document, and the literary style of the period does not contribute to clarity.

He entitled his comprehensive discussion, "Sur la Lesion Dite Stenose Congenitale de L' aorte Dans La Region De L' Isthme". This memoir concerning congenital stenosis of the aorta in the region of the ithmus was published in five parts, all in the Revue of Medicine, vol 23, 1903 (14).

Part A listed twenty-seven observations of stenosis in the adult and Part B included twenty-eight cases of stenosis in the newborn, all from the literature. Part C included clinical and physiological considerations, D pathological anatomy and E pathogenesis.

The classification most often referred to is part D. In E he reviewed the theories of etiology and emphasized two types, the *infant type* arising on the basis of an embryological defect, and an *adult type* arising at the site of insertion of the ductus and related to involution of ductus tissue. He illustrated a hypothetical explanation. This has been redrawn (Fig. 68).

In Part D he noted in general the lesion presented differently in the newborn and adult and each group corresponded to a distinct anatomical type. He accepted the fact that there are exceptional or unusual instances in the newborn or adult types which ordinarily belong to the other group. This part can be summarized, although with difficulty.

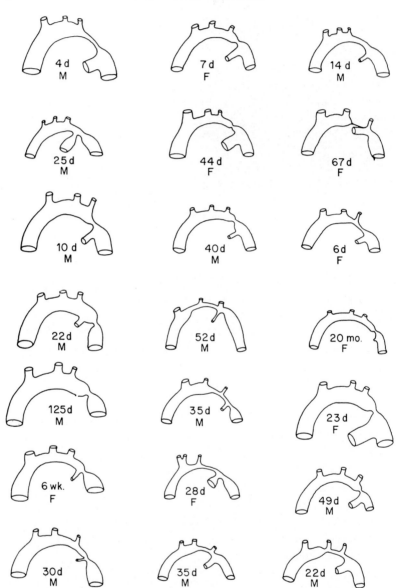

Figure 67. The great variety of ductus-coarctation anatomy was shown by Calodney and Carson (26). When areas of tubular hypoplasia of the aorta are also involved the simple infantile and adults classifications are applied with difficulty.

From Calodney, M.M. and Carson, M.J.: *J Pediatr, 37*:46, 1950.

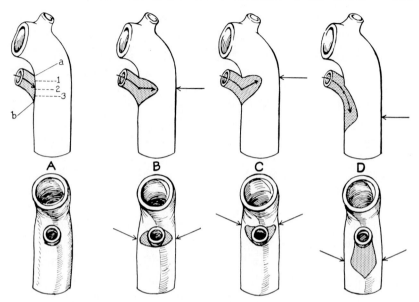

Figure 68. The schematic and hypothetical confluence of the ductus arteriosus and the aorta according to Bonnet[14]. This was designed to explain some of the anatomical variations of coarctation of the aorta. He wrote:

> its tissue is stippled. Above, the region is seen in the profile and an arrow, bent or not, indicates the direction which the ductus tissue (aborde) approaches and invades the aortic wall. The arrow indicates the area of the aorta which will be narrowed. Below, the region is seen from the front (en face). The ductus is cut level with the aorta, into which its tissue does or does not continue. The arrows indicate the level of future stenosis.

From Bonnet, L.M.: *Rev Med Paris, 23*:108, 1903.

1. The Type Commonly Found in the Newborn.

This is characterized by abnormal narrowing of the aorta immediately upstream from the ductus. The degree of narrowing varies considerably, without complete obliteration. The change in size is progressive with maximum narrowing between the left subclavian artery and the ductus. Usually there is stenosis only at this point, but sometimes diminution of calibre starts more proximally to the subclavian. The state of the ductus varies with age and "according to individual conditions the nature of which escapes us." The ductus may continue as a full canal into the thoracic aorta and the aorta is only a feeble tributary.

2. The Type Ordinarily Found in the Adult.

He shows an exterior view of the constriction of the aorta distal to the subclavian "as if the aorta had been squeezed by a ligature." He noted the concavity is most pronounced on the convex side of the aorta which produces a deep furrow above and posteriorly.

When incised the walls appear brought together as by a complete or incomplete ligature and he noted longitudinal folds on the interior surface in one case. The opposite walls may be fused, or there may be a circular diaphragm with or without an orifice.

The stenosis can appear like (a) it was produced by constriction of a single thread or (b) the aorta was choked by a collar instead of a thread.

The ductus ligament is always inserted in the stenosed region, most frequently below the stenosis. In general, he noted (a) it was unusual for the narrowing to correspond to the superior border of the ligament, (b) sometimes it was in the same axis, but (c) most often the stenosis is below the ligament or more or less at the level of the inferior edge.

3. Cases in Which There Were Inversion of the Two Types.

He noted the type uually formed in the newborn had seven exceptions, and of these four had the *usual adult type.*

In the adult there was one exception, a case of the usual newborn type with a rudimentary aortic ithmus and a wide ductus arteriosus continuing into the descending aorta.

4. Cases in Which There Were Irregular Forms.

There were three irregular forms with (a) the stenosis above the left subclavian, (b) the stenosis and the ductus both opposite the subclavian and (c) the narrowing starts after the left carotid and continues further distally and has a maximum below the isthmus. The ductus entered opposite the subclavian.

He then engaged in speculation, reinforcing this by ingenious schematic diagrams. His subscript and discussion are shown. A is the normal insertion.

FIRST: The ductus tissue can (B) enter the aortic wall with a more or less horizontal direction without being clearly either higher or lower. The maximum retraction of the aorta will occur at the center of the orifice of the canal of the ductus. The ligamentum will be found later at the same level as the stenosis.

SECOND: It can also (C) lie chiefly in the aortic segment which corresponds to the superior part of the ductus orifice and the maximum ductus tissue will be above the center of the ductus orifice. The vestigal lumen of this will be just below the stenosis.

Also, it can lie predominantly in the aortic segment which corresponds to the inferior part of the ductus orifice. The point marking the vestige of this orifice will be immediately above the stenosis.

THIRD: It can even (D) lie below this orifice. The circumference of the aorta containing the maximum ductus tissue will be found below the whole orifice. Later, the ligametnum will be completely above the stenosis.

The classification of Bonnet is not always applicable, especially when areas of tubular hypoplasia are present.

The most useful modern clasiffication, based upon the state of the ductus, its relation to the site of coarctation and the inference of collateral circulation is that of Johnson, Ferencz, Wiglesworth and McRae (28).

Coarctation of the Aorta

I. Ductus arteriosus closed
  (1) with collateral circulation
  (2) without (or with inadequate) collateral circulation*
    (incompatible with life)

II. Ductus arteriosus open

  A. Proximal to coarctation
    (1) with collateral circulation
    (2) without (or with inadequate) collateral circulation*
      (incompatible with life)

  B. Distal to coarctation
    (1) with collateral circulation
        (a) pressure maintained by collateral circulation adequate to prevent flow from pulmonary artery to aorta.
        (b) pressure maintained by collateral circulation inadequate to prevent flow from pulmonary artery to aorta.
    (2) without collateral circulation*

*While the absence of a collateral circulation may not be demonstrated by clinical or pathologic means, it is at least a hypothetic possibility.

However, since this discussion is concerned only with the ductus aspects of coarctation of the aorta, a very simple scheme is adequate. The patent ductus has its origin (a) above the constriction, (b) at the point of constriction and usually in such a way that the hemodynamic relation of the ductus-aorta anastomosis is not clear or (c) the ductus joins the aorta below the coarctation. In this category, complete obstruction of the arch or even interruption of the arch above the ductus (29, 30, 31) may be considered as varieties with the same etiological basis, an embryological defect at the junction of the arch system with the dorsal aorta. The abnormality is variable in site and severity.

The hemodynamics of the ductus-coarctation complex are fairly well known in a qualitative way, although quantitative measurements are difficult. When the ductus is above the coarctation, the usual formula for ductus and pulmonary artery flow apply, but even here while systemic flow is calculated, the relation to peripheral flows above and below the coarcted segment are not known. In the absence of a patent ductus total peripheral resistance is elevated (32) and peripheral blood flows in the legs, as measured by plethysmography (33) is about normal. The pulse pressure in femoral arteries is grossly diminished, the femoral pulse is palpated with difficulty, but the mean pressure is nearly normal.

In the fetal situation, the problem is complicated by the requirement of placental flow, and speculation replaces information. If it is assumed the fetal lung has abnormal resistance to blood flow due to (a) its collapsed state and (b) the fetal type pulmonary arteries which show medial hypertrophy and small lumen to wall ratio (34), resistance would be required to a greater extent if hypertension in the aortic arch exists during fetal life.

Since apparently normal infants are born with coarctation and the ductus above it, it must be presumed placental flow takes place in a normal flow -low pressure system that includes the placenta. Since the placenta is a low resistance large flow system, the circulation through infant collaterals is indeed adequate for growth and maturation of the fetus. Whether the placental flow is greater or less or equal to the average flow would seem to depend upon accidental acquisition of information with respect to preductal coarctation during a study of placental flow, or to the study of fetal hemodynamics after aortic constriction has been made below the ductus.

In the situation of preductal coarctation the placental flow would likely approximate that of the normal fetal situation, and venous blood flow to the placenta under the usual systemic pressure and arterial blood returns to the left heart through the umbilical vein, ductus venosus and foramen ovale. It is not clear whether hypertension exists in the aortic arch or what contribution flow through the aortic isthmus makes to placental flow since this is not known in the human in the normal situation. The pulmonary arterial system should show high resistance and possibly increased medial hypertrophy.

The coarctation-ductus problem is made difficult by the question of the collateral circulation, the auxiliary vascular flow from the upper segment of the aorta which is to some degree isolated from the aorta and aortic circulation below this. There is more speculation than data available, and there are few studies such as Olney and Stephens (35) who observed the collateral vessels present by opacification during retrograde aortogram. Observing two groups separated on the basis of presence or absence of decompensation, it was noted that while in the majority of both groups the coarctation was distal to the insertion of the ligamentum, the heart failure group had little collateral circulation discernible. Statements have been made regarding the probable absence of functional collateral vessels in the infantile coarctation, the patent ductus opening below the aortic constriction. It is clear from the study other factors are involved since both in the group with a paucity of opacified collaterals and in the group with well-defined collaterals, the ligamentum, the previous ductus arteriosus, entered the aorta above the constriction. Since the group with cardiac decompensation was young, four and one-half months to four and one-half years, it is easy to conclude that when older, with the advent of collateral circulation, heart failure would not have supervened. It is also easy to conclude that with the open ductus below the constriction and good flow and pressure to the placenta and lower torso, collateral circulation is not required and the stimulus for an alternate collateral circulation does not exist. However, this postcoarctation flow is venous blood with both oxygen saturation and oxygen pressure, PO_2, diminished, and in other situations represents an independent for arterial blood flow.

The variation of constriction of the aorta above, below or at the site of the ductus has been demonstrated in such detail by Calodney and Carson (26) that the terms adult and infantile coarctation are meaningless, especially as these types may occur in the same patient.

The aortic arch has several derivatives, as shown in detail by Barry (36). The part of the greater curvature lying between the subclavian and the first intercostal artery represent the original eighth, ninth and tenth aortic segments. The part of the arch between the left carotid and the left subclavian is derived from the fourth left aortic arch and the third through the seventh segments of the left dorsal aortic root. Any segment or more than one may have an abnormality of development, and there can be areas more commonly involved. The degree of constriction at any place and the position of the ductus in relation to this produce the anatomical and hemodynamic status.

In this context local hypoplasia or coarctation may or may not be related to ductus insertion, but may be an abnormality of development. While it seems unreasonable to ascribe one pathological state to an embryological defect in some segments of the aorta but defects in another area to another cause due to proximity to the ductus arteriosus, the problem posed is probably not yet solved. As shown in isolation of the left subclavian artery from the aorta isolated aortic segments may persist, and isolated segments may also be hypoplastic.

Of great interest, considering the early suggestion of Craigie, Bonnet and the histological studies relating to the association of the ductus insertion and this lesion is the rarity of coarctation in a right aortic arch (37, 38). The incidence of the right aortic arch is believed to be 0.1 percent (39). While the incidence of a right ductus arteriosus in these cases is not known, the relation of a right ductus and a right arch coarctation is extraordinarily uncommon. The histology of the ductus-aorta interdigitation should be the same on the right side as on the left side, and the incidence would be the same if the same causal effect were present. While presumably the segmental makeup of a right aorta is the same as on the left, either explanation, (a) ductus tissue in the aorta or (b) a congenital anomaly related to the eighth, ninth or tenth dorsal root segments has not been adequately studied in coarctation in the right arch.

Coarctation between the right subclavian and the ductus was reported in a ten week old infant who had in addition dextrocardia and transposition of the great vessels (40). The coarctation was of the *infantile type,* with a large patent ductus which continued as the descending aorta.

Interest in constriction of the aorta has been increased by the observation of Gillman and Burton (41) that increased oxygen tension perfusing a preparation of the ductus-aorta of neonatal guinea pigs not only caused closure of the ductus but also constriction of the aorta. However, this occurred only in the preductal area and it is not known whether ductus tissue was present in this site. Other species were also studied, and responses were similar but variable except in the dog where neither the ductus or the aorta seemed responsive to oxygen, although they contracted with noradrenalin.

It seems unlikely, however, that this constriction of the aorta is related to the development of coarctation of the aorta.

The studies of Balis, Chan and Conen (47) suggest ductus tissue is not involved in the formation of the lesion of the media characteristic of coarctation of the aorta. They conclude that from the histopathological viewpoint this is a congenital malformation best defined as a medial myoproliferative lesion which is accompanied by progressive increase of fibroelastic tissue.

Thus, in spite of 130 years of observation and study of the pathogenesis of coarctation, problems persist.

The appropriate time for surgery varies with the associated clinical problem, the only rule being it is better too soon than too late.

The relation of chronic aortic arch hypertension to (a) formation or rupture of aneurysmal dilatation of intracranial arteries is not clear. (b) Systemic hypertension is considered one of the high risk factors in coronary disease in the adult. With greater emphasis on prevention the factor of aortic root hypertension must be considered a hazard to early involvement of coronary arteries in this disease, especially since the diastolic pressure may be quite elevated. The coronary vessels in aortic coarctation have not been studied in detail. The relation of left ventricular pressure and the elevated end-diastolic pressure seen so frequently in the infant to mycardial fibrosis also is not clear. However Skosey et al. (43) have shown aortic obstruction in rats produces elevation of connective tissue collagen within a few days.

There is considerable evidence that the normal closure of the ductus may be related to the onset of heart failure in the infant with coarctation. This sequence presumes coarctation was present at birth and was not induced by ductus closure.

REFERENCES

1. Craigie, D.: Instance of obliteration of the aorta beyond the arch, illustrated by similar cases and observations. *Edinb Med Surg J, LVI:* 427, 1841.
2. Skoda, J.: Protokoll der sections-sitzung fur physiologie and pathologie, am 19 Oct. Wochenblatt der Ztschr der K.K. Gesellsch, der Aerzte z Wien, 710, 1855.
3. Jordan, Joseph: A case of obliteration of the aorta. *North of Eng Med Surg J, Lond, 1:*101, 1830-31.
4. Reynaud, A.: Observation d'une obliteration presque complite de l' aorte, suivie de quelquis reflexions, et precedee de l'indication des facts analagues. *J Hebd Md, 1:*161, 1828.
5. Rokitsansky von, G.: Regelwidrige enge, verengerung, obliteration der arterien, *Lehrbuch pathologischen Anatomie,* p 337, 1855.
6. Nixon, Robert: Case of constriction of the aorta with disease of its valves, and an anomalous tumor in the right hypochondrium. *Dublin J Med Clin Sci, 5:*386, 1834.
7. Muriel, William: Case of contracted aorta. *Guys Hosp Rep, 7:*453, 1842.
8. Rees, G.A.: The heart of a child, presenting an open state of the ductus arteriosus. *Trans Pathol Soc Lond, 1:*203, 1847.
9. Dumontpallier, M.: Retrecissement aortique au niveau de l' abouchement du canal arteriel. *Mem Soc Biologie, 111:*273, 1856.
10. Peacock, T.B.: Heart with an open ductus arteriosus. *Lancet, II:* 475, 1861.
11. Pezzi, C. and Agostoni, G.: Considerazioni anatomiche, patogenetiche e cliniche sulla stenosi aortica situata fra l'arcoela porzione discendente. *Cuore circ, 12:*525, 1928.
12. Bremer, J.L.: Coarctation of aorta and aortic isithmus. *Arch Pathol, 45* 425, 1948.

13. DeBoer, A., Grana, L., Potts, W.J. and Lev, M.: Coarctation of the aorta—A clinical pathological study. *Arch Surg, 28*:801, 1961.
14. Bonnet, L.M.: Sur la lesion dite stenose congenitale de l'aorte dans la region de l'isthme. *Rev Med Paris, 23*:108, 335; 418; 481, 1903.
15. Wielenga, G.: *De Relatie Tussen Coarctation Aorta en Iigamentum Arteriosum.* Thesis, Leiden, 1959.
16. Wielenga, G. and Dankmeijer, J.: Coarctation of the aorta. *J Pathol Bacteriol, 95*:265, 1968.
17. Brom, A.G.: Narrowing of the aortic isthmus and enlargement of the heart. *J Thorc Cardiovasc Surg, 50*:166, 1955.
18. Costa, A.: Obliterazione dell aorta all imbocco dell aorta destra; rottura della prima intercostae aortica. Cassifizione e patogenes; delle atresie e stretture dell aorta. *Arch Pat Clin Med, 9*:305, 1930.
19. Bakker, P.M.: *Morfogeness en Involutie Van de Ductus Arteriosus by de Mens.* Thesis, Leiden, 1962.
20. Clagett, O.T., Kirklin, J.W. and Edwards, J.W.: Anatomic variations and pathological changes in coarctation of the aorta. *Surg Gynecol Obstet, 98*:103, 1954.
21. Edwards, J.E., Christenson, N.A., Clagett, O.T. and McDonald, J.R.: Pathologic considerations in coarctation of the aorta. *Proc Staff Meet Mayo Clinic, 23*:324, 1948.
22. Kromer, Han Wiesb., Die Aortenuarbe Der Aorta Thoracica. J.F. Bergmann, 19, p. 8 (Freiburg 1, Br.) 1913.
23. Ingham, D.W.: Coarctation of the Aorta. *N Y State J Med, 39*:1865, 1939.
24. Kesson, C.W.: Coarctation of the aorta in the neonatal period. *Proc R Soc Med, XLI*:449, 1948.
25. Morgan, John: Evidence of nongenetic origin of coarctation of aorta. *Can Med Assoc J, 100*:1134, 1967.
26. Calodney, M.M. and Carson, M.J.: Coarctation of the aorta in infancy. *J Pediatr, 37*:46, 1950.
27. Gross, R.E.: Coarctation of the aorta. *Circulation, 1*:41, 1950.
28. Johnson, A.L., Ferencz, C., Wiglesworth, F.W., McRae, D.L.: Coarctation of the aorta complicated by patency of the ductus arteriosus. Physiologic considerations in the classification of coarctation of the aorta. *Circulation, IV*:242, 1951.
29. Evans, W.: Congenital stenosis (coarctation), Atresia and interruption of aortic arch. Study of 28 cases. *Q J Med, 2*:1, 1933.
30. Moller, J.H. and Edwards, J.E.: Interruption of aortic arch. Anatomic patterns and associated cardiac malformations. *Am J Roentgen, 95*:557, 1965.
31. Chiemmongkoltip, P., Moulder, P.V. and Cassels, D.E.: Interruption of the aortic arch with aortico-pulmonary septal defect and intact ventricular septum in a teenage girl. *Chest, 60*:324, 1971.
32. Steward, H.J. and Bailey, R.L., Jr.: Cardiac output and other measure-

The Ductus Arteriosus

ments of the circulation in coarctation of the aorta. *J Clin Invest,* 20:145, 1941.

33. Wakim, K.G., Slaughter, O. and Clagett, O.T.: Studies of the blood flow in the extremities in cases of coarctation of the aorta: Determinations before and after excision of the coarctate region. *Proc Staff Meet Mayo Clinic,* 23:347, 1948.

34. Civin, W.H. and Edwards, J.E.: The postnatal structural changes in the intrapulmonary arteries and arterioles. *AMA Arch Pathol, 51*:192, 1951.

35. Olney, M.B. and Stephens, H.B.: Coarctation of the aorta in children. *J Pediatr, 37*:639, 1950.

36. Barry, A.: The aortic arch derivaties in the human adult. *Anat Rec,*

37. Felson, B.F., Palayero, M.T.: The two types of right aortic arch. *Radiology, 81*:745, 1965.

38. Grossman, M. and Jacoby, W.J.: Right aortic arch and coarctation of the aorta. *Dis Chest, 56*:158, 1969.

39. Hastreiter, A.R., D'Cruz, I.A. and Cantez, T.: Right sided aorta. *Br Heart J, 28*:722, 1966.

40. Sinclair, J.G., Cooley, R.N., Schreiber, M.H. and Stoeckle, H.E.: Transposition of great vessels, isolated dextrocardia, coarctation of the aorta, patent ductus passing to the descending aorta, and cleft palate in a ten weeks infant. *Tex Rep Biol Med, 16*:166, 1958.

41. Gillman, R.B. and Burton, A.C.: Constriction of the aorta by raised oxygen tension. *Circ Res, XIX:*755, 1966.

42. Balis, J.W., Chan, A.S. and Conen, P.E.: Morphogenesis of human aortic coarctation. *Exper Molecular Path 6*:25, 1967.

43. Skosey, J.L., Zak, R., Aschenbrenner, V. and Rabinowitz, M.: Biochemical correlates of cardiac hyperttrophy. *Circ Res,* Aug., 1972.

Thirteen

PULMONARY HYPERTENSION

P ULMONARY HYPERTENSION RELATED TO PATENCY of the ductus arteriosus may be classified into three main categories, related to age and projected course.

I. Pulmonary hypertension in the newborn and first year which shows no evidence of diminution and or normal involution of vascular resistance. In the second year the resistance and pressure are fixed or increasing. Such patients are hypertensive from birth and remain so unless surgical closure of the ductus occurs early.

II. Transitional Group

A. There is normal regression of pulmonary resistance. While moderate hypertension may have been present early, this group becomes the usual clinical patent ductus with a lft to right shunt. There may be abnormal involution of pulmonary vasculature from the fetal type with a very large pulmonary flow in early infancy contributing to heart failure.

B. There is moderate hypertension from birth but this is not fixed or rapidly progressive. Closure of the ductus during the first one to two years produces regression of resistance and pressure and in a few years the electrocardiogram and hemodynamic values are normal. This group is similar to group I, but less severe, and surgery is less urgent.

C. A ductus manifested early by a left to right shunt slowly develops vascular disease, pulmonary hypertension and (a) diminution or absence of the normal ductus shunt and lessened pulmonary flow, (b) evidence of right ventricular hypertrophy and (c) sometimes a venous shunt and cyanosis of the feet, best seen in the toes, where clubbing may occur. The disease is progressive.

There is some objection to the concept of progressive vascular resistance, but (a) this can be produced in animals, (b) it occurs following large shunts produced surgically, as in a large Potts anastomosis for palliation of Tetralogy of Fallot, and it is (c) occasionally documented clinically chiefly in patients who have been studied but who have a medical care hiatus of several years and then return hypertensive and often inoperable.

III. Severe hypertension, bidirectional shunting and regional cyanosis are present when the patient is first seen. This is the usual clinical situation and the previous medical status is not known or is fragmentary and speculative. There are instances where the history states the patient has been blue since birth, but this is usually without reliable confirmation.

The usual age when the hypertensive ductus presents with symptoms is older than symptoms occurring with other types of pulmonary hypertension and later than in the large ventricular septal defect with bidirectional shunting.

The sex ratio in the literature examined relative to the large ductus and pulmonary hypertension seems to be about the same as in the usual patent ductus, with a predominance of females.

It is believed by some that although these patients originated in group I, hypertensive since birth, early correction of the defect, either ductus or ventricular septal defect, would not have influenced the course of the hypertension. These suggest the basic problem is primary pulmonary hypertension and that any defect present is incidental to chronic progressive vascular disease of the lung of unknown origin.

It would appear the distinction between patency with regression of the anatomical basis for increased resistance and acquisition of normal pressure and increased ductus flow and patency with non-regression of fetal vasculature is some functional or anatomic peculiarity of late fetal life. The status of the pulmonary vessels and the ductus seem delineated before birth. The ductus which is destined to remain patent is deficient in the necessary anatomical closure constituents at birth and the lung small vessel-high resistance anatomy which will persist is likewise present at birth. If a ductus shunt is present, progression of the vascular changes may occur if the aorta-pulmonary artery vessel is large and if it remains equal to one half of the diameter of the aorta.

STRUCTURAL CHANGES IN LUNG VESSELS

The pulmonary vesssels and their characteristics were described and defined by Brenner (1) in 1935.

1. *Elastic* arteries are those which lie outside the lung and those exceeding 1000 μ in external diameter—*elastic pulmonary arteries.*

2. *Muscular* arteries are about 100 and 1000 μ in diameter with a distinct muscular media and internal and external limiting elastic laminae.

3. *Arterioles* are vessels lined by a single elastic lamina and with no media and arising from a small muscular pulmonary artery.

4. *Venules*—pulmonary venules are of the same structure as arterioles but are distinguished from them by their connection with veins.

5. *Veins* exceed 100 μ in external diameter.

The pathological criteria for hypertensive pulmonary vascular disease was defined by Heath and Edwards (2) in 1958. Some modification has been proposed, but these grades of severity are usually accepted:

GRADE 1. THE STAGE OF RETENTION OF FETAL-TYPE PULMONARY ARTERIES. The definitive histological features lie in the pulmonary arteries. This grade is the earliest ever found in large post-tricuspid shunts.

GRADE 2. STAGE OF MEDIAL HYPERTROPHY WITH CELLULAR INTIMAL PROLIFERATION. Cellular intimal proliferation is seen in both the smallest muscular pulmonary arteries, less than about 300 μ in diameter, and in the arterioles. It is restricted to these small arterial vessels, and there is no intimal reaction elsewhere in the pulmonary vasculature.

GRADE 3. STAGE OF PROGRESSIVE FIBROUS VASCULAR OCCLUSION. There is progressive intimal fibrosis in the small muscular pulmonary arteries and pulmonary arterioles with a change in the nature of the intimal proliferation and an extension of it into medium-sized arteries (300 to 500 μ).

GRADE 4. THE STAGE OF PROGRESSIVE GENERALIZED ARTERIAL DILATION WITH THE FORMATION OF COMPLEX "DILATATION LESIONS". (a) plexiform lesions; (b) veinlike branches of hypertrophied, usually occluded, muscular pulmonary arteries; (c) angimatoid lesions and (d) cavernous lesions.

GRADE 5. STAGE OF CHRONIC DILATATION WITH FORMATION OF NUMEROUS DILATATION LESIONS AND PULMONARY HEMOSIDEROSIS. In grade 5, all four types of dilatation lesion previously described are found and give rise to thin-walled, dilated vessels which ramify throughout the lung rendering it highly vascular.

GRADE 6. STAGE OF NECROTIZING ARTERITIS, Necrotizing arteritis occurs rarely but nevertheless has been described in cases of atrial septal defect, ventricular septal defect, mitral stenosis and idiopathic pulmonary hypertension. It is usually associated with a very high pulmonary artery blood pressure.

Brewer (3) depicted a reconstruction by serial sections of fibrous occlusion and formation of new pathways to alveoli.

The patient studied was 26 years old at death. At age twenty-one she had profuse hemoptysis for three days and three other episodes in the last year of her life. She became dyspneic and had cyanosis of limbs, sometimes the legs only, although there was clubbing of the fingers. Of great interest was the presence of loud systolic and

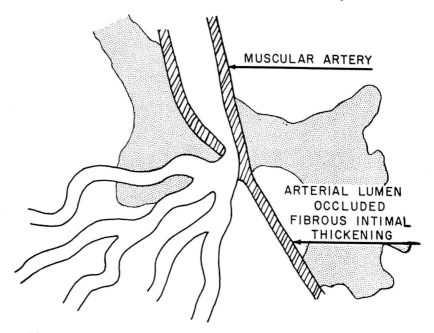

Figure 69. Reconstruction by serial section of an area of fibrous intimal occlusion and dilated vessels arising proximal to the point of occlusion. These apparently new vessels reach alveolar capillaries. The patient was twenty-six years old, and a murmur of *CHD* was present at age six months. No real difficulty until age twenty-one years when she had hemoptysis. Redrawn from Brewer, D.B.: *J Pathol Bacteriol, 70*:299, 1955.

diastolic murmurs in the third interspace sometimes fusing into a typical continuous murmur of patent ductus arteriosus.

She had a very high pulmonary pressure, 130/85 mm Hg with bi-directional shunt at the ductus level, the oxygen saturation in the right brachial artery 95 percent and in the femoral artery 82.5 percent. There was increased saturation in the pulmonary artery, 76.5 percent with the right ventricle 63 percent.

Death followed ligation of a very large short ductus of 3 cm in diameter. Atheroma were present in the pulmonary artery. A placque adjacent to the ductus could be construed as representing previous left to right shunt.

In all specimens the vessels showed striking changes:

1. Medial thickening, splitting of internal elastic membrane and intimal thickening.

2. In some small arteries, disorganization and thinning of the wall, sometimes affecting only part of the circumference.

3. Unusual structures were present with small muscular arteries communicating with thin walled vascular spaces. The reconstruction of one of these by serial sections has been redrawn (Fig. 69). These vessels become smaller and ultimately give rise to alveolar capillaries.

4. The primary event was believed to be widespread occlusion of small muscular arteries, with the lumen filled with fibrous tissue either old and organized or more cellular and loose. It was suggested breaches in the media where elastic lamina had disappeared and muscle replaced by fibrous tissue resembled healed polyarteritis nodosa and the healing of necrotizing arteritis associated with severe pulmonary hypertension.

5. The anomalous thin walled vessels develop because of the obstruction and are either dilatation of previous minute vessels or represent formation of new rout to alveolar capillaries.

Figure 70 illustrates the changes in the pulmonary vessels associated with pulmonary hypertension, reversal of flow and cyanosis of the toes. Larger vessels show an intimal placque, and an instance of thrombosis and beginning recanalization. A plexiform lesion with fibrous occlusion of a vessel and small vessels arising near the area of occlusion is also apparent.

Short (4) illustrated a clinical x-ray facet of constriction or occlusion of arterial branches by means of magnified arteriogram (Fig. 71).

The extremes of opinion represented by those who believe (a) pulmonary hypertension continues from birth, or (b) is acquired by large high pressure shunts through the pulmonary vascular bed are illustrated by two group of patients, those (a) blue since birth and (b) those with disappearance of the continuous murmur typical of patent ductus arteriosus. Both groups are small, suggesting

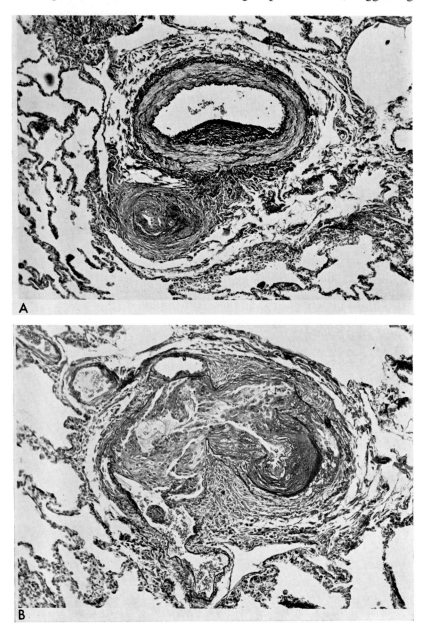

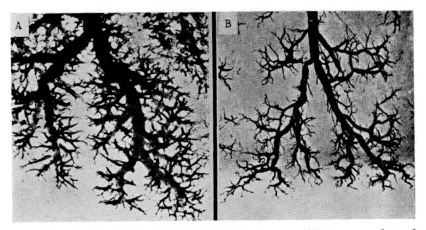

Figure 71. Magnified arteriogram (X5) showing diffuse narrowing of arteries and arterioles in pulmonary hypertension, right, in contrast to the normal lung, left, narrowing caused by contracture does not show arterial blacking and pruning caused intimal proliferation and obstruction.
From Short, D.S.: *Lancet,* 2:12, 1957.

either of the extremes are unusual and an intermediate situation usually prevails.

1. Hypertensive—Blue Since Birth

There are a few reports of persistence of high pulmonary vascular resistance after birth causing persistence of the fetal flow from pulmonary artery to aorta. In most cases the history of cyanosis since birth is related to a statement by the mother, and faint blueness in early infancy is notoriously difficult to document. Frequently there will be a complaint of blueness in an infant without heart disease. In early infancy, before the neonatal polycythemia disappears, crying produces a plethoric appearance by suffusion of superficial venous plexus which is present especially over the upper lip. This gives the appearance of circumoral cyanosis. Polycythemia

Figure 70. L.S., age fourteen years. Lung biopsy. A. (Gomori Trichrome X135) A small pulmonary artery contains an organized occlusive thrombus which is partially recanalized. A somewhat larger artery contains a fibrous intimal placque. B. (Gomori Trichrome X200) A plexiform arterial lesion showing multiple small and irreguar vascular channels. The vessels originate proximal to fibrous intimal occlusion (see Fig. 71).

may persist longer than usual and add to the interval of apparent cyanosis. It is difficult to document arterial oxygen saturation by arterial blood samples, since with crying venous shunting may occur at the foramen ovale level (5).

There are fourteen reports of the patent ductus pulmonary hypertension syndrome with cyanosis since birth. These are, in general, not documented by arterial oxygen saturation determinations. Cases which seem acceptable are in Table XI. No doubt others have been omitted.

TABLE XI
BLUE SINCE BIRTH

Dammann, J.F., Jr., et al.............. Case 1 Case 2	Case 1. 36 yr old F.—cyanosis since birth Case 4. 30 yr old F. Increasing cyanosis, dyspnea and fatigability since birth. Dammann, J.F., Jr., Berthrong, M. and Bing, R.J. Reverse ductus; presentation of syndrome of patency ofductus arteriosus with pulmonary hypertension and shunting of blood flow from pulmonary artery to aorta. *Bull Johns Hopkins Hosp, 92*:128, 1953.
Limon Lason, R., et al............ Case 3	Case 8. 15 yr old F. Blue since birth. Saturation, Ao 73.3%, PA 57.4%; Pressure, Ao 123/72, PA 136/68. Limon Lason, R., Bouchard, F., Rubio Alvarez, V, Cahen, P. and Novelo, S.: Cateterismo en conducto arterioso atipco. *Arch Inst Card Mexico, 20*:147, 1950.
Gardiner, J.M............................. Case 4	Three patients with hypertension and all three mothers had rubella during pregnancy. Case 3 had cyanosis since birth. Patent ductus arteriosus with atypical signs. *Med J Aust, 2*:41st year, 1954.
Campbell, M., Hudosn, R. .... Case 5	F., 32 yr, blue since birth. Patent ductus arteriosus with reversible shunt due to pulmonary hypertension. *Gulys Hosp Rep, 100*:26, 1951.
Holman, E., et al......................... Case 6	16 yr old—cyanosis since birth. Holman, E., Gerbode, F. and Purdy, A.: The patent ductus. *J Thor Surg, 25*:111, 1963.
Anderson, R.C., et al................. Case 7 Case 8 Case 9	Case 4. Case 9. 16 mos—blue with crying since birth Case 10. Anderson, R.C., Adams, P. Jr. and Varco, R.L.: Patent ductus with reversal of flow. Clinical study of ten children. *Peds, 18*/3:410, 1956.
Smith, G. .... Case 10	Age 19 yr—blue since birth. Patent ductus arteriosus with pulmonary hypertension and reversible shunt. *Brit Heart J, 16*:233, 1954.
Bouchard, F............................. Case 11	Moderate cyanosis since birth Op: 20 mm long, 15 mm diameter (16 yrs old) Autopsy: ductus only, placques up to branches 3 to 4 mm diameter. Media hypertrophic in pulmonary arterioles.

La persistans du canal arteriel in cardopathies congenitales. Ed. P. Soulie, p. 215, L Expansion Scientifique
Francaise, 1952.

Abrams, H.L. .... Tachypnea soon after birth, clubbing of toes and leg
Case 12   cyanosis by 9 mos. Died of intractable failure. Au-
topsy: patent ductus arteriosus only.
Persistance of fetal ductus function after birth.
Circulation, 18:206, 1958.

v. Schroetter, H. .... 15 yr old F.—cyanosis, palpitation and shortness of
Case 13   breath since birth. Swelling of the legs and paralysis
of left vocal cord. Autopsy: ductus dilated to size of
main branches of the pulmonary artery and the aortic
ostium had a diameter of 35 mm. The left recurrent
nerve was tightly wedged between the aorta and ductus
and was atrophic and discolored over 10 mm.
Ueber eine selbene enseitrger recurrens laehmung zuglech beitragzur symptomatologie und diagnose
des offenen ductus Botalli (unilateral paralysis of recurrens in patent ductus Botalli).
H Zietsch f klin med, 43:160, 1901.

Bruins, C. .... Bruins entitled a paper "Terminal cyanosis in a patient
Case 14   with an open ductus Botalli". However she was only
4 yrs and postmortem showed a large patent ductus
arteriosus with vascular changes in the lungs, reversal
of flow and what he called terminal cyanosis. This
occurrence at age 4 yrs is so remarkable that the status
at an early age might be questioned. While this case
does not absolutely fit the category blue since birth,
since this statement is not made, she falls into the
group of very early hypertension with pulmonary
vascular pathology and reversal of flow.
Terminal cyanosis in a patient with an open ductus
Botalli. *Maandschr Kindergeneesk, 19*:368, 1951.

2. Disappearance of a Murmur in the Pulmonary Hypertension Syndrome

The same problem of early documentation of the presence of a
ductus murmur which has disappeared occurs as in the history of
blueness since birth. The murmur problem is made more complex
by the necessity of having a statement based upon auscultation by
a physician and later then repeated by the mother in a history. The
problem involves several questions: (a) was the murmur present
in infancy or early childhood and possibly not discussed because of
a possibility that it was functional and might disappear, (b) was
the murmur systolic only or (c) the typical continuous murmur
of a patent ductus arteriosus.

Adequate documentation of the disappearance of a ductus
murmur presumably due to the development of pulmonary hyper-

tension requires (a) continuous observation by the same physician until this event occurs. This is unlikely at this time since the patient will be referred to surgery before a great change occurs. (b) Availability of previous medical records or abstracts of these with an unequivocal and acceptable description of a typical ductus murmur. A frank grade two or more long systolic murmur maximum in the second interspace with accentuation of S_2, should be acceptable as evidence of a previous left to right shunt in a patient with a later proven open ductus and systemic hypertension in the pulmonary artery.

There are eight reports of disappearance of a ductus murmur presumably related to acquisition of high pulmonary pressure, and no doubt other patients have had this sequence occur. But it is uncommon, and the rarity of this sequence has been the subject of some discussion. The cases acceptable are listed in Table XII.

TABLE XII

DISAPPEARANCE OF A CONTINUOUS MURMUR

Gordon, H.J., et al Case 1	Born 1928, age 6 mos—enlarged heart; 1938, age 10 yrs—systolic and diastolic murmurs in pulmonary area, S_2 loud; 1947, age 19 yrs—no murmurs, cyanosis of left hand greater than right; 1953—operation—died. Ductus: 2 cm wide; .8 cm long. Gordon, H.J., Donoso, E., Kuhn, L.A., Ravitch, M.M. and Himmelstein, A.: Patent ductus arteriosus with reversal of flow. *New Eng J Med, 251*:923, 1954.
Campbell, M. Case 2	Case 18. Female with enlarged heart at 29 yrs, fair conditions up to 36 yrs. Age 39 yrs—cyanosis left arm and feet. Some notes and prognosis on pulmonary hypertension. *Brit Heart J, 17*:511, 1955.
Campbell, M., Hudson, R. Case 3	Female, 39 yrs—classical mill wheel murmur 10 yrs before. The disappearance of the continuous murmur of patent ductus arteriosus. *Guys Hosp Rep, 101*:32, 1952.
Lukas, D.S., et al Case 4	Female, 24 yrs—typical ductus murmur at 10 yrs. At 24 yrs accentuated P2 and cyanosis and only a harsh low pitched systolic murmur in 3rd and 4th left interspace. Saturation: 73% right arm; 56% left arm. Lukas, D.S., Aranjo, J. and Steinberg, I.: The syndrome of patent ductus arteriosus with reversal of flow.
Harris, P. Case 5	Female, 43 yrs—heart found to be abnormal at 8 yrs. Age 9 yrs—systolic murmur in pulmonary area and loud P2. Age 25 yrs—a harsh murmur heard throughout systole and diastole, but mainly in diastole, in the pulmonary area. Patent ductus arteriosus with pulmonary hypertension. *Brit Heart J, 17*:85, 1955.

Burchell, H.B., et al........................Case 5. Machinery murmur at 18 yrs. F., age 30 had
    Case 6   a grade 3 systolic murmur and thrill at 3rd left inter-
space and a grade 1 continuous murmur; 10 mos later
feet were cyanosed but hands were not. Pulmonary
artery pressure 150/90, femoral artery 135/85. While
absence of a previous machinery murmur not specifically stated such a murmur seems impossible.
Burchell, H.B., nad Swan, H.J.C. and Wood, E.H.:
Demonstration of differential effects no pulmonary
and systemic arterial pressure by variation in oxygen
content of inspired air in patients with patent ductus
arteriosus and pulmonary hypertension. *Circulation,*
8:681, 1953.

Limon Lason, R..........................Age 13 yrs, typical patent ductus arteriosus. Age 23
    Case 7   yrs this status changed with swelling and cyanosis of
toes, segmented cyanosis. Pulmonary artery pressure
126/86, abdominal aorta O_2 saturation 80%.
In Pulmonary Circulation. Ed. W. Adams and I. Veith,
Grune & Stratton, N.Y., 1959.

Jose, A.D., et al ....18 yrs, ductus with left to right shunt. Surgery, ductus
    Case 8   13 to 14 mm closed. In 6 mos, murmur reappeared,
but disappeared over 5 yrs. Pulmonary artery pressure
rose to systemic level 106/55 and pulmonary resistance
to 64 percent of systemic, a false saccular aneurysm
found at surgery. Pathology showed gross narrowing
or occlusion of many small or medium sized vessels.
Jose, A.D., Ferencz, C., Sheldon, H. and Bahnson,
H.T. Progressive rise in pulmonary vascular resistance
in a patient with ductus arteriosus. Case report. *Bull*
Johns Hopkins Hosp, 108:280, 1961.

Clinical Aspects of the Hypertensive Ductus

The clinical aspects of the patent ductus associated with severe pulmonary hypertension can be reviewed rather briefly since the presenting complaints, the etiological history, the cardiac and circulatory findings and the auxiliary and laboratory information are somewhat stereotyped.

The most common differential diagnosis is a ventricular septal defect with pulmonary hypertension. This distinction is not always possible on a clinical basis, even if an x-ray and electrocardiogram are available. If the pulmonary disease has progressed to the point of a reversal of shunt, an accentuation of cyanosis in the feet and toes indicates a venous shunt at the ductus level and is diagnostic of a large patent ductus.

A loud S_2 in the second interspace in the presence of cyanosis usually suggests pulmonary hypertension and venous shunting either at the ventricular or ductus level. In corrected transposition, the booming second sound is the aortic valve closure, and can be misleading.

The history is seldom one specific of patency. There is no previous information of a continuous murmur. There is often a history of a cardiac murmur in early childhood with no noticeable voluntary restriction of activity at that time. The older patient of ten to twenty years will complain of increasing fatigue and dyspnea. Sometimes an episode of hemoptysis will frighten a patient with pulmonary hypertension and precipitate medical consultation.

Precordial pain, anginal in type, may occur intermittently. It is not clear whether gross right ventricular hypertrophy contributes to coronary insufficiency of the right ventricle, or whether an elevated right ventricular end-diastolic pressure diminishes coronary flow to contribute to anginal pain. Some believe distension of the pulmonary arteries cause chest pain which clinically closely simulates anginal episodes but could be differentiated since nitroglycerine did not give relief.

The physical findings are mild hyperpnea or dyspnea at rest, and real or probably cyanosis of the toes. Right ventricular hypertrophy is indicated by a parasternal lift and the pulmonary hypertension by a grossly accentuated S_2 in the second left interspace. Right ventricular hypertrophy in the infant is uniformly present if the ventricle is palpable in the epigastrium at the xiphoid.

Hypertrophy and enlargement of the left ventricle or biventricular hypertrophy are identified with more difficulty by physical examination. The electrocardiogram is helpful in indicating previous left to right shunt by left atrial hypertrophy.

Murmurs are not diagnostic. They are variable even with mild exercise. They have been reported as (a) systolic only, ejection in type or occuring later in systole; (b) separate grade one or two systolic and diastolic murmurs; (c) diastolic only, suggesting a pressure gradient in diastole; or (d) a diminundo diastolic murmur following a loud second sound and representing pulmonary insufficiency. This is an ominous sign suggesting inoperability.

These signs may be followed within a few years by (a) increasing dyspnea and cyanosis, (b) episodes of acute pulmonary distress with x-ray infiltrates probably representing infarction and hemorrhage, (c) increasing arrhythmia usually multiple premature ventricular contractions and (d) frequent periods of hospitalization before demise.

A diastolic murmur which represents dilatation of the pulmonary artery and annulus with ensuing pulmonary regurgitation is decrescendo, soft and characteristic. With subsequent lowering of the pulmonary diastolic pressure, a diastolic flow through the ductus from the aorta may be established giving evidence on catheterization of a left to right shunt. This is quite misleading if interpreted as an indication of operability. Phasic bidirectional shunt has been demonstrated.

It seems possible pulmonary valve insufficiency may be so severe and the pulmonary artery diastolic pressure so low that even with severe and inoperable pulmonary vascular disease a left to right shunt can occur during diastole. The patient of Harris (6) had a pulmonary artery pressure of 140/10.

In addition, Rosenthal (7) reported a female age thirty-six:

> with a history of frequent cyanosis and increasing dyspnea. When seen, she had generalized cyanosis, clubbing, polycythemia and right ventricular hypertrophy by x-ray and electrocardiogram. Of great interest was a loud diastolic murmur and thrill in the second left intercostal space, where S_2 was accentuated.
> An isolated large patent ductus was shown during right and left heart catheterization. He suggested that the murmur arose by decompression of an aneurysmally dilated pulmonary artery into the aorta during diastole.

He noted there were two previous reports of a diastolic murmur and thrill in patients with a hypertensive ductus syndrome, ages forty-two years and sixteen years (8, 9). Rodbard (10) had suggested aortic flow may have a Bernoulli effect, and therefore could reverse a small gradient to give a right to left shunt. In the fetal lamb asynchrony of ventricular contraction contributes to paradoxical pulmonary artery to aorta against a pressure gradient (11).

The literature related to pulmonary hypertension as a facet of the patent ductus arteriosus reached maximum during the decade 1950 to 1960. Since 1965 this has not been a consistent subject for either medical or surgical reports. This is a reflection of (a) the ductus is treated surgically early in infancy or childhood upon recognition and (b) the formidable aspects of systemic hypertension are well known and the inoperable status of some patients accepted.

The reports of surgical closure of the ductus with hypertension vary with the classification of hypertension accepting as the most severe those with reversal of flow and unsaturation or cyanosis distal to the ductus.

Anderson et al. (12) in 1956 collected forty-five cases from the literature and studied ten more. Of the ten three had surgery with one successful outcome in a year old infant. In the series of forty-five, twenty-two had surgery with good results in only four, three of whom were children. This review suggests this syndrome is less malignant early and age groups require separate consideration in relation to surgery. In the forty-five cases collected, only six were under fifteen years, and two under six years.

Anderson and Coles (13) reviewed nine cases age one to six and one-half years, with pulmonary hypertension. All had surgical correction, with death one month postoperatively in one who had associated defects mitral and aortic stenosis. The mean pulmonary artery pressure was above 60 mm Hg in all except one, which was probably in error, since there was gross unsaturation in the femoral artery. Restudy of six patients showed pulmonary artery pressure and resistance had returned to normal.

Anabtawi, Ellison and Ellison (14) entitled a paper *Natural History of Pulmonary Hypertension in Surgically Treated Patent Ductus Arteriosus.* They tried to determine the incidence of pulmonary hypertension in the patent ductus and the role of division of the vessel on reversibility. One hundred consecutive patients were studied with pressure measurements before or at the time of surgery with temporary occlusion or division.

This series of unselected cases would seem to give a reasonable summary of the clinical status of an average group of patients with patent ductus arteriosus.

The categories of pulmonary artery pressure were related to peak systolic pressure. (a) Less than 30 mm Hg was considered normal; (b) 31 to 35 mm Hg, mild; (c) 56 to 75 mm Hg, moderate and (d) over 76 mm Hg, severe. The distribution of cases by age and pulmonary artery pressure are shown in Figure 72.

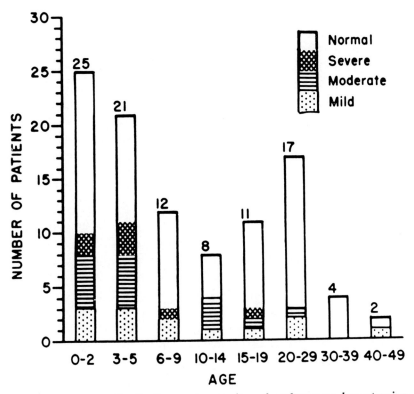

Figure 72. Age distribution and severity of pulmonary hypertension. Classification of severity by systolic pressure was less than 30 mm Hg, normal; 31 to 55, mild; 56 to 75, moderate; and over 75, severe.
By permission of the American Heart Association, Inc. From Anabtawi, I.N., Ellison, R.G. and Ellison, L.T.: *Circulation,* Suppl *31 & 32,* 1965.

There were twenty-two patients with residual hypertension following temporary or permanent occlusion, seven of whom were severe. A study of these one to four years after surgery showed six of seven, mild; two of eight, moderate and one of seven, severe to have normal pulmonary artery pressure. Thus 10 percent of 100 cases had residual hypertension. While this seems high, it is probably representative of an average patent ductus arteriosus population.

It is of interest that in an analysis of thirty cases of pulmonary hypertension with hemodynamic data and a peak systolic pressure of over 60 mm Hg there were eighteen females and twelve males, a sex ratio rather different from the usual three to one (15).

In these thirty cases a mortality of 17 percent occurred, all in those with a right to left shunt. A drop in pressure was usually found in those restudied although not always to normal values. This group included three with a right to left shunt prior to operation.

It is quite possible the mortality would be less in 1972 due to change in techniques. But the conclusion would be the same, that the group with left to right shunt only and the group with major left to right and only slight or intermittent right to left shunt would have surgery. The third group, with predominant right to left shunt are probably inoperable.

However, even in group three a trial closure below seven to eight years is probably desirable. If the pulmonary artery pressure rises and the pressure in the aorta falls on occlusion of the ductus the procedure can be discontinued at low risk (Fig. 73).

Even in the presence of pulmonary hypertension at systemic level and cyanosis Burchell et al. (16) found that increase of oxygen in inspired air varied the degree of pulmonary artery to aorta flow and might be useful as an index to possible surgical repair. If pulmonary vascular resistance has a substantial vasoconstrictive component partially relieved by oxygen, surgery might be attempted, especially in the younger age group, probably under five to six years.

The ultimate fate of the patient with a large patent ductus arteriosus, reversal of flow and cyanosis and who is inoperable because of grade five or six pulmonary catastrophe seems to vary between sixteen and forty years, with the greatest problem in the twenty to thirty year group.

The role of unilateral pulmonary artery banding for production of nonpulsatile flow in one lung as proposed by Moulder et al. (17) has not been fully evaluated. Seven patients were reported and an additional three operated upon. While these patients had large ventricular septal defects, except one, the pulmonary vascular problem is the same. Of these patients one died suddenly in another city and no examination was possible. One died of a brain abscess. The remaining eight seem reasonably comfortable although with mild symptoms and mild cyanosis. One is thirty years of age, married, an office worker with an adopted child. However, she was

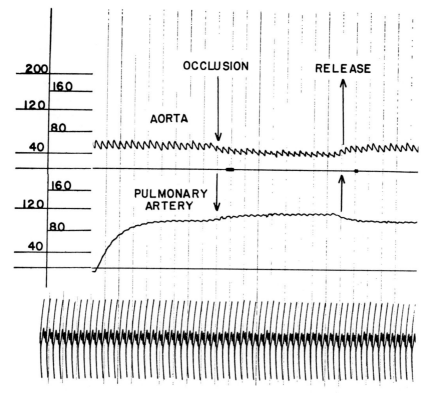

Figure 73. In occlusion of the ductus at surgery the aortic pressure decreases and the pulmonary artery pressure increases. The patient is inoperable and effort at closure should be abandoned.

twenty years old, dyspneic and cyanotic at the time of banding of the right pulmonary artery.

Progressive obstruction to blood flow at the small artery and arteriole level appears to be the basis of irreversible vascular disease, contraindication to surgery and a lethal prognosis. At some point of obstruction scattered thrombotic episodes occur.

Necrotizing arteritis is described in the late, Grade 6, vascular lesions.

Studies of the ultrastructure of the lesions suggest intimal occlusion may arise from portion of smooth muscle cells of the media. Such tudies were reported by Hatt et al. (18) in 1959 and by Esterly, Glagov and Ferguson (19) in 1968.

If early occlusive features are thus not real fibrosis, the possibility of some reversibility should exist, if the inciting cause, hypertension, could be alleviated by banding of the main pulmonary artery. This procedure seems lethal in the presence of systemic pressure in the pulmonary system.

Although not completely substantiated, unilateral banding, usually of the right branch, at least offers a possibility of unilateral improvement and increase of blood flow to the banded side.

Cyanosis

Pulmonary hypertension associated with wide patency of the ductus arteriosus may produce cyanosis. Ehara (20) reports that in this circumstance there may be decreased diffusing capacity and thickened alveolar basement membrane, and an increase of alveolar-arterial PO_2 gradient could occur. The demonstrable cause, however, is venous admixture with shunting of pulmonary venous blood to the aorta through the ductus. Venous admixture within the lung parenchyma by vessels that bypass an alveolar capillary network has been demonstrated.

Spencer (21) described vessels arising from arteries and joining veins in a patient with primary pulmonary hypertension and a patient age six years who had a patent ductus arteriosus, suggesting the possibility of venous-arterial intrapulmonary shunt as a contribution to cyanosis.

Cyanosis may include full body cyanosis. Shepard et al. (22) reported a seven and one-half year old boy in whom it was estimated that about 28 percent of the systemic blood flow to the upper part of the body, an area supplied by branches of aortic arch, was contributed by retrograde flow via a large patent ductus. Cyanosis may be absent from the right arm and present in the left and lower extremities. This depends upon the anatomy of the aortic arch and a variable retrograde venous flow in to the arch of the aorta. This is particularly variable with exercise. The variations are shown in Figure 74.

The clinical feature of the usual ductus-pulmonary hypertension syndrome is cyanosis and clubbing of the toes in contrast to the minimum or absent cyanosis in the fingers. The clinical diagnosis is made more obvious by comparing fingers and toes in all patients with an accentuated second sound in the second interspace, with a

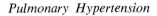

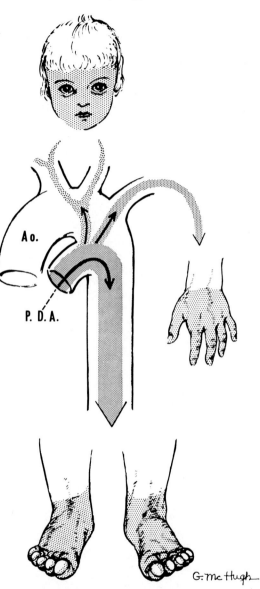

Figure 74. Schematic illustration of the origin of cyanosis in the presence of a patent ductus arteriosus, pulmonary hypertension and some reversal of flow with venous blood entering the aorta. The greater shunt is to the descending aorta, producing cyanosis and clubbing of the toes. But some flow may occur retrograde upward into the aortic arch and vessels arising from it.

nontypical murmur and right ventricular hypertrophy. It is of interest that occlusion of the aorta below a ductus, even when there is cyanosis, appears to reverse or diminish the venous shunt and increase oxygenation, as in Figure 75.

Polycythemia may be slight in a younger child with hematocrit, hemoglobin and red blood cells only at the upper limit of normal for the age.

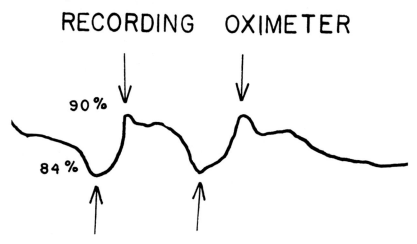

RECORDING OXIMETER

OCCLUSION AND RELEASE OF AORTA

DISTAL TO DUCTUS

Figure 75. An oximeter earpiece recorded rapid changes in arterial saturation as the ear supplied by a branch of the carotid artery. With a baseline of about 84 percent, occlusion of the aorta below the ductus-aorta junction and consequent elevation of pressure in the arch and pulmonary artery, saturation in the arch increased. Therefore, (a) higher pressure increased pulmonary flow through high resistance vessels and oxygenation improved and (b) there was no increase in retrograde venous blood into the arch.

Arterial oxygen saturation may be misleading and nearly normal. Simultaneous right brachial and femoral artery samples are diagnostic, but difficult to obtain except with indwelling needles. This technique is not satisfactory for bedside study in the younger crying child.

In the presence of pink fingers and cyanosis of the toes it is tempting to believe bone marrow hyperplasia should occur in the areas supplied by blood with less oxygen saturation and lowered PO_2. However, studies by Stohlman, Rath and Rose (23) and Schmid and Gilbertson (24) indicate bone marrow of the sternum and ilium showed the same marked degree of normoblastic hyperplasia. A hormonal factor, such as erythropoitein must be considered.

Prognosis of Increasing Pulmonary Hypertension

While the categories of (a) blueness since birth and (b) disappearance of a ductus murmur are difficult to document in relation to the pulmonary hypertension and the ductus arteriosus, there is rather profuse documentation of the onset of cyanosis. This literature is replete with case reports of persistent shortness of breath and beginning cyanosis. Even hemoptysis has occurred as early as six years. A more common age for onset of cyanosis, by history at least, is ten to twenty-five years. The patent ductus pulmonary hypertension, reversal of flow and cyanosis with increasing dyspnea may last for many years. Heath and Whitaker (25) refer to a married woman fifty-eight years old who had chronic disease and polycythemia to the point of 25.0 gms of hemoglobin. Ordinarily, however, there will be desperate difficulties in the twenty to forty year age.

There is an intermediate position between the extremes of (a) hypertensive since birth and (b) acquired hypertension in relation to the patent ductus arteriosus. This group has progression of hypertension and reversal of flow, and cyanosis occurs later.

Controversy persists in relation to the possibility that a large flow typical ductus initiates vascular changes sufficient to produce hypertension to a point where it will perpetuate and augment itself. There is evidence that maximum distension of pulmonary arteries during systole evoke afferent impulses beat by beat, with reactive constriction. The mechanism may be reflex mediated through the nervous system (26).

ALTITUDE. There is increasing evidence that incidence may vary with geographic location in relation to altitude. Dexter (27) suggested this possibility in 1952. Penazola et al. (28) gave more

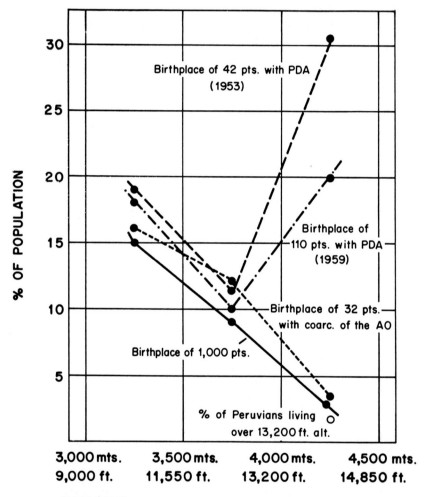

Figure 76. The incidence of coarctation of the aorta does not seem to be affected by altitude. This is of interest in relation to the ductus-coarctation problem. From Alzamora-Castro, V. and Battilana, G., Abugattas, R. and Sialer, S. *Am J Cardiol,* 5:761, 1960.

substance to this possibility when they reviewed the pulmonary circulation at high altitudes and noted an increasing incidence of patency of the ductus with altitude, and suggested incidence at high altitudes was 0.72 percent. Others had noted this increased incidence. Alzamora-Castro et al. (29) observed a higher incidence of patent ductus arteriosus in patients from high altitudes. While the population decreased with altitude the incidence of patency increased (Fig. 76).

A study of patency related to cardiac consultation at the Cardiology Institute in Mexico City (30), altitude 7,347 feet above sea level, reported an incidence of 3.69 percent in 568 referrals zero to four years of age with a decreasing incidence up to fifty years.

This 3.69 percent of the zero to four year group cannot be contrasted exactly with the incidence seen in infants with heart disease in the first year of life. But the data suggests considerable mortality in the first few years, probably in the first eighteen months, since formidable and lethal heart failure associated with an isolated patent ductus is uncommon in the older child.

There are important implications to reports of an increased incidence at high altitude. There are well established physiological consequences to breathing diminished oxygen, since all investigators have observed ductus contraction with breathing air of increased oxygen and relaxation with 15 or 10 percent oxygen. With hypoxic breathing pulmonary arteriolar contraction occurs, resistance to blood flow increases and pulmonary artery pressure rises (31).

The inference would then be that (a) while the ductus lacks or partially lacks the oxygen stimulation for functional closure, (b) some degree of pulmonary hypertension also ensues. It is implied that either diminution of functional closure or pulmonary hypertension, or both act to influence and retard anatomical closure produced by intimal and subintimal proliferation of tissue. The development of *intimal mounds* associated with the mechanism of structural closure, starts before birth (32) and therefore lowered PO_2 (a) either effects the fetal ductus to inhibit this growth or (b) proliferation is strongly depressed after birth.

No information is available concerning patency in animals

living at high altitudes, as sheep, llamas and in mammals other than man. It seems reasonable to expect this.

The opinion that pulmonary hypertension associated with a patent ductus is persistent since birth and analogous to primary pulmonary hypertension can be substantiated in some instances by patients who are reported to be *blue since birth*. Although blueness since birth is difficult to evaluate, there are, as noted, fourteen cases in the literature where this statement would seem to apply.

Likewise there are a few reported cases where acquisition of severe hypertension has occurred as indicated by the disappearance

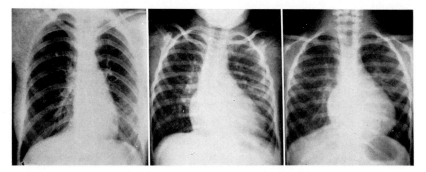

Figure 77. Three cases of patent ductus arteriosus with pulmonary artery pressure at systemic level. In case 1 there was reversal of flow. The enlarged left atrium from a previous left to right shunt is seen in case 3. The pulmonary segment is not prominent in these instances of the hypertensive ductus.

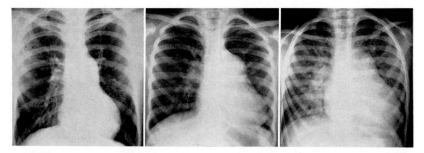

Figure 78. The contrast in silhouette in three instances of VSD with pulmonary hypertension and reversal of flow in case 1 and 2 is striking. At this time it was thought that when the systolic ejection thrust was below the pulmonary artery the vessel dilated much more than when this flow occurred at the pulmonary artery bifurcation. Further study of this concept did not substantiate it.

of a continuous murmur. While these extremes are not numerous, they do exist, and the *disappearance of a continuous murmur* group indicates augmentation of hypertension. There are at least eight cases in this group.

In view of the paucity of reports of either category, the great majority of patients with patent ductus arteriosus appear in an intermediate position, either with normal or only slightly elevated pressure or with slowly increasing vascular changes which are not sufficiently severe to either (a) reverse flow through the ductus or

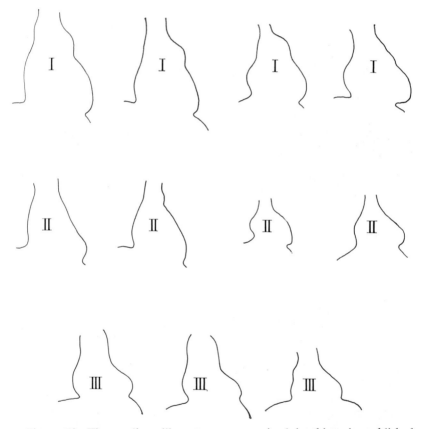

Figure 79. The cardiac silhouette was examined in thirty-six published reports of patent ductus arteriosus and pulmonary hypertension. Type I and II, marked or moderate enlargement of the pulmonary artery on the A-P view predominated. Type III with no real distension and even a concavity in the region of the pulmonary artery was seen rarely in the cases reviewed.

(b) cause disappearance of a continuous murmur without showing cyanosis.

However, Landtman and Hjelt (33) believe most of all cases of patent ductus arteriosus show hypertrophy of the media of the pulmonary vessels and thickening of the intima and adventitia. No significant changes have been found in capillaries (34).

CARDIAC SILHOUETTE IN HYPERTENSION. Sometimes the cardiac silhouette does not show a distended pulmonary artery in the presence of pulmonary hypertension of systemic level. Figure 77 illustrates this. All patients had an isolated large patent ductus, all had systemic pressures and all are dead. It was thought at this time that when the early shunt and pressure thrust came from

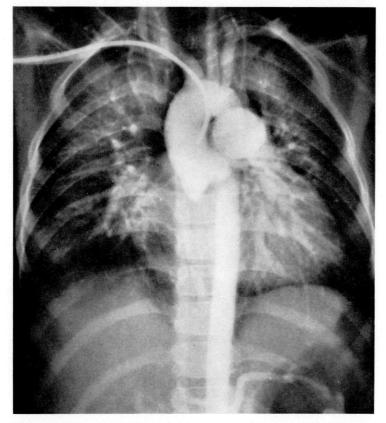

Figure 80. Even when the pulmonary artery is not striking in the x-ray, opacification shows the gross enlargement.

below, as in the Eisenmenger complex with ventricular septal defect, the pulmonary artery was more distended and prominent as in Figure 78. However, this may not be so. The cardiac silhouette was examined in thirty-nine published reports of the hypertensive ductus (35) and these silhouettes can be noted (Fig. 79). Moderate to marked prominence of the pulmonary artery was the predominant silhouette. The absence of this x-ray feature does not preclude this diagnosis. Even when the pulmonary artery is not too evident, opacification shows gross enlargement (Fig. 80).

Probably of more importance radiologically, if it were possible, would be microangiograms of the pulmonary vasculature to show multiple areas of narrowing and occlusion as in Figure 71.

In the presence of systemic hypertension evidence of increased pulmonary flow at a time recent enough to demonstrate persistent left atrial enlargement by x-ray as in Figure 81 or electrocardiogram encourages thoracotomy and trial occlusion of the ductus.

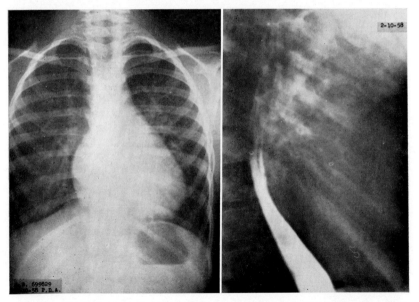

Figure 81. L.B., age six years. Patent ductus arteriosus with pulmonary hypertension and identical pressures on catheter pullout from left carotid-aorta-ductus-pulmonary artery. Peripheral pulmonary vascularity reduced. However, the left atrium is seen well on the A-P view and by esophogram. Trial closure was followed by complete closure with a good result.

212 *The Ductus Arteriosus*

REFERENCES

1. Brenner, O.: Pathology of the vessels of the pulmonary circulation. *Arch Intern Med, 56*:211, 1935.
2. Heath, D. and Edwards, J.E.: The pathology of hypertensive pulmonary vascular disease. *Circulation, XVIII:*533, 1958.
3. Brewer, D.B.: Fibrous occlusion and anastomosis of the pulmonary vessels in a case of pulmonary hypertension associated with patent ductus arteriosus. *J Pathol Bacteriol, 70:*249, 1955.
4. Short, D.S.: The arterial bed of the lung in pulmonary hypertension. *Lancet, 2:*12, 1957.
5. Prec, K.J., Cassels, D.E.: Oximeter studies in newborn infants during crying. *Pediatrics, 9:*756, 1952.
6. Harris, P.: Patent ductus with pulmonary hypertension. *Br Heart J, 17:*85, 1955.
7. Rosenthal, R.: Diastolic murmurs in patent ductus arteriosus with flow reverse. *Arch Intern Med, 114:*760, 1964.
8. Johnson, R.E., Wermer, P., Kuschner, M. and Cournand, A.: Intermittent reversal of flow in a case of patent ductus arteriosus; a physiologic study with autopsy findings. *Circulation, 1:*1293, 1950.
9. Hultgren, H., Selzer, A., Purdy, A., Holman, E. and Gerbode, F.: The syndrome of patent ductus arteriosus with pulmonary hypertension. *Circulation, 8:*15, 1953.
10. Rodbard, S.: Study of hydraulics is simulated patent ductus arteriosus. *Circ Res, 3:*613, 1955.
11. Morris, J.A., Bekey, G.A., Assoli, N.S., and Beck, R.: Dynamics of blood flow in the ductus arteriosus. *Am J Physiol, 208:*471, 1965.
12. Anderson, R.C., Adams, P.J. and Varco, R.: Patent ductus with reversal of flow—clinical study of 10 patients. *Pediatrics, 18:*410, 1956.
13. Anderson, I.M. and Coles, H.M.T.: Patent ductus with pulmonary hypertension. *Thorax, 10:*338, 1955.
14. Anabtawi, I.N., Ellison, R.G. and Ellison, L.T.: Natural history of pulmonary hypertension in surgically treated patent ductus arteriosus. Suppl to *Circulation, XXXI* and *XXXII,* April, 1965.
15. Ellis, F.H., Jr., Kirklin, J.W., Callahan, J.A. and Wood, E.H.J.: Patent ductus arteriosus with pulmonary hypertension: an analysis of cases treated surgically *J Thorc Surg, 31:*268, 1956.
16. Burchell, H.B., Swan, H.J.C. and Wood, E.H.: Demonstration of differential effects on pulmonary and systemic arterial pressure by variation in oxygen content of inspired air in patients with patent ductus arteriosus and pulmonary hypertension. *Circulation, VIII:*681, 1953.
17. Moulder, P.V., Harrison, R.W., Cassels, D.E., Long, E.T., Covell, J.W., Rams, J.J. and Daicoff, G.R.: Therapeutic enigma of unilateral pulmonary artery coarctation in pulmonary hypertension. *Ann Surg, 162:*702, 1965.

18. Hatt, P., Raniller, C. and Grosgogeat, 4.: Les ultrastructures pulmonaires et le regime de la petite circulation, II. Au cours des cardio-
pathies congenitales comportant une augmentation du debit sanguin
intrapulmonaire. *Path et Biol, 7*:715, 1959.

19. Esterly, J.A., Glagov, S. and Ferguson, D.J.: Morphogenesis of the intimal hyperplasia of small arteries in experimental pulmonary hypertension: an ultrastructural study of the role of smooth muscle cells.
Am J Pathol, 52:325, 1968.

20. Ehara, H.: Pre and post operative assessment of cardiopulmonary function in patent ductus arteriosus. *J Jap Assn Thorc, Surg, 14*:38, 1966.

21. Spencer, H.: Primary pulmonary hypertension and related vascular
changes in the lung. *J Pathol Bacteriol, LXII*:75, 1950.

22. Shepard, J.T., Weidman, W.H., Burke, E.C. and Wood, E.H.: Hemodynamics in patent ductus arteriosus without a murmur. *Circulation, XI*:404, 1955.

23. Stohlman, F., Rath, C.E. and Rose, J.C.: Evidence for a humeral regulation of erythropoiesis. *Blood, 9*:721, 1954.

24. Schmid, R. and Gilbertson, A.S.: Fundamental observations on the
production of compensatory polycythemia in a case of patent ductus
arteriosus with reversed blood flow. *Blood 10*:247, 1955.

25. Heath, D.H. and Whitaker, W.: Hypertensive pulmonary vascular disease. *Circulation, XIV*:323, 1956.

26. Whitteridge, D.: Afferent nerve fibers from the heart and lung in the
cervical vagus. *J Physiol, 107*:496, 1948.

27. Dexter, L.: Congenital defects of the heart in high altitudes. *N Engl J
Med, 247*:851, 1952.

28. Penazola, D., Arias-Stella, J., Sime, F., Recavarren, S. and Marticorena,
E.: The heart and pulmonary circulation in children at high altitudes.
Pediatrics, 34:568, 1964.

29. Alzamora-Castro, V., Battilana, G., Abugattas, R. and Sialer, S.: Patent
ductus arteriosus and high altitude. *Am J Cardiol, 5*:761, 1960.

30. Chavez, I., Espino Vela, J., Limon, R. and Dorbecker, N.: La per-
sistencia del conducto arterial. Estudio de 200 cases. *Arch Inst
Cardiol Mex, 23*;687, 1953.

31. Fishman, A.P.: Respiratory gases in the regulation of pulmonary circulation. *Physiol Rev, 41*:214, 1961.

32. Potter, Edith L.: *Pathology of the Fetus and Infant,* second ed. Chicago,
Year Bk Med, 1961.

33. Landtman, B. and Hjelt, L.: Pulmonary vascular changes in patent
ductus arteriosus. *Ann Paediatr Fenn, 3/1*:37, 1957.

34. Turunen, M. and Stjernvall, L.: Submicroscopic structure of the pulmonary capillaries in patent ductus arteriosus. *Acta Chir Scand,
117*:131, 1959.

35. Cardiac Silhouette in Patent Ductus Arteriosus with Pulmonary Hypertension.

(1) Tsugi, H., et al.: Surgical treatment of high pressure patent ductus arteriosus. *Circulation, 27/4(II):*652, 1963.

(2) Dailey, F.H., Genovese, P.D. and Behnke, R.H.: Patent ductus arteriosus with reversal of flow in adults. *Ann Intern Med, 56:*865, 1962.

(3) Storstein, O., Humerfelt, S., Muller, O. and Rasmussen, H.: Studies in catheterization of the heart in cases of patent ductus arteriosus Botalli. *Acta Med Scand, 141:*419, 1952.

(4) Shepard, J.T., Weidman, W.H., Burke, E.C. and Wood, E.H.: Hemodynamics in patent ductus arteriosus without a murmur. *Circulation, 11:*404, 1955.

(5) Silver, A.W., Kirklin, J.W., Ellis, F.H. and Wood, E.H.: Regression of pulmonary hypertension after closure of patent ductus arteriosus. *Proc Staff Meet Mayo Clinic, 29:*293, 1954.

(6) Johnson, R.E., Werner, P., Kuschner, M. and Cournand, A.: Intermittent reversal of flow in a case of patent ductus arteriosus: A physiologic study with autopsy findings. *Circulation, 1:*1293, 1950.

(7) Douglas, J.M., Burchell, H.B., Edwards, J.E., Dry, T.J. and Parker, P.L.: Systemic right ventricle in patent ductus arteriosus. Report of a case with obstructive pulmonary vascular lesions. *Proc Staff Meet Mayo Clinic, 22:*413, 1947.

(8) Ulrich, H.L.: Report of a case of patent ductus arteriosus with some unusual features. *Acta Med Scand* (suppl), *196:*160, 1947.

(9) Dotter, C.T. and Steinberg, J.: Angiocardiography in congenital heart disease. *Am J Med, 12:*639, 1952.

(10) Gordon, A.J., Donoso, E., Kuhn, L.A., Rabitch, M.M. and Himmelstein, A.: Patent ductus arteriosus with reversal of flow. *N Engel J Med, 251:*293, 1954.

(11) Heath, D. and Whitaker, W.: Hypertensive pulmonary vascular disease. *Circulation, 14/3:*323, 1956.

(12) Gonzalez-Cerna, J.L. and Lillehei, W.C.: Patent ductus arteriosus with pulmonary hypertension simulating ventricular septal defect. *Circulation, 18:*871, 1958.

(13) Adams, P., Jr., Adams, F., Varco, R.I., Dammann, J.F., Jr. and Muller, W.: Diagnosis and treatment of patent ductus arteriosus in infancy. *Pediatrics, 12:*664, 1953.

(14) Vsoh, J.A.: Patent ductus arteriosus with pulmonary hypertension. *Br Heart, J, 15:*423, 1953.

(15) Adams, F.H., Diehl, A., Jorgens, J. and Veasy, L.G.: Right heart catheterization in patent ductus arteriosus and aortic-pulmonary septal defect. *J Pediatr, 40:*49, 1952.

(16) Dammann, J.F. and Ferenz, C.: The significance of the pulmonary vascular bed in congenital heart disease. *Am Heart J, 52:*210, 1956.

(17) Evans, W. and Short, D.S.: Pulmonary hypertension in congenital heart disease. *Br Heart J, 20/4:*529, 1958.

(18) Campbell, M.: Patent ductus arteriosus, some notes and prognosis on pulmonary hypertension. *Br Heart J, 17:*511, 1955.

(19) London, F., Stevenson, T.D., Morrow, A.G. and Haller, J.A.: Patent ductus arteriosus with reverse flow. *South Med J, 50:*160, 1957.

(20) Sandblom, P. an dEkstrom, G.: Surgical treatment of wide patent ductus arteriosus. *Acta Scand, 102:*167, 1951.

(21) Meyers, G.S., Scannel, J.G., Wyman, S.M., Dimond, E.G. and Hurst, J.W.: Atypical patent ductus arteriosus with absence of the usual aortic-pulmonary pressure gradient and of the characteristic murmur. *Am Heart J, 41:*819, 1951.

(22) Edwards, J.E. and Burchell, H.B.: Effects of pulmonary hypertension of the tracheobronchial tree. *Dis Chest, 38:*272, 1960.

(23) Emslie Smith, D., Hill, G.W. and Lowe, G.: Unilateral membranous pulmonary venous occlusion, pulmonary hypertension and and patent ductus arteriosus. *Br Heart J, 17:*79, 1955.

(24) Bothwell, T.H., Van Lingen, B., Whidborne, J., Kaye, J., McGregor, M. and Elliott, G.A.: Patent ductus arteriosus with partial reversal of the shunt. *Am Heart J, 44:*360, 1952.

(25) Winchell, P., Redington, J. and Varco, R.L.: Patent ductus arteriosus in the adult with partial reversal of flow. *Dis Chest, 34:*181, 1958.

(26) Braun, K., Milwidsky, H., Izak, G. and Schor, S.: Pulmonary hypertension in patent ductus arteriosus relieved by surgery. *Angiology, 5:*329, 1954.

(27) Ye, P.N., Lovejoy, F.W., Joos, H.A., Nye, R.E. and Beatty, D.C.: Studies of pulmonary hypertension, the syndrome of patent ductus arteriosus with marked pulmonary hypertension. *Am Heart J, 48:*544, 1954.

(28) Dammann, J.F. Berthrong, M., and Bing, R.J.: Reverse ductus: A presentation of the syndrome of patency of the ductus arteriosus with pulmonary hypertension and a shunting of blood flow from pulmonary artery to aorta. *Bull John Hopkins Hosp, 92:*128, 1953.

(29) Campbell, M. and Hudson, R.: Patent ductus arteriosus with reversal shunt due to pulmonary hypertension. *Guys Hosp Rep, 100:*26, 1951.

(30) Campbell, M. and Hudson, R.: The disappearance of the continous murmur of patent ductus arteriosus. *Guys Hosp Rep, 101:*32, 1952.

(31) Holman, E., Gerbode, F. and Purdy, A.: The patent ductus. *J Thorc Surg, 25:*111, 1963.

(32) Anderson, R.C., Adams, P., Jr. and Varco, R.L.: Patent

ductus arteriosus with reversal of flow. Clinical study of ten children. *Pediatrics, 18/3*:410, 1956.

(33) Lukas, D.S., Araujo, J. and Steinberg, I.: The syndrome of patent ductus arteriosus with reversal of flow. *Am J Med, 17*:298, 1954.

(34) Harris, P.: Patent ductus arteriosus with pulmonary hypertension. *Br Heart J, 17*:85, 1955.

(35) Reid, J.M., Stevenson, J.G., Coleman, E.N., Barclay, R.S., Welsh, T.M., Fyfe, W.M. and Inall, J.A.: Moderate to severe pulmonary hypertension accompanying patent ductus arteriosus. *Br Heart J, 26*:600, 1964.

(36) Smith, G.: Pulmonary hypertension and reversal shunt. *Br Heart J, 16*:233, 1954.

(37) Whitaker, W., Heath, D.H. and Brown, J.W.: Patent ductus arteriosus with pulmonary hypertension. *Br Heart J, 17*:121, 1955.

(38) Steinberg, I.: Roentgenography of patent ductus arteriosus. *Am J Cardiol, 13*:698, 1964.

(39) Rees, S.: The chest radiograph in pulmonary hypertension with central shunt. *Br J Radiol, 41*:172, 1958.

Fourteen

PATHOLOGY

P ATHOLOGICAL ABNORMALITIES OF THE DUCTUS ARTERIOSUS might be classified as (a) absence or duplication of the vessel, (b) abnormality of position, (c) anomaly or abnormality of the terminations of the vessel (d) of shape or volume of the vessel itself and (e) abnormalities of the vessel itself or its lumen produced by physiological or pathological modification (1). The last two of these categories are most frequently associated with pathology since the first three are related to embryological abnormalities.

In the last category, pathology is related to (a) prenatal closure, (b) thrombosis of the vessel, (c) rupture and hemorrhage of the ductus, (d) aneurysms, either of the ductus itself or of the pulmonary artery or aorta and associated with a patent ductus. (e) Dissecting aneurysms of the patent ductus may occur with or without rupture and hemorrhage. (f) Degenerative changes, including the formation of atheroma or calcification are more common above thirty years. (g) Infection is almost exclusively bacterial endarteritis. (h) Pathological changes produced by altered physiology are related to the problem of the *ductus lung,* the effects of increased flow and especially concomitant pulmonary hypertension on the pulmonary vasculature. Some aspects of this problem remain controversial.

Pathology produced by altered physiology must be considered also in relation to the heart itself. These changes are a reflection of hemodynamics altered by patency, and are related to chamber dilatation of hypertrophy.

Thrombosis has at times been considered as a probable mechanism of closure of the ductus arteriosus, but further observation has indicated this is not the usual method of closure. However, many instances of thrombosis of the ductus have been reported, and there are occasional reports in current literature.

The early reports were concerned chiefly with thombosis in the newborn period or in early infancy when bacteriological studies were not yet available. Infection seems probable in most of the cases reported from information presented by clinical protocol or by autopsy.

Virchow (2) said the ductus begins to obliterate by muscular contraction of its walls, and as the blood flow becomes slow and stagnant a thrombus forms if the lumen does not obliterate completely. Incomplete obliteration aids formation of a thrombus at the aortic end, which may continue into the aorta, and in ductus aneurysms blood may enter from the aorta, stagnate and form a thrombus. Rauchfuss (3) a few years later published several case histories of thrombosis of the ductus. He attributed thrombosis to a primary infection of the blood before involution of fetal passages. The patients were infants under the age of one month, and most of them had frank sepsis with peripheral embolization. Many such cases were reported by different authors, the reports gradually diminishing in numbers as newborn sepsis became less frequent. In addition to the reports of infection and thrombosis in infancy, there were a number of caes in which thrombosis appeared where infection did not seem to play a role (4). Sometimes the thrombus would be small and partially occluding the lumen of what otherwise would have been a patent ductus. Such thrombi are quite adherent to the wall of the ductus, and either the infected or noninfected thrombus can protrude into the lumen of the pulmonary artery or aorta. While there was associated congenital heart disease, thrombosis of the ductus has been reported which extended into the aorta, left common carotid and peripherally through the left subclavian artery (5).

Although thrombosis occurs in a ductus otherwise normal in size, the most frequent occurrence is in the ductus which has an aneurysm or an aneurysmal dilation. Westhoff (6) classified these into three kinds. (a) The spherical or spindle-shaped aneurysm, (b) the funnel-like aneurysm, although this is regarded by some as a traction aneurysm of the aorta with dilatation caused mainly by aortic tissue, and (c) the evenly dilated ductus. The latter two may or may not have a thrombus present, but the spherical dilatation which usually occurs in the middle portion of the vessel, although occasionally toward one end and then most commonly the pulmonary end, almost always contains a thrombus. This occurrence is not so rare, as indicated by the study of Jager and Wollenman (7). In this study of closure of the ductus they also found several instances of organized or unorganized thrombus in the lumen of the ductus. Thrombus formation may in many instances be a normal occurrence, presumably occurring when blood flow is small or stagnant. That unusual amounts of some substance in the vessel wall, like thromboplastin, might be present is speculative.

While the occurrence of a small or even occluding thrombus in the funnel or cylindrically dilated ductus may not be of special significance, the occurrence of the spherical dilatation in the center of the ductus, which may be relatively large, is of some interest. In these aneurysms the ostia to the pulmonary artery or to the aorta may be small or the aneurysm with its thrombus may be completely impermeable at one or both ends (8,9,10,11,12). It seems likely that the normal histological process toward closure occurred at the extremities and this process was delayed toward the center of the vessel or prevented by the presence of a large thrombus, which is usually but not always present in this type of aneurysm.

The possible mechanisms of production would seem to be (a) a large duct to begin with, which normally during functional life contained much blood, with occlusion of the ends trapping sufficient blood to form a clot, or (b) occlusion at the pulmonary end, with aortic pressure applied to thinner than normal walls bulging them with blood under stasis, followed by partial closure of the aortic end. Whatever its origin, this combination of aneurysm and thrombosis in the newborn or early infancy is the most frequent occurrence of either thrombosis or aneurysm. Gerard (1) believed these swellings and clots later resorbed and the ductus became a normal ligament. Certainly the incidence in infancy is much greater than in older ages, and since there is no reason for them to cause death unless infected, most of them must indeed disappear.

Aneurysmal dilatation of the ductus may be associated with infection in the wall, an arteritis which may be termed *ductitis*.

Infected ductus with arteritis and destruction of the wall was described by Hamilton and Abbott (13) and Schlaepfer (14), and endarteritis occurs in all instances of bacterial infection. Some of the aneurysms with rupture can properly be called mycotic aneurysms on the basis of the infection present. Periarteritis nodosa in the ductus area with aneurysmal dilatation and thrombosis has been reported (15).

Aneurysms of the ductus are not confined to infancy, and may occur in the older child or adult. In the case of Hoffman (16):

> a 42 year old female, it was believed related to syphillis and there was a syphlitic meso-aortitis. The aneurysmally dilated ductus was filled with thrombi which projected into the pulmonary artery. The aortic media in the region of the aneurysm was destroyed and replaced by connective tissue, the elastic fibers were missing and the intima was partly sclerotic.

Mackler and Graham (17) have reviewed the problem of the ductus aneurysm in relation to surgery since, if large, they form rounded shadows and can be confused with mediastinal tumors. The distinguishing feature is that tumors of the upper mediastinum usually lie in the posterior portion and are neurogenic in origin, while an aneurysm of the ductus is more anterior. Ductus aneurysms were reported by Graham (18), Holman and Gerbode (19) and others.

Because of the position of the recurrent laryngeal nerve under the ductus at its insertion in the aorta, aneurysmal dilatation in this area may exert pressure on the nerve, pressing it between the dilated duct and the aorta and producing left vocal paralysis (20,21) although this did not occur in the cases reported by Graham (18). Schroetter (22) described such an instance where the large patent ductus had compressed the left recurrent laryngeal so that it had become discolored and atrophied for a length of 10 mm. When clinical signs of patency are present and there is hoarseness which laryngoscopy indicates is due to left vocal cord paralysis the ductus may be of unusual size or aneurysmal near it aortic junction.

In addition to dilatation of the ductus, other pathology can occur in its walls. Esser (23) reported two instances of rupture of the ductus in the newborn and Busse (24) reported instances of hemorrhage in the wall of the ductus which did not communicate with its lumen, and suggested these may be related to rupture. Such hemorrhage may be considerable. Mycotic aneurysm was noted twice by Blumer and McAlenney (25) in twenty-eight autopsied cases of the patent ductus and has been described by others (26,27).

Roeder (28) wrote about rupture of the ductus arteriosus in 1900, and there are other case reports (29,23). The problem of rupture was reviewed by Molz (30) and except for infection, appears to be in relation to hematoma in the ductus wall in the newborn or early infancy.

In addition to aneurysms of the ductus itself, these may be found in either of the great vessels in association with a patent ductus arteriosus. Aneurysms of the aorta at the insertion of the ductus are reported less frequently than are those of the pulmonary artery. Foulis (31) described a twenty-two year old female with an aneurysm of the aorta on the posterior wall exactly opposite the ductus orifice. This was one inch by one-half inch, and was partly filled and the walls hardened. There was concomitant vegetations on the valves, and material extended from an aneurysmal sac on the left lateral wall into and occluding the pulmonary ductus opening. Reid (32) reported a patient sixty years old in whom the ascending portion of the aorta was somewhat dilated and had yellowish spots on its inner surface. But the aorta became dilated three times its normal size just beyond the origin of the left subclavian artery, the diameter becoming normal at the diaphragm. From the upper and right side of the dilated portion of the descending arch an aneurysmal pouch more than one inch long projected to the right and inserted into the left branch of the pulmonary artery one quarter of an inch beyond the bifurcation. This pouch could contain "the point of the thumb, from the aortic side, while the opening into the pulmonary artery was the size of the carotid artery." The inner surface of the pulmonary artery had several yellow spots near the opening into it and others were present a little above the pulmonary valves. The communication was exactly at the site of the ductus arteriosus.

There are other similar cases. Altschule (33) also reported aneurysmal dilation of the aorta at the point of origin of the ductus with the pulmonary ostium of the ductus closed. Hutchinson (34) in 1922 reported an aneurysm of the ductus with the pulmonary end closed, which ruptured into the lung. The case of Hebb (35) also appears to represent a blind aneurysm, which was filled with brown fibrinous clot, and lay against the left bronchus and pulmonary artery. The main pulmonary artery was aneurysmal, the size of a *turkey's egg,* and remarkably atheromatous so that the right pulmonary artery was partially occluded and the left branch completely occluded. The thickening was due to a concentric fibrosis of its walls and this obliterated the lumen.

In 1954 Birrell (36) noted the closure of the pulmonary end of the ductus and an aneurysm of the ductus 2.0 by 11.5 by 1.5 cm filled with thrombus. In a nine week old infant a ductus aneurysm was thrombosed, but much fibrous tissue was present. He speculated that such aneurysms may be quite common but are not seen in older children or adults since they fibrose and regress like a normal ductus.

This tendency for the pulmonary end of the ductus to close and to be related to many of the ductal aneurysms was illustrated by Kneidel (37) in a postmortem angiogram of an aneurysm of the ductus.

An instance of a true aneurysm of the aorta in this region showed a large aneurysm of the arch of the aorta from which the ductus arose and opened into the pulmonary artery in the usual way.

Closure of the pulmonary end of the ductus only is not too uncommon, for Jager and Wollenman (7) found this in two instances in seventy-one cases in their study of the closure of the ductus. These were the cylindrical type ductus and not associated with an aneurysm.

While aneurysms of the aorta other than in the region of the ductus may be dismissed as coincident rather than related to the ductus, closely related dilatation must have some significance. The more marked funnel-shaped ductus is considered by some to be more in the nature of traction diverticula of the aorta rather than true aneurysms of the aorta related to patency of the ductus are few. The final criteria must be the histological study of the aortic-ductus junction.

In contrast to the limited number of aneurysms of the aorta related to a patent ductus, the literature regarding the association of the patent ductus and disease of the pulmonary artery is greater. This possibly reflects the relative frequency of a predominant pulmonary artery to aorta flow or aorta to pulmonary flow.

The pathology of the pulmonary artery in association with patency of the ductus arteriosus may be divided into five general categories: (a) aneurysm of the artery, more or less restricted to the area of insertion of the ductus or sometimes more peripheral and unilateral or bilateral, or generalized diffuse dilation of the pulmonary artery and its branches; (b) atheromatous formation with or without aneurysm formation, rather restricted; (c) a patch of intima thickened by fibrous, collagenous and elastic tissue opposite an orifice of the ductus and related to ejection trauma, a jet lesion; (d) atheromatous formation near the orifice of the ductus or with increasing age and larger ducts and associated flows and pressure more diffusely scattered in the pulmonary vascular system and its branches; and (e) diffuse arterial or arteriolar changes peripherally, either associated with atheromatous formation of the larger vessels or with minimum large vessel pathology. Since these changes are associated with augmented blood flow and usually hypertension, they are associated with abnormal hemodynamics and are more important physiologically than the isolated or multiple atheromatous placques in the larger pulmonary vessels. It seems likely that the two pathological changes have a similar etiology and hence are usually associated with each other, although the older literature contains only reports of gross dilatation and atheroma in the larger pulmonary arteries without study of the more peripheral arterial and arteriolar vessels.

A distinction should probably be made between the more or less primary dilatations of the pulmonary artery, even coincident with a small patent duct, and aneurysmal dilation probably related etiologically with patency of a larger ductus.

Aneurysmal dilatation of the pulmonary artery may occur as a primary malformation in the absence of a patent ductus. It has been suggested that this occurs as a result of imperfect division of the truncus aortis communis, more of this forming the pulmonary artery than usual. This *idopathic dilatation*, however, is usually associated either with increased pulmonary flow due to an associated lesion or to pulmonary hypertension. This diagnosis is difficult to accept on the basis of physiological or angiocardiographic examination only, and in the absence of surgical exploration or autopsy. Since the condition may occur as an isolated anatomic or anatomic hemodynamic syndrome, it is difficult to determine under what circumstances the association with a patent ductus is responsible for the formation of (a) aneurysmal dilatation of the pulmonary artery and (b) commonly associated pulmonary hypertension.

It seems certain that when these are associated with a cardiac lesion, the concurrent large flow plays some role in their formation. But when the same and apparently identical anatomical lesion has no such pulmonary artery pathology, there are probably unrecognized factors involved. For instance a dilated and atheromatous pulmonary artery has been reported in association with an atrial septal defect (38). It is believed this is the result of the greatly increased pulmonary artery blood flow which can occur with this defect, but such changes do not always occur, even with the same size lesion. And the pulmonary artery may be dilated and atheromatous even if the pulmonary flow is not augmented by an intracardiac defect in the presence of hypertension.

Consequently, while caution must be exercised in the interpretation of pulmonary artery pathology in association with patency of the ductus arteriosus, there are many case reports and reviews of the literature indicating this association. The relation of aneurysms to the patent ductus was reviewed by D' Aunoy and Von Haan (39). They noted in young persons aneurysms are much more frequent in the pulmonary artery than in the aorta. In 1934 they collected eighty-seven cases and found that in these a patent ductus was associated in twenty instances and in five of these there was bacterial infection and in another luetic infection. Costa (40) found congenital defects present in 46.5 percent of instances of pulmonary artery aneurysm and in 20 percent there was a patent ductus arteriosus. In 1950 Lindert and Correll (41) tabulated thirty reported cases of pulmonary aneurysm associated with patent ductus arteriosus. These included a case they reported in a sixty-seven year old female. One third of the patients had bacterial endodarteritis. Aneurysms may be coincident with arachnodactyty (42).

The site of aneurysms of the pulmonary artery is usually the main pulmonary trunk, but they may be more peripheral. If rupture occurs in the pulmonary trunk, hemorrhage into the pericardium is likely (43, 44). Rupture into the left pleural cavity has occurred. Rarely rupture may be into a bronchus (45). The aneurysm is usually single, although multiple dilatations may occur, especially in the presence of bacterial endarteritis and embolization. The size varies from a *nut* to an *orange*. Because of its thin wall dissection in the substance of the wall is not likely, and rupture occurs. The aneurysmal sac is frequently filled with a laminated clot. The aneurysm with rupture described by Moench (46) was especially large, over three inches in diameter.

An aneurysm of the ductus can occur postoperatively, as reported by Kerwin and Jaffe (26) and Das and Chesterman (47). This followed occlusion of a ductus by tape at each end. A dissecting aneurysm occurred which infiltrated the lung.

While fusiform dilatation of the pulmonary artery is not uncommon, atheroma formation in the absence of underlying disease is rare. Atheromatous placques may occur at the site of the jet lesion near the insertion of the ductus into the pulmonary artery. In older patients these may be numerous and occur along the artery and branches, especially when pulmonary hypertension is present.

Degenerative changes take place in the walls of the vessel and at the site of its insertions. In addition to the normal degenerative process related to transformation of a vessel with a lumen into a solid ligament, these changes may be accelerated or abnormal and pathological. Calcium may be deposited in the ductus or ligament (48). These are more abnormal in the aorta or pulmonary artery, and occur at or near the site of junction of the ductus with these vessels. This occurs more frequently at the aortic end and sclerotic placques appear in the aortic wall, often opposite the ductus opening, and are assumed by Holman (49) to represent the point of impact of the ductus flow when it is reversed and flows from pulmonary artery to aorta. He collected a series of cases which showed this jet effect, and argued that in these cases the flow was in this abnormal direction. Others have reported these lesions.

The large number of cases which Holman collected suggests that either continuous or intermittent flow into the aorta occurs more frequently than usually supposed. These placques are found more frequently in older patients. Weiss (50) reported a hollow depression at the point of attachment of the ductus and aorta in a thirty-three year old female and at this point there was a large calcified placque with small nodular projections. Murray (51) in 1888 has noted calcification of the wall at the aortic end of a patent and infected ductus in a thirty-six year old.

Since calcified placques in the aorta occur with increasing age, calcification in the aorta near areas of turbulence are perhaps to be expected. It is difficult to determine at about what age x-ray or pathological reports of such calcification should be considered abnormal. Calcification in the aorta identifiable by x-ray begins at about fifty years. For instance, Brady and Randell (52) noted calcification at each ostia, but also calcereous deposits scattered throughout the aorta, and in the patient of White (53) who was in her sixty-sixth year there was marked sclerosis and calcification at the aortic opening of the ductus, but also generalized in the aorta.

The pressure differential between ductus flow into the pulmonary artery is greater than this differential into the aorta, and the impact of a jet stream on the wall of the pulmonary artery is greater. This lesion would be expected with greater frequency, in view of the predominant direction of flow and the relatively greater force of the flow into the low pressure pulmonary artery blood stream.

While calcification of the ductus or of placques near the origin of insertion of the ductus occurs more frequently in older patients, it has been reported in infants (54) and sometimes a tendency to accelerated calcification is seen in infants. If the calcification is sufficiently large it can be seen by x-ray, and calcification in this area is an important point in diagnosis in doubtful situations.

While there has been histological study of the insertion of the ductus or ligament into the aorta this insertion into the pulmonary artery has received little attention. Samek (55) studied the insertion into the aorta in fifty bovines. While this review does not include comparative anatomy or pathology, it is of interest that Samek found, in contrast to observations in equines, that in bovines the area of insertion of the ligament into the aorta is depressed for a considerable distance around the point of insertion, which may project slightly into the lumen of the aorta above the floor of the depression. Frequently the area of insertion of the ligament showed a variation in color between the intima at this point and the intima further away. The intima may be milky white, hard and compact, and at the point of insertion hard and shiny. Histologically these areas contained osseous tissue in various stages of formation, sometimes containing bone marrow and nucleated red cells. Samek found eivdence of calcification regardless of the age of the animals, and suggested that calcification was physiological, associated with metaplasia of connective tissue at the point of traction by the ductus or ligamentum arteriosum.

If the tendency to calcification in the area of termination of the ductus in the aorta is normal, then calcification should not be considered pathological but a variation of the normal. However, for practical purposes x-ray identification of calcification in this region is unusual, and until the more or less constancy of this finding is demonstrated in the human, it must be considered pathological and abnormal. Figure 82 shows calcification in a patent ductus in a postmortem specimen, female age thirty-two years.

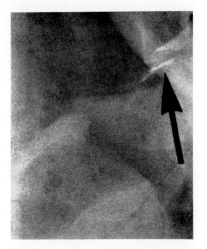

Figure 82. Postmortem specimen. Calcification of the ductus in a female, age thirty-two years, who died of the malformation.

INFECTION

While thrombosis, aneurysm and rupture of the ductus arteriosus occur, they represent unusual types of pathology. The major portion of cardiovascular pathology subsequent to a patent ductus is related to (a) infection and (b) heart disease or lung disease secondary to increased blood flow and impaired function as a result of the side effects of the extracardiac arteriovenous fistula, the patent ductus arteriosus.

The threat of incidence of infection in a patent ductus arteriosus cannot be ascertained in the antibiotic era of medicine. Treatment of all infections is rather routine therapy. Dental hygiene has improved and auxiliary care during tooth extraction with penicillin prophylaxis is now customary, since the common infecting agent in bacterial endocarditis or endarteritis is streptococcus viridans. However, the older literature gives good information regarding incidence of ductus infection.

In Abbott's (56) 1000 cases of congenital malformations of the heart nine-two had patent ductus arteriosus. The bibliography of these cases by Bauer and Astbury (57) indicate that about 30 percent died of bacterial endarteritis. The series collected by Bullock, Jones and Dolley (58) excluded patients below four years, and in the remaining group over 50 percent of the mortality was due to bacterial endarteritis. Gross (59) suggested an incidence of infection of about 25 percent.

Infections in the patent ductus may be restricted to the wall of the duct itself in its early stages, subacute bacterial endarteritis. Early implantation of infection may occur at or near the pulmonary end (60). Hamilton and Abbott (13) reviewed this aspect in 1915, finding that the wall of the pulmonary artery adjacent was involved in all eleven cases reviewed. In three cases vegetations involved the wall of the aorta opposite the ductus ostia, suggesting flow had impinged there related to reversal of flow. The infection spreads in a serpiginous way into the pulmonary artery (61) and may reach the pulmonary valves (62). By this time there has been gross systemic bacteremia and pulmonary embolization with small infarcts. Occurrence of systemic petechial phenomenon early in the disease indicates or suggests transmission of emboli through the ductus and distribution peripherally by the aorta. Petechiae confined to the lower body and extremities therefore suggests an infected ductus. Upper body petecriae also associated with infection of the ductus can be explained only by (a) the petechiae are due to local lodgement of bacteria only, as in mengococcus bacteremia for instance; (b) small emboli from pulmonary artery infection are lung passing; (c) there has been retrograde flow of ductus blood into the arch intermittently or (d) bacterial endocarditis in the mitral or aortic valve has occurred secondary to systemic bacteremia.

As with subacute bacterial endocarditis the incidence of primary ductus infection in childhood is low. In intracardiac infection the incidence under age ten years represents only 14 percent of 100 cases collected from the literature.

Since 1945 the criteria for surgical interference has broadened and includes the nonsymptomatic ductus. Allowing the transition period of 1945 to 1950 for prophylactic and surgical regimes to become crystallized, series reported since 1950 are numerically inadequate for comparison of incidence. The eradication of bacterial endarteritis depends upon surgical closure of all isolated patent ductus arteriosus before the age of five years, and preferrably by one to two years. Since age plays such an important role in the incidence of bacterial infections of the cardiovascular system, figures weighted with younger age groups minimize the threat of infection superimposed upon the ductus, and statistics based mainly upon studies in adults overemphasize this complication.

There are few reports of infection occurring subsequent to operation, although Humphreys (63) recorded an instance of staphyloccmus infection in a recanalized ductus several months after surgery.

The cause of the age differential in relation to bacterial endarteritis is not clear, but there are two likely explanations: (a) the incidence of a source of infection, especially dental caries and dental infection increases with age, and (b) degenerative changes related to hemodynamic trauma increase with age and placques and changes in the intima provocative for bacterial implantation increase. Both of these aspects of pathology accelerate concurrently to encourage major infections.

Bacteriology

In a group of 100 cases collected from the literature (Table XIII), streptococcus viridans was the infecting organism in 78 percent. Other organisms may cause infection, with staphylococcus

TABLE XIII

REVIEW OF 100 INSTANCES OF DUCTUS ENDARTERITIS

Author	Age	Sex	Strep Viridans	Pneumococci	Staph Aureus	Staph Albus
Horder (1)	42	F		1		
Hamilton & Abbott (2)	19	F		1		
Schlaepfer (3)	8	F	1			
Philpott (4)	6	F	1			
Matusoff (5)	11	F	1			
Trimble & Larson (6)	15	F	1			
Blumer & McAlenney (7)	8	M	1			
(7)	16	F	1			
(7)	37	F	1			
(7)	19	M	1			
Gordon & Perla (8)	13	M	1			
Brown (9)	12	M	1			
Perry (10)	35	F	1			
Hines & Wood (11)	18	F	1			
Chester (12)	29	F	1			
Finn (13)	23	F	1			
Sinkford & Cassels (14)	10	M	1			
Graybiel, et al (15)	22	F	1			
Fleury (16)	17	—	1			
Grenet & Levent (17)	—	—	1			
Kelson & White (18)	21	M	1			
Heyman (19)	38	F	1			
Jones, et al (20)	13	F			1	
Gibb (21)	51	M				1
Dayton & Lindskog (22)	25	F	1			
Johnson, et al (23)	21	M	1			
Harrington (24)	15	F	1			
Hartwell & Tilden (25)	12	F	1			
Nixon, et al (26)	9	F	1			
Shapiro & Keys (27)	16	F	1			
Touroff (28)	29	F	1			
(28)	29	F	1			
(28)	51	F	1			
(28)	18	F	1			
(28)	29	F	1			
(28)	63	F	1			
(28)	24	F	1			
(28)	20	F	1			
(28)	9	M	1			
(28)	31	M	1			
(28)	33	M	1			
Bettman & Tannebaum (29)	18	F	1			
Harper & Robinson (30)	28	F	1			
Neuhof (31)	30	F	1			
Tubbs (32)	19	F	1			
(32)	17	F	1			
(32)	10	F	1			
(32)	29	F	1			
(32)	22	F	1			
(32)	26	M	1			

Table XIII

Author	Age	Sex	Strep Viridans	Pneumococci	Staph Aureus	Staph Albus
(32)	33	M	1			
(32)	15	F	1			
Cunningham (33)	5	F	1			
East (34)	26	F	1			
Shallard (35)	7	F		1		
Trent (36)	34	F	1			
Fleet & Powell (37)	10	F		1		
Vessel & Kross (38)	25	F	1			
Ziegler (39)	17	F				1
Gilchrist & Mercer (40)	27	F	1			
Jones (41)	16	F			1	
Rees (42)	7	F	1			
Pinniger (43)	18 days	F			1	
Gross & Longino (44)	—	—	12			
Ekstrom (45)	22	F	1			
(45)	10	F	1			
Hamburger & Stein (46)	21	M	1			
(46)	15	M	1			
Chiles, et al (47)	8	M	1			
Holman, etal (48)	11	F				1
Starer (49)	25	F	1			
Margulis (50)	29	F	1			
Bonham-Carter, et al (51)	4	F	1			
Das & Chesterman (52)	26	F			1	
Clatworthy & McDonald (53)	—	—	1			
Blumenthal, et al (54)	8	F	1			
(54)	7	F	1			
(54)	11	M	1			
(54)	12	M			1	
(54)	6	F			1	
(54)	6	F			1	
Ross, et al (55)	30	F			1	
(55)	5	F				1
(55)	23	F				1
(55)	4	F			1	
TOTAL			78	5	9	5

Table XIII
Also included is 1 instance of gonococcus infection in a 15 year old male (50), 1 instance of H. influenza infection in a 23 year old male (32) and 1 infection with a fungus, actinomyces in a 25 year old female (48).

aureus, 9 percent, pneumococcus and staphylococcus albus each 5 percent, and one instance each of gonococcus and influenza. One case of a fungus infection occurred, an aerobic gram-positive member of the actinomyces group. It is of interest that only eighteen patients were males, and in this endarteritis group the ratio of female to male was over 5 to 1 (77).

This corresponds closely to the high incidence of alpha streptococcus intracardiac infection.

While it is not customary to divide infections of the ductus into (a) subacute infection and (b) acute infection, this classification would seem applicable to bacterial endarteritis. The fulminating recent infection due to highly pathogenic or resistant organisms may be termed acute bacterial endarteritis, although the distinction is vague and arbitrary.

Infections due to higher bacterial forms or to fungi are very infrequent. This would be described as mycotic endarteritis. There are a small number of reports of such intracardiac infection.

The vegetations which form are similar to those which form on infected valves, composed chiefly of fibrin with luxuriant bacterial growth. Because of their position emboli which form are carried into the pulmonary branches and infarction occurs, either large and symptomatic or small, microscopic and asymptomatic, the equivalent of the peripheral petechiae. These occur about the same time, two to four weeks after nonspecific symptoms, fever and malaise begin. Spectacular pathology and the fulminating clinical course of rampant infection in the ductus arteriosus are rarely seen because of administration of drugs. The natural history of the clinical, bacteriological and pathological aspects of the infected ductus and ultimate complications of it is found in the preantibiotic literature. Spontaneous healing of endarteritis due to streptococcus viridans with closure of the ductus has been reported (64).

The vegetations may take any form, and may grow so abundantly that the ductus may be closed, with the disappearance of the murmur and hemodynamic abnormalities. Rarely they may protrude from the aortic orifice (65) when distal peripheral embolization may be pronounced. Gross systemic and lung infarction occurs. By this time the cardiac murmurs may be multiple and valvular infection has occurred. The heart is dilated and large, and the patient septic and very ill. Multiple abscesses in the lung may occur.

In relation to infection and thrombosis of the left pulmonary artery, and massive lung infarction and as a striking illustration of advances in surgery, the case of Cope and Ellison (66) must be cited:

A 35 year old female had fever, hemoptysis and physical signs and x-ray evidence of pathology in the left lung. A grade 1 systolic murmur only was heard at the second left interspace. One week later a characteristic continuous murmur was heard in the same area. Clinical deterioation continued, and on surgical exploration there was (1) massive infarction of the left lung, (2) thrombosis of the left pulmonary artery which was enlarged, firm and nonpulsatile, and during pneumonectomy was seen filled with a thrombus, portions of which were removed and (3) a large ductus with severe periductal inflammation.

It seems likely, as the authors point out, that vegetations occluded the ductus and prevented the typical murmur. With severe embolization the ductus cleared sufficiently to allow blood flow and production of the ductus murmur.

The origin of the rather prompt cardiac dilatation which occurs with infection of a patent ductus is not clear. A heart which has been relatively normal in size or has shown only slight or moderate enlargement in the presence of a small or average sized ductus will enlarge rapidly and signs of heart failure will appear. Presumably, this is not caused by fever and accelerated rate only, and either a toxic myocarditis or coronary embolization should be present. In the untreated cases reported in the older literature, death appears to have occurred as a combination of overwhelming sepsis and cardiac decompensation.

Touroff (67) and others (25, 68, 69, 70) demonstrated many of the facets of the relation of infection to the patent ductus. Colony counts were done on pulmonary artery and systemic artery blood cultures before and after closure of the infected ductus. With closure the pulmonary artery and peripheral blood became bacteria free or the count was markedly reduced and the infection readily controlled. In other observation (71, 72, 73) surgical closure of the ductus alone, without medication, was sufficient to cure subacute bacterial endarteritis. It must be assumed that infection was limited to the ductus and there were no valvular or pulmonary artery vegetations.

There is no easy explanation for the association of the open ductus and infection within it. The effect of closure upon the infection emphasized the strong affinity of this open vessel for localization of bacterial infection. Various speculations have been presented. (a) The oxygen rich arterial blood flowing through the ductus encourages bacterial growth, after initial lodgement on plicated walls. It has been suggested that bacterial endocarditis is less frequent in the presence of cyanosis, and more highly aerobic conditions encourage bacterial growth.

(b) Excessive and augmented blood flow contributes to bacterial lodgement and growth. For instance, if in the usual or average patent ductus the ductus flow is 30 to 40 percent of the aortic flow, the total flow or the bacteria passing through the vessel susceptible to infection is greater than in any area except lungs, left atrium and ventricle, the valves in the left heart and the ascending aorta. There is the possibility of recirculation of bacteria through the ductus when the flow from the aorta is large and the chance of lodgement is enhanced to this degree. There has not been so far any study of recirculation of the blood sample or foreign material repeatedly through the ductus, since blood tagged in any way is quickly contaminated by mixture with venous blood in the pulmonary artery.

Persistent pulmonary embolization during antibiotic therapy does not necessarily mean the antibacterial treatment is ineffective since sterile emboli and infarcts may recur before organization of vegetations occurs. While this event is of concern, embolic phenomena gradually subside if the clinical course is otherwise good and the blood sterile.

Miscellaneous Pathology

Pathology related to anatomical position resulting from unusual patterns of embryology are classified as problems in anatomy. These include the ductus contribution to the vascular ring, the ductus in abnormal aortic arches, the ductus as a segment of the peripheral pulmonary artery when the proximal part is absent, and the subclavian artery as a direct continuation of the ductus.

It is conceivable that the ductus could be involved in noninfectious arteritis or in leukemic or tumor infiltrates. The status of a patent ductus in collagen disease states is not known.

Jacobi and Rascoff (74) described a two week old infant with stenosis of the esophagus with a septum 0.3 cm thick between the segments. There was an aberrant patent ductus passing over the site of the esophageal anomaly. It passed behind the distal end of the esophagus, across the fibrous cord of the esophagus and in front of the right bronchus. It is implied that the esophageal anom-

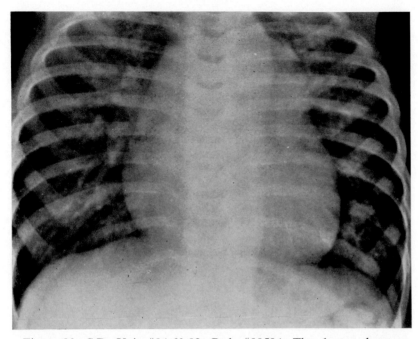

Figure 83. C.D. Unit #84-63-82, Path #88594. The ductus shows an intact internal elastic membrane which is rather thick. The media presents a layering architecture but examined more closely it shows considerable disruption of tissue and cellular elements. The elastic tissue stain shows a poor lamellar architecture with a mixture of smooth muscle, elastic tissue and collagen. The collagen is greatly decreased and the elastic fibers are somewhat disrupted. Smooth muscle does not make continuous layers but is interdigitated with the elastic tissue. The adventitia is made up of collagen and small vessels with some elastic tissue within it. Verhoef-van Giesen elastic tissue stain reveals a line of cleavage extending along the inner media just beneath the internal elastic membrane. This line of cleavage is surrounded on each side by dense elastin fibers and on H & E section a ground substance is within the line of cleavage.

aly was related to the external pressure of the aberrant ductus.

Lobar emphysema has been reported associated with a patent ductus by Leape, Ching and Holder (75). This developed while under observation and apparently was due to obstruction of a lobar bronchus by a dilated right pulmonary artery. Lobar emphysema has been reported previously in isolated patent ductus arteriosus, and dilatation of pulmonary arteries seems to be one mechanism.

An instance of patent ductus arteriosus was seen in a twenty month old girl who had all of the features of Marfan's disease.

Surgical closure of the ductus with a biopsy was accomplished without any vascular complications. Figure 83 shows the grossly dilated aorta and pulmonary artery, and the histology is described. Presumably the line of cleavage described is related to the underlying vascular disease.

There may be other pathology related to hemodynamics. For instance Wells (76) showed the opening of the ductus into the pulmonary artery with a mound of intimal disease surrounding it. He described this as protrusion of the intima of the pulmonary artery.

REFERENCES

1. Gerard, G.: An anatomical study of the arterial canal. *J anatomie Physiologie, 36*:1, 1900.
2. Virchow, Rudolf: Gesammelte abhand and lungenzur wissenschaftlichen medizin meidinger. Frankfort alm, from chapter IV, Thrombose und embolie (Gefaessentzuendung and septische infection). Die thrombosen der Neugeborenen, p. 591 (Thrombosis in the newborn), 1856.
3. Rauchfuss, C.: Ueber thrombose des ductus arteriosus Botalli. *Arch J Pathol Anat etc Berl, XVIII*:376, 1859.
4. Jager, B.V.: Noninfections thrombosis of patent ductus arteriosus; report of a case. *Am Heart J, 20*:236, 1940.
5. Wolf, I.J. and Levinsohn, S.A.: Arterial occlusion in the left upper extremity of a mongoloid idiot with congenital heart disease (Tetralogy of Fallot). *Am Heart J, 18*:241, 1939.
6. Westhoff, Franz: Dissertation Gottingen (Hofer). Ueber das sogenznnte aneurysma des ductus arteriosus Botalli, 1873.
7. Jager, B.V. and Wollenman, J., Jr.: Anatomic study of closure of the ductus arteriosus. *Am J Pathol, XVIII*:595, 1942.
8. Renault, J.: Deux cas de aneurysome du canal arteriel. *Bull Soc Anat Par, X/V*:238, 1870.
9. Voss, M.: *Ein Aneurysma des Ductus Arteriosus Botalli.* Diss Kiel p. 18, 1900.
10. Schattmann, P.: *Ueber Aneurysmenbildung am Ductus Arteriosus Botalli.* Diss, p. 40, Bresl, 1919.
11. Parise, M.: Dilatation fusiform—aneurisme du canal arteriel. *Bull Soc Anat, 12*:95, 1837-38.
12. Dry, D.M.: Congenital aneurysmal dilatation of ductus Botalli. *Proc Pathol Soc Phil, 37*:49, (1916) 1917.
13. Hamilton, W.F., and Abbott, M.E.: Patent ductus arteriosus with acute pulmonary endarteritis. *Trans Assoc Am Physicians, 29*:294, 1914.
14. Schlaepfer, C.: Chronic and acute arteritis of the pulmonary artery and of the patent ductus arteriosus. *Arch, Intern Med, 37*:473, 1926.

15. Lyon, R.A. and Kaplan, S.: Patent ductus arteriosus in infancy. *Pediatrics, 13*:357, 1954.
16. Hoffman, B.: *Ueber Einen Todesfall and Herzdekompensation Mit Aneurysma des Ductus Botalli.* Diss Berlin, p. 20, 1934.
17. Mackler, S. and Graham, E.A.: Aneurysm of the ductus Botalli as a surgical problem. *J Thorc Surg 12*:719, 1943.
18. Graham, E.: Aneurysm of the ductus arteriosus with the consideration of its importance to the thoracic surgeon. *Arch Surg, 41*:324, 1940.
19. Holman, E., Gerbode, F.P.: The patent ductus. *J Thorc Surg, 25*:111, 1953.
20. Guggenheim, H.: Aneurysma des ductus arteriosus mit rupture. *Frank z Pathol, 40*:436, 1930.
21. Berger, M., Ferguson, C., Hendry, J.: Paralysis of the left diaphragm, left vocal cord, and aneurysm of the ductus arteriosus in a 7 week old infant. *J Pediatr, 56*:800, 1960.
22. v. Schroetter, H.: Ueber eine selbene sursache einseitrgerrecurrens laehmung zuglech ein beitragzur symptomatologie und diagnose des offenen ductus Botalli. (unilateral paralysis of recurrens in patent ductus Botalli) *H. Zietsch Klin Med, 43*:160, 1901.
23. Esser, J.: Die ruptur des ductus arteriosus Botalli. *Arch Kinderheilkd, 33*:398, 1902.
24. Busse: Zur normalen und pathology. Anatomic des ductus Botalli. *Korbl Schweiz Aexzte, 48*:457, 1918.
25. Blumer, G., McAlenney, P.: The relationship of patent ductus arteriosis to infectious endocarditis in the duct itself, the pulmonary artery, the aorta and the heart valves. *Yale J Biol Med,3*:483, 1931.
26. Kerwin, A.J. and Jaffe, F.A.: Post operative aneurysm of the ductus arteriosus with fatal rupture of a mycotic aneurysm of a branch of the putmonary artery. *Am J Cardiol, 111*:397, 1959.
27. Scheef, S.: Rupture of mycotic aneurysm of Botallos duct and roentgen demonstration of enlarged duct in infant. *Arch Klind, 117*:234, 1939.
28. Roeder, H.: Die ruptur des ductus arteriosus Botalli. *Arch Kind, 30*: 157, 1900.
29. Fritz, E.: Ruptur des ductus arteriosus Botalli. *Dent Zschr Gerichtl Med, 21*:365, 1933.
30. Molz, G.: Ruptur der ductus Botalli bei einorer neugeborenen. *Z Allg Pott, 102*:566, 1961.
31. Foulis, J.: On a case of patent ductus arteriosus with aneurysm of the pulmonary artery. *Edinb Med J, XXX*:17, 2 pl, 1884-85.
32. Reid, John: Four cases of aneurism of the arch of the aorta, and a case of diaphragmatic hernia. *Edinb Med Surg J, 53*:95, 1840.
33. Altschule, M.D.: Aneurysm of arch of aorta due to persistence of portion of ductus arteriosus in adult. *Am Heart J, 14*:113, 1937.
34. Hutchinson, R.: A case of aneurysm of the ductus and atheroma of pulmonary artery. *Trans Pathol Soc Lond, XLIV*:45, 1893.

36. Birrell, J.H.W.: Three aneurysms of the ductus arteriosus in the newborn. *Australas Ann Med, 3*:37, 1954.
37. Kneidel, J.H.: A case of aneurysm of the ductus arteriosus with post mortem roentgenologic study after instillation of barium paste. *Am J Roent 62*:223, 1949.
38. Apert, E. and Baillet, P.C.: Association of generalized atheroma of pulmonary artery and its branches and open Bottalus duct in a 13 year old girl. *Arch Med Enf, 35*:147, 1932.
39. D'Aunoy, R. and Von Haan, E.: Aneurysm of the pulmonary artery with patent ductus arteriosus (Botallo's duct): Report of two cases and review of the literature. *J Pathol Bacteriol, 38*:39, 1934.
40. Costa, A.: Morfologia e patogenesi degli aneurismi dell arteria polmorare (Sopra in caso di voluminosi aneurismi multipli del tronco e dei grossi e medi rami, su base malformativa.) *Arch Patol Clin Med, viii*:257, 1929.
41. Lindert, M.C.F. and Correll, H.L.: Rupture of pulmonary aneurysm accompanying patent ductus arteriosus. *JAMA, 143*:888, 1950.
42. McKusick, V.: The cardiovascular aspects of Marfan's syndrome: A heritable disorder of connective tissue. *Circulation, XI*:321, 1955.
43. Durno, L. and Brown, W.L.: A case of dissecting aneurism of the pulmonary artery; patent ductus arteriosus; rupture into the pericardium. *Lancet, 1*:1693, 1908.
44. Fleming, H.A.: Aorto-pulmonary septal defect with patent ductus arteriosus and death due to rupture of dissecting aneurysm of the pulmonary artery into the pericardium. *Thorax, 11*:71, 1956.
45. Yuskis, Anton: Aneurysm of the right pulmonary artery: with rupture into bronchus and patent ductus arteriosus. *Calif West Med, 58*:272, 1943.
46. Moench, G.L.: Aneurysmal dilatation of pulmonary artery with patent ductus arteriosus—Death from rupture of aneurysm into pericardial sac. *JAMA, 83*:1672, 1924.
47. Das, J.B. and Chesterman, J.T.: Aneurysms of the patent ductus arteriosus. *Thorax, 11*:295, 1956.
48. Husebye, O.W.: Calcified ductus Botalli persistens. *Acta Radiol, 32*:173, 1949.
49. Holman, Emile and Gerbode, F.: The patent ductus arteriosus. *J Thorc Surg, 25*:111, 1953.
50. Weiss, Edward: A calcified placque of the aorta at the entrance of a patent ductus arteriosus: point in diagnosis. *Am Heart J 7*:114, 1931.
51. Murray, H.M.: Patent ductus arteriosus in a woman 36. *Trans Pathol Soc Lond, 39*:67, 1888.
52. Brady, J.G. and Randell, A.: Patent ductus arteriosus; case report of a woman 65 years 11½ months of age. *Ohio State Med J, 31*:597, 1935.

53. White, P.D.: Patent ductus arteriosus in a woman in her 66th year. *JAMA, 91*:1107, 1928.

54. Childe, A.E. and MacKenzie, E.R.: Calcification in the ductus arteriosus. *Am J Roent, 54*:370, 1945.

55. Samek, E.: Formation of bony and osseous covering in wall of bovine aorta in region of obliterated ductus Botalli. *Pathologica, 20*:294, 1928.

56. Abbott, M.E.: *Atlas of Congenital Cardiac Disease.* New York, Am Heart, 1936.

57. Bauer, D. and Astbury, E.C.: Congenital cardiac disease: Bibliography of the 1000 cases analyzed in Maude Abbott's atlas with an index. *Am Heart J, 27*:688, 1944.

58. Bullock, L.T., Jones, J.C. and Dolley, F.S.: The diagnosis and the effects of ligation of the patent ductus arteriosus: A report of 11 cases. *J Pediatr, 15*:786, 1939.

59. Gross, R.E.: The patent ductus arteriosus. Observations on diagnosis and therapy in 525 surgically treated cases. *Am J Med, 12*:478, 1952.

60. Tubbs, O.S.: The effect of ligation on infection of the patent ductus arteriosus. *Br J Surg, 32*:1, 1944.

61. Trimble, W.H. and Larsen, R.M.: A case of patent ductus arteriosus with primary bacterial pulmonary endarteritis. *Am Heart J, 6*:555, 1931.

62. Hines, D.C. and Woods, D.A.: Patent ductus arteriosus complicated by endocarditis and hemorrhagic nephritis. *Am Heart J, 10*:974, 1935.

63. Humphreys, G.H.: Ligation of the patent ductus arteriosus. *Surgery, 12*: 841, 1941.

64. Chiles, N.H., Smith, H.L., Christensen, N.A. and Geraci, J.E.: Cardiac Clinics CXLI. Spontaneous healing of subacute bacterial endarteritis with closure of patent ductus arteriosus. *Staff Meet Mayo Clinic, 28*:520, 1953.

65. Trimble, W.H. and Larsen, R.M.: A case of patent ductus arteriosus with primary bacterial endarteritis. *Am Heart J, 6*:555, 1930-31.

66. Cope, J.A. and Ellison, R.G.: Infected patent ductus arteriosus with massive lung infarction. *J Thorc Surg 34*:190, 1957.

67. Touroff, S.W.: Blood cultures from pulmonary artery and aorta in a patent ductus arteriosus. *Proc Soc Exper Biol Med, 49*:568, 1942.

68. Manges, M.: Infective pulmonary endarteritis occurring with patent ductus arteriosus; observations on pregnancy and heart disease. *NY Med J, 104*:581, 1916.

69. Flett, D.M. and Powell, W.M.: Acute bacterial endarteritis. *JAMA, 131*:397, 1946.

70. Vesell, H. and Kross, I.: Patent ductus arteriosus with subacute bacterial endarteritis. *Arch Intern Med, 77*:659, 1946.

71. Touroff, A.S.W. and Vesell, H.: Subacute streptococcus viridans endarteritis complicating patent ductus arteriosus: Recovery following surgical treatment. *JAMA, 115*:1270, 1940.
72. Touroff, A.S.W., Vesell, H. and Chasnoff, J.: Operative cure of subacute streptococcus viridans endarteritis superimposed on patent ductus arteriosus. Report of the second successful case. *JAMA, 118*:89, 1942.
73. Ziegler, R.E.: Cure of subacute bacterial endarteritis by surgical ligation in a patient with patent ductus arteriosus complicated by the presence of multiple cardiac defects. *Am Heart J, 31*:231, 1946.
74. Jacobi, M. and Rascoff, H.: Congenital esophageal stenosis associated with aberrant ductus arteriosus. *Am J Dis Child 42*:1149, 1931.
75. Leape, L.L., Ching, N. and Holder, T.M.: Lobar emphysema and patent ductus arteriosus. *Pediatrics, 46*:97, 1970.
76. Wells, H.G.: Persistent patency of the ductus arteriosus. *Am J Med Sci, 136*:381, 1908.
77. 100 Cases of Ductus Endarteritis
    (1) Horder, T.: Infective endocarditis. *Q J Med, 2*:289, 1909.
    (2) Hamilton, W.F. and Abbott, M.E.: Patent ductus arteriosus with acute infective pulmonary endarteritis. *Trans Assoc Am Physicians, 29*:294, 1914.
    (3) Schlaepfer, K.: Chronic and acute arteritis of the pulmonary and of the patent ductus arteriosus. *Arch Intern Med, 37*:473, 1926.
    (4) Philpott, N.W.: Two cases of cardiovascular anomaly. 1. Vegetative pulmonary endarteritis complicating persistent ductus. 2. Hyperplasia of the aorta. *Ann Intern Med, 2*:948, 1928-29.
    (5) Matusoff, I.: Congenital mirror image dextrocardia with situs inversus, patent ductus arteriosus and subacute bacterial inflammation. *Am J Dis Child, 39*:349, 1930.
    (6) Trimble, W.H. and Larsen, R.M.: One case of patent ductus arteriosus with primary bacterial endarteritis. *Am Heart J, 6*:555, 1930-31.
    (7) Blumer, G. and McAlenney, P.: The relationship of patent ductus arteriosus to infections processes in the duct itself, in the pulmonary artery, the aorta and the heart valves. *Yale J Biol Med, 3*:483, 1931.
    (8) Gordon, H. and Perla, D.: Subacute bacterial endarteritis of the pulmonary artery associated with patent ductus arteriosus and pulmonic stenosis. *Am J Dis Child, 41*:98, 1931.
    (9) Brown, J.: Patent ductus arteriosus with infective endocarditis. *Lancet, 1*:82, 1933.
    (10) Perry, C.B.: Patent ductus arteriosus. *Lancet, 1*:82, 1933.
    (11) Hines, D.C. and Woods, D.A.: Patent ductus arteriosus complicated by endocarditis and hemorrhagic nephritis. *Am Heart J, 10*:974, 1934-35.

(12) Chester, W.: Patent ductus Bottalli with subacute bacterial endocarditis and recovery. *Am Heart J, 13*:492, 1937.

(13) Finn, J.L.: Thrombosis of patent ductus arteriosus associated with septicemia due to streptococcus viridans. *Trans Soc Philadelphia,* March 11, 1937. *Arch Pathol, 24*:399, 1937.

(14) Sinkford, Stanley M. and Cassels, Donald E.: The treatment of bacterial endocarditis. *Pediatr Clin North Am, 11/2*:483, 1964.

(15) Braybiel, A., Strieder, J.W. and Boyer, N.H.: An attempt to obliterate the patent ductus arteriosus in a patient with subacute bacterial endarteritis. *Am Heart J, 15*:621, 1938.

(16) Fleury, J.: Malignant streptococcic endocarditis lenta grafted on permeable arterial canal after extractions of teeth; dental origin of malignant endocarditis. *Arch Mal Coeur, 32*:464, 1939.

(17) Grenet, H., Levent, R.: Endo cardite maligne developple sur une cardiopathie congenitale (persistance du canal arteril). Fr. Joly et Combes-Hamell. *Bull Mem Soc Med Hosp Par,* Mar-Dec. 1939, p. 824.

(18) Kelson, S.R. and White, P.D.: A new method of treatment of subacute bacterial endocarditis. *JAMA, 113*:1700, 1939.

(19) Heyman, J.: Subacute bacterial endocarditis successfully treated with sufanilamide. *JAMA, 114*:2373, 1940.

(20) Jones, J.C., Dolley, F.S. and Bullock, L.T.: The diagnosis and surgical therapy of patent ductus arteriosus. *J Thorc Surg, 9*:413, 1940.

(21) Gibb, W.: Acute bacterial endarteritis of a patent ductus arteriosus. *NY State J Med, 41*:1861, 1941.

(22) Dayton, A.B. and Lindskog, G.E.: Patent ductus arteriosus complicated by subacute bacterial endarteritis. *Yale J Biol Med, 15*:259, 1942.

(23) Johnson, J., Jeffers, W.A. and Margolies, A.: The technique of the liagtion of the patent ductus arteriosus. *J Thorc Surg, 11*:346, 1942.

(24) Harrington, S.: Patent ductus arteriosus with bacterial endarteritis. *Proc Staff Meet Mayo Clinic, 18*:217, 1943.

(25) Hartwell, A.S. and Tilden, I.L.: Aneurysm of the pulmonary artery. *Am Heart J, 26*:692, 1943.

(26) Nixon, J.W., Bondurant, W.W. and Roan, O.: Ligation of a patent ductus arteriosus with probable endarteritis: Apparent cure. *Ann Intern Med, 19*:1003, 1943.

(27) Shapiro, M.J. and Keys, A.: The prognosis of untreated patent ductus arteriosus and the results of surgical intervention. *Am J Med Sci, 206*:174, 1943.

(28) Touroff, A.S.: The results of surgical treatment of patency of the ductus arteriosus complicated by subacute bacterial endocarditis. *Am Heart J, 25*:187, 1943.

(29) Bettman, R.B. and Tannenbaum, W.: Ligation of patent ductus arteriosus in the presence of an apparent bacterial endocarditis. *Ann Intern Med, 21*:1035, 1944.
(30) Harper, F. and Robinson, M.E.: Occlusion of infected patent ductus arteriosus with cellophane. *Am J Surg, 64*:294, 1944.
(31) Neuhof, H.: Indications for pericardiotomy with special reference to the exposure of an infected patent ductus. *J Thorc Surg, 13*:374, 1944.
(32) Tubbs, O.S.: The effect of ligation on infection of the patent ductus arteriosus. *Br J Surg, 32*:1, 1944.
(33) Cunningham, N.C.: Patent ductus arteriosus. *Med J Aust, 2*: 158, 1945.
(34) East, T.: Ligation of the patent ductus arteriosus. *Br Heart J, 7*:95, 1945.
(35) Shallard, B.: Patent ductus arteriosus. *Med J Aust, 2*:353, 1945.
(36) Trent, J.C.: Surgical therapy of the patent ductus arteriosus. *Arch Surg, 51*:106, 1945.
(37) Fleet, D.M. and Powell, W.M.: Acute bacterial endarteritis. *JAMA, 131*:397, 1946.
(38) Vessel, H. and Kross, I.: Patent ductus arteriosus with subacute bacterial endarteritis. *Arch Intern Med, 77*:659, 1946.
(39) Ziegler, R.F.: The cure of subacute bacterial endarteritis by surgical ligation in a patient with patent ductus arteriosus complicated by the presence of multiple congenital cardiac defects. *Am Heart J, 31*:231, 1946.
(40) Gilchrist, A.R. and Mercer, W.: Infective endarteritis of the pulmonary artery. *Lancet, 2*:267, 1947.
(41) Jones, J.C.: Complications of the surgery of patent ductus arteriosus. *J Thorc Surg, 16*:305, 1947.
(42) Rees, C.E.: A cause for the restablishment of communication following ligation of patent ductus arteriosus. *Calif Med, 68*:35, 1948.
(43) Pinniger, J.L.: Aneurysm of the ductus arteriosus. *J Pathol Bacteriol, 61*:458, 1949.
(44) Gross, R. and Longino, L.: Observations from 412 surgical treated cases. *Circulation,3*:125, 1951.
(45) Ekstrom, G.: The surgical treatment of patent ductus arteriosus. *Acta Chir Scand,* (suppl. 169-172) 142, 1952.
(46) Hamburger, M., and Stein, L.: Streptococcus viridans subcute bacterial endocarditis. *JAMA, 149*:542, 1952.
(47) Chiles, N.H., Smith, H.L., Christensen, N.A. and Geraci, J.E.: Spontaneous healing of subacute bacterial endocarditis with closure of patent ductus arteriosus. *Proc Mayo Clinic, 28*:19, 1953.
(48) Holman, E., Gerbode, F. and Purdy, A.: The patent ductus.

J Thorc Surg, 25:111, 1953.
(49) Starer, F.: Analysis of 50 cases of persistent ductus arteriosus. *Br Med J, 1*:971, 1953.
(50) Margulis, A.R., Figley, M.M. and Stern, A.M.: Unusual roentgen manifestations of patent ductus arteriosus. *Radiology, 63*: 334, 1954.
(51) Bonham-Carter, R.G., Walker, C.H.M., Daley, R., Matthews, M.B. and Medd, W.E.: Patent ductus arteriosus with abnormal aortic valve. *B Heart J, 17*:255, 1955.
(52) Das, J.B., and Chesterman, J.T.: Aneurysms of the patent ductus arteriosus. *Thorax, 11*:295, 1956.
(53) Clatworthy, H.W., Jr. and McDonald, V.G., Jr.: Optimum age for closure of patent ductus ateriosus. *JAMA, 167/4*:444, 1958.
(54) Blumenthal, S., Griffith, S.P. and Morgan, B.D.: Bacterial endocarditis in children with heart disease. *Pediatrics, 26*:993, 1960.
(55) Ross, R.S., Feder, F.P., and Spencer, F.C.: Aneurysms of previously ligated patent ductus arteriosus. *Circulation, 23*:350, 1961.

Fifteen

CLINICAL ASPECTS OF EMBRYOLOGY — ATYPICAL ANATOMY

V ARIABILITY EXISTS IN THE MORE OR LESS ORDERLY TRANS-
FORMATION OF THE AORTIC ARCHES into the predominant left arch,
left ductus configuration accepted as normal or at least usual
in man.

Some possible developmental variations may be drawn schematically. In these the vessels of the arch will be shown somewhat
what perfunctorily except when an integral part of the vascular
abnormality. The basic embryology and resultant atypical anatomy
are shown for most of the possible combinations of the fourth and
sixth arches.

The ductus may be bilateral, as in the basic system of two
aortic arches, one arising from each arch and extending to each
pulmonary artery. Figure 84 is the basic system and Figure 85 is
the anatomic representation of this.

Figures 86 and 87 represent the usual left aortic arch, left ductus
in a schematic and in a more realtistic anatomical way. Figure 88
shows a right aortic arch and a right ductus.

The basic arch abnormality is seen in Figure 89 and the anatomical situation in Figures 90 and 91. This abnormality was shown
by Quain (1) and has been redrawn in Figure 92. The view is
somewhat posterior and the pulmonary artery and ductus have been
displaced to show the anatomy. Turner (2) reported this in 1862
with an explanation of the embryology (Fig. 93).

The situation may occur with a normal left arch, and the right

244

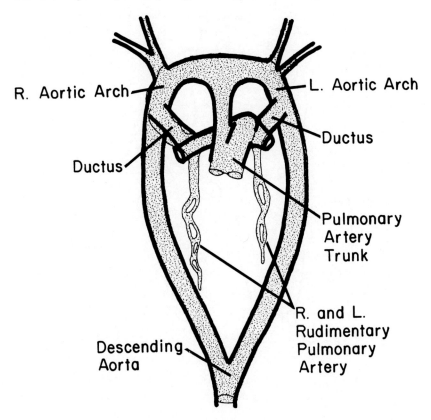

Figure 84. The basic embryology of the right and left aortic arches and the right and left 6th or pulmonary arch. The branchial phase persists, the right pulmonary arch has not separated from the right dorsal aorta.

aortic root persists. A right ductus inserts into this and the right subclavian arises from it (Fig. 94). The anatomical situation is seen in Figure 95. The distinction between a persistent aortic root, either right or left with a subclavian arising from it and a subclavian as the last branch of an aortic arch with a ductus is made with difficulty. The embryology is similar, the vessel size is different.

In Figures 96 and 97 the ductus is in a normal position on the same side as a right arch. The left subclavian as the last branch of the arch crosses midline behind the esophagus and indents it in an esophogram in a lateral view.

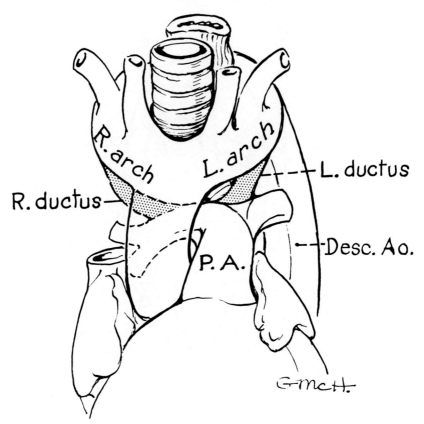

Figure 85. Anatomical representation of the double aortic arch and right and left ductus arteriosus.

The possible resorption of the proximal part of the right or left aortic arch with the ductus insertion on this side is shown chiefly for completeness (Fig. 98, Fig. 99). This could be the basis of the long ductus which is occasionally described from an arch to the opposite pulmonary artery.

The position of the ductus or ligamentum on a left aortic arch when the right subclavian arises as the last branch of the left aorta is not clear (Fig. 100, Fig. 101). Two clinical instances are shown in Figure 102 and Figure 103. In the first, a ligament inserted into an area of hypoplasia of the aorta in which there was almost complete obstruction by a narrow coarctation. There was also some severe aortic stenosis, in a nineteen year old male. The

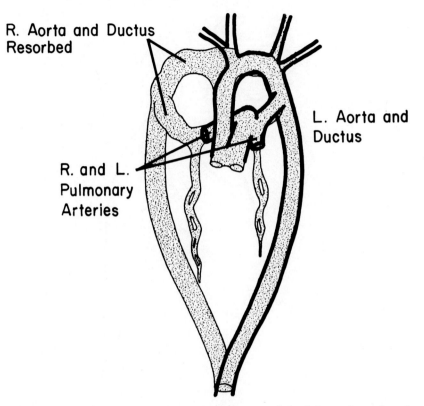

R. Aorta and Ductus Resorbed

L. Aorta and Ductus

R. and L. Pulmonary Arteries

Figure 86. The usual and normal persistance of the left aortic arch and left ductus. The right arch and ductus has disappeared, except the base of the right arch as the innominate.

anomalous right subclavian arose just above the ligament and began its course across the mediastinum to the right shoulder and arm. The left subclavian arose just above this and was large.

Figure 103 shows a rather large patent ductus with an anomalous right subclavian arising as the last branch of the arch just above the ductus. The left subclavian was the next proximal branch of the aorta, just above the anomalous right subclavian.

While perhaps this anatomy is not entirely or strictly a ductus problem, the right subclavian as the last branch of the aorta arises as a remnant of the right aortic arch when this arch absorbs high, above the rudimentary right subclavian rather than low and leaving the innominate artery pattern.

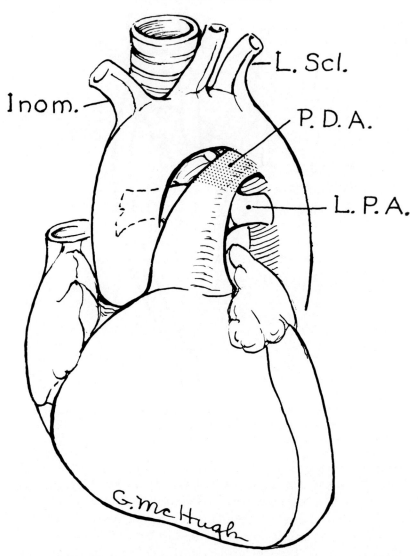

Figure 87. Anatomic representation of the normal left arch and ductus.

The question arises how does the anomalous right subclavian obtain a position above the ductus.

It would be plausible to say the changes in the arch occurred before the sixth pulmonary arch was complete, before the ductus was formed. However, the sequence of events in the aortic arch system is such that this is not correct since the resorption of the

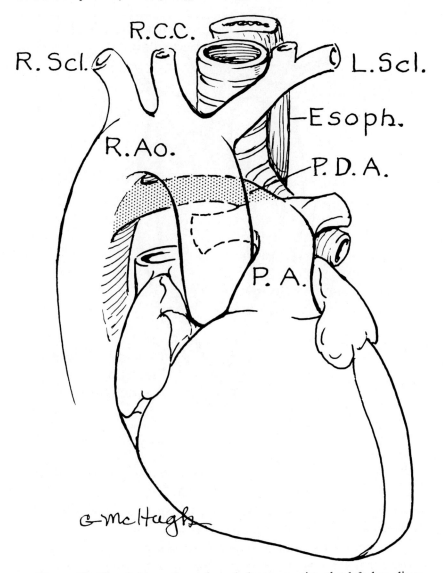

Figure 88. The right aortic arch and ductus persist, the left has disappeared.

proper segment of the right aortic occurs rather late after the pulmonary arch is formed.

A similar question occurs in visualizing the left subclavian, arising as the seventh segmental artery migrating by differential

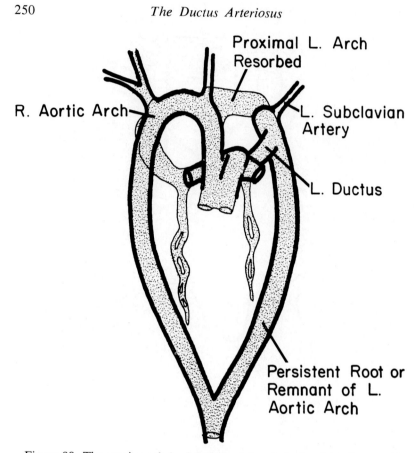

Figure 89. The aortic arch is right. The left subclavian is the last branch of the right aortic arch. A left ductus inserts into this. Since the posterior root of a left aortic arch arises in the same way the distinction between the two lies in the size of the posterior vessel.

growth past the anomalous right subclavian to lie above this vessel in its usual position on the aortic arch.

The adjustments in the position of vessels in the arch system are therefore subtle and must be related to differential growth and merging of the remnant of the right arch into the left to give the position of the anomalous right subclavian above the ductus. It may lie at or below the ductus, but this position is rare.

It is of interest that the embryology of the anomalous subclavian was proposed by Wood (3) in 1859.

It has been stated by Quain (1) that the right subclavian, as the

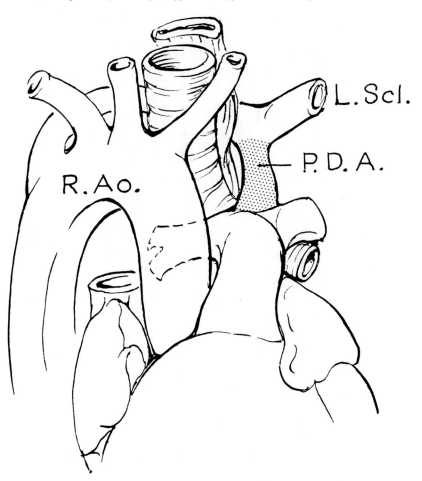

Figure 90. Anatomic representation of Figure 89. A left ductus inserts into a vessel arising as the last branch of a right aortic arch. This can be either a persistent posterior root of the left arch or a left subclavian.

last branch of the left arch, is a common anomaly and occurs in the general population once in 250.

The ductus may continue directly into the left subclavian. The proposed embryology is a persistent right aortic arch, but disappearance of the left arch except for the area of joint insertion of the ductus and the subclavian (4) as in Figure 104. This assumes the left arch disappears only after migration of the segmental artery which forms the subclavian nearly to its final position above

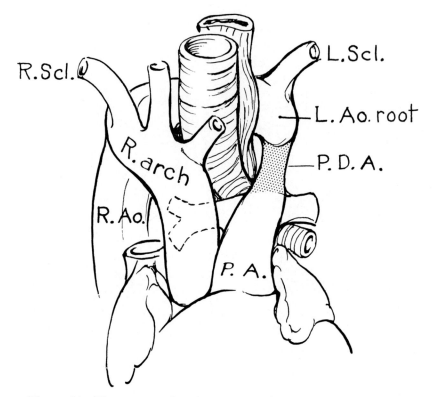

Figure 91. The same embryology occurs, but the posterior vessel is large and is the posterior root of the left aortic arch. A left ductus inserts into this. A vascular ring is formed.

the ductus. A right ductus or ligament to the right arch may or may not be present, but probably is not.

If there is no functioning ductus arteriosus in late fetal life, the fetal circulation is indeed complex.

This ductus abnormality occurs most frequently in tetralogy of Fallot with a right aortic arch. The clinical situation has been seen several times and was depicted at surgery in Figure 105 in an eight year old child.

Presumably this isolation of the subclavian from the aortic arch could also occur on the right, with a left arch present.

If the anomaly occurred on the same side as the arch, the theory of its origin would be difficult to substantiate. While not precisely the same, Potter (5) showed a newborn with a left aortic arch and

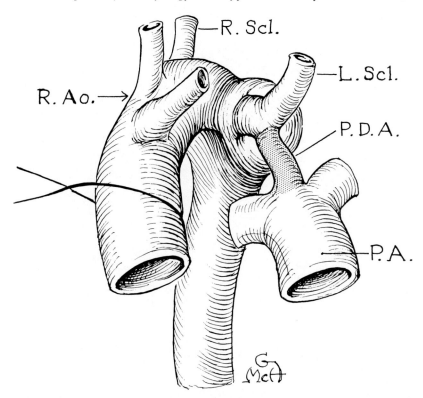

Figure 92. This anatomic situation was identified by Quain (1) The view is rather posterior and the pulmonary artery has been displaced to show the ductus and posterior root of the left aortic arch, and the left subclavian artery.

From Quain, R. London, Taylor & Walton, p. 550, 1844.

a left ductus which crossed the aorta anterior to it but did not connect with it and ended as branches to the pectineal area. The status of the left subclavian was not stated.

There are instances of atypical anatomy or position of the ductus which are not easily explained as anomalies of the aortic arch system.

There are instances of ductus origin in the aortic arch proximal to the left carotid artery. The case of Hara and Johnson (6) has been redrawn in Figure 106. Poynter (7) also lists an instance of this.

Clinically the signs are similar to those of a patent ductus, but

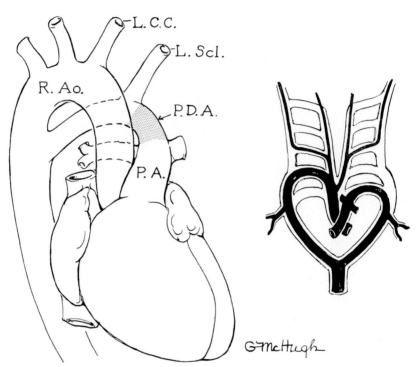

Figure 93. Turner (2) reported this in 1862 with an explanation of the embryology.

From Turner, W. *Br Foreign Med Chir Rev, 30*:173, 1862.

there is no ductus in the usual anatomical position below the left subclavian.

The position is too high on the aortic arch to be a remnant of a common trunk, an aortico-pulmonary window. But it cannot be the usual ductus since it is above the left subclavian and the left carotid.

It is suggested that a ductus could be placed on this position by a minor malformation of the aortic arch system. If the segment of the proximal aorta between the third arch, which becomes the carotid, and the fourth, which contributes to the arch of the aorta persisted and the proximal part of the third arch did not form or was resolved, the ductus lies proximal to the left carotid, as in Figure 107.

More difficult to understand is an aortic-pulmonary communi-

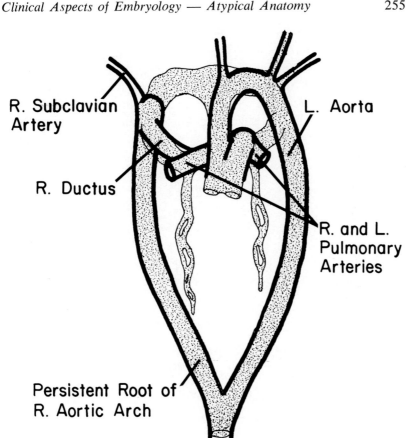

Figure 94. Insertion of a right ductus arteriosus into the persistent root of the right arch or the right subclavian as the last branch of a left aortic arch. The embryology is similar.

cation high on the ascending aorta but just proximal to the right innominate (Fig. 108). There was an associated vascular anomaly in the right lung (Fig. 109).

Since the innominate is present and in the normal embryology of the aortic arches must represent a proximal segment of the fourth right arch, the possibility this is the right aortic root associated with a short ductus is not likely.

This vessel was 2 mm in length and 4 mm in diameter and arose on the posteromedial aspect of the aorta just before the innominate.

A section was obtained during surgery. The vessel wall appears to be quite homogeneous without the usual lamellar architecture seen in large artery walls. Endothelium is generally one cell layer thick, but in one or two areas is somewhat thicker. The media is rather thick with uniform scattering of cell nuclei. Elastic tissue stain reveals a uniform green coloration throughout the entire thickness of the media indicating dense elastin deposition. Under somewhat higher power, 400 magnification, lamellar structure is apparent but with the lamella so close together that under the lower

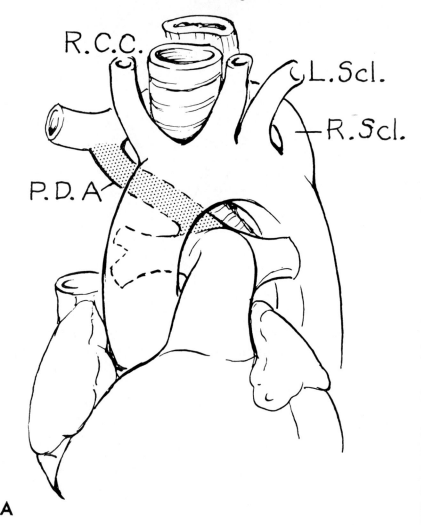

A

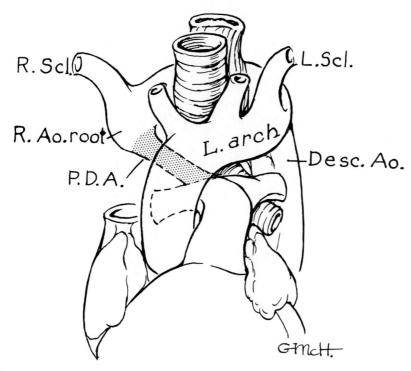

B

Figure 95. A. The right subclavian arises as the last branch of a left aortic arch. A right ductus arteriosus inserts into this. B. The posterior vessel is the right aortic root. The distinction between a persistent right aortic root and the right subclavian as the last branch of the left aortic arch.

power they fuse into a more homogeneous looking tissue. The impression was that this is not pulmonary artery, aorta and is compatible with the structure of a ductus in early life. (Courtesy of Dr. F. Straus, Department of Pathology)

This aortic-pulmonary communication was (a) abnormally placed for an aortic-pulmonary artery window, the remnant of the truncus arteriosus, and it had length (b) in the presence of a normal right inominate artery as the first branch of a left aortic arch, this should not be the root of a right aortic arch with a ductus. (c) It is abnormally placed for a right sided ductus. (d) The histology is neither aorta nor pulmonary artery.

Some clinical aspects were of interest. The patient was eight

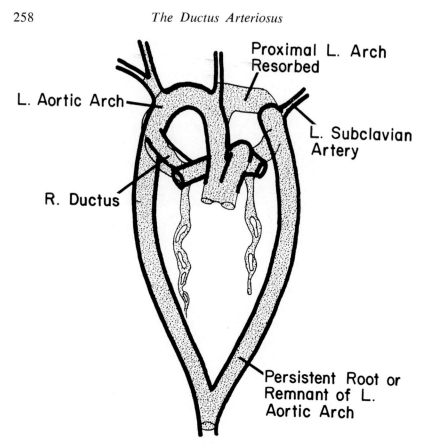

Figure 96. The left subclavian is the last branch of a right aortic arch.

months of age. (a) The murmur was a typical murmur of an aortic pulmonary artery communication, although more prominent than usual on the right. While there was some respiratory variation, it was clear that there was an auscultatory gap, a pause between the first sound and the start of the murmur, even though the A-V shunt occurred much earlier anatomically than the ductus-pulmonary artery site where the ductus murmur usually originates. (b) The hemodynamics pre and postoperative are given. It is of interest that the angiomatous appearance of the right lung did not contribute to increased pulmonary flow after repair. (c) Considering the anatomy of the venous shunting in the right lung through the diffuse A-V fistula expected cyanosis was absent and the arterial saturation 94 percent, a normal value for Van Slyke analysis.

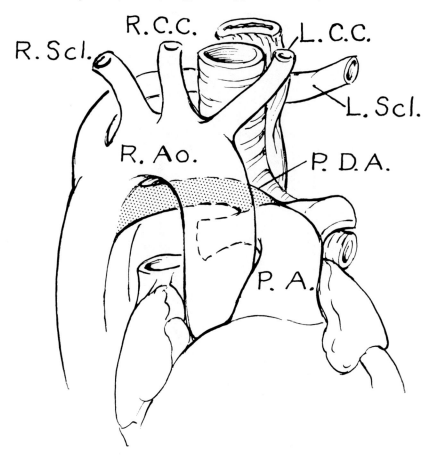

Figure 97. An anatomical representation of the left subclavian as the last branch of a right aortic arch. The ductus is on the same side as the arch.

In 1884 Combes and Christopherson (8) reported an instance of abnormality of the arch and ductus arteriosus more difficult to explain. Their drawing has been faithfully copied in Figure 110. There was an obvious right aortic arch. The pulmonary artery arose normally and divided into right and left branches, and the right pulmonary artery entered the right lung. The left had two parts, one entered the left lung, and the other joined the aorta opposite the right subclavian, although their drawing shows it somewhat lower. "Obviously, this corresponded to the ductus arteri-

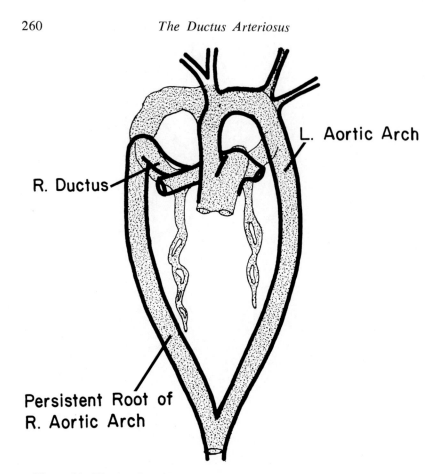

R. Ductus

L. Aortic Arch

Persistent Root of
R. Aortic Arch

Figure 98. The last branch of a normal left arch is the distal root of the right arch. Instead of continuing as the right subclavian it terminates in a right ductus or ligamentum. The left ductus is not shown, but could be present.

osus but strangely enough before it terminated in the aorta the left subclavian artery sprang from it."

The origin of these vessels have alternate explanations: (a) the base of both of these vessels is a remnant of a rudimentary left arch. This requires an explanation of the long left subclavian behind the esophagus. This vessel acts, like the left subclavian, as the last branch of a right aortic arch. It also requires an explanation of the long ductus and its peculiar course to a common insertion of the left subclavian. It is clearly not a right ductus. A root of the left arch may contribute a significant part of this vessel, the ductus re-

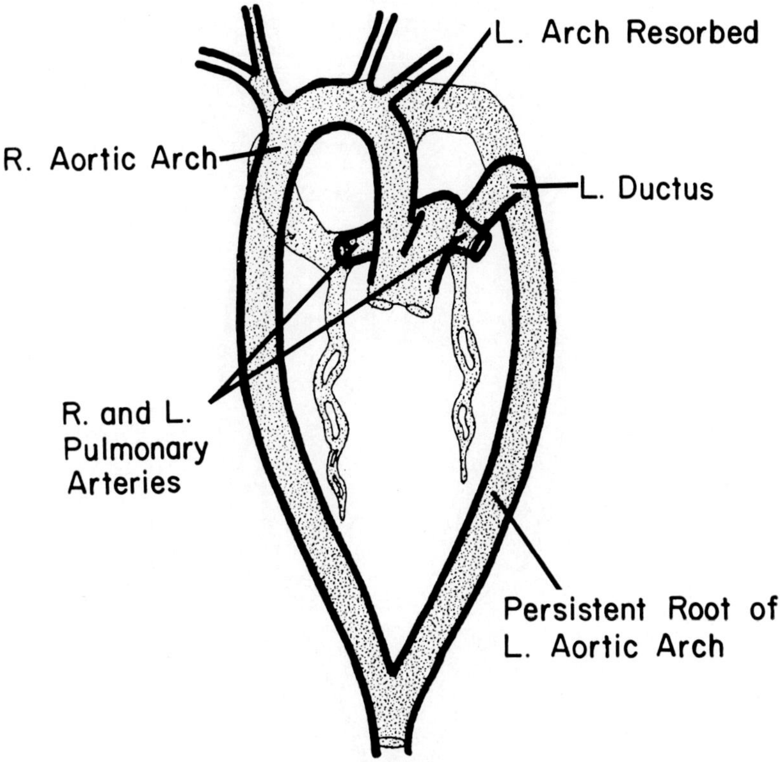

Figure 99. The right aortic arch persists. The distal portion of a left arch is present but instead of terminating as the left subclavian artery ends with confluence with a left ductus arteriosus.

maining its usual length, or a long root of the left arch persists, and at the same time the left subclavian remains as the last branch of the right arch. And lastly, (b) it is possible to invoke the possibility of a persistent base of a controversial fifth arch on the left.

The anatomical problem suggests that all ductus abnormalities are not easily compatible with the schematic diagrams of the fourth and sixth branchial arch systems.

A case cited (9) as the left subclavian artery arising from a patent ductus arteriosus would seem also to represent (a) a right aortic arch, (b) a persistent posterior root of the left arch with the left subclavian and (c) a large patent ductus arteriosus with a

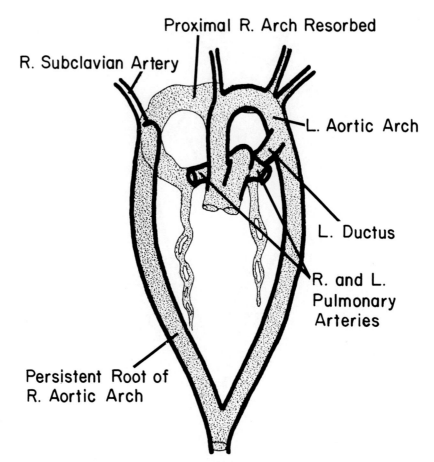

Proximal R. Arch Resorbed

R. Subclavian Artery

L. Aortic Arch

L. Ductus

R. and L. Pulmonary Arteries

Persistent Root of R. Aortic Arch

Figure 100. Schematic diagram to show origin of the right subclavian as the last branch of a normal left aortic arch.

diameter of 12 cm (7mm) "joining the descending aorta behind the esophagus on the fifth thoracic verterbra." This is assuming the entire vessel, from the origin at the bifurcation of the main pulmonary artery to the aorta, is all ductus. This vessel from the aorta through the left subclavian must be a persistent posterior left aortic root with a large but usual ductus arteriosus inserting at the area of origin of the left subclavian. Embryologically it would seem impossible for the left subclavian artery to arise from the middle of a ductus. There was a large ventricular septal defect in addition.

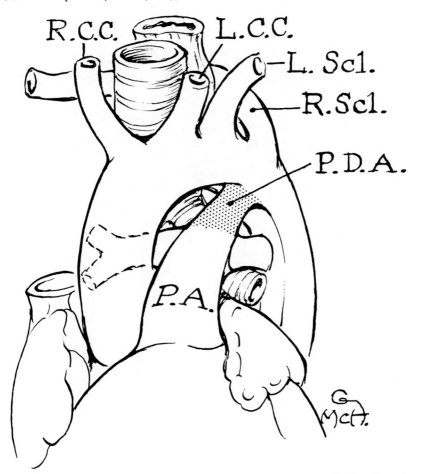

Figure 101. Anatomy of the right subclavian arising as the last branch of a normal left aortic arch.

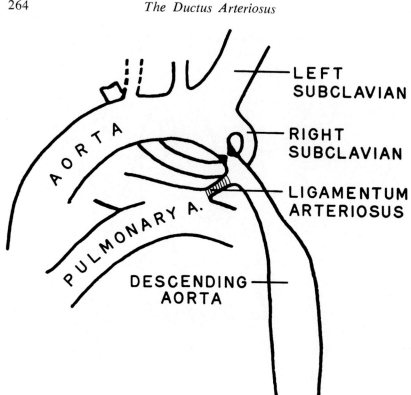

Figure 102. J.G. Unit #97-15-56, age nineteen years. The right sub-clavian arises above the ductus ligament which terminates near a narrow coarctation in a long segment of narrowing of the aorta. At surgery there was no lumen seen at the site of coarctation.

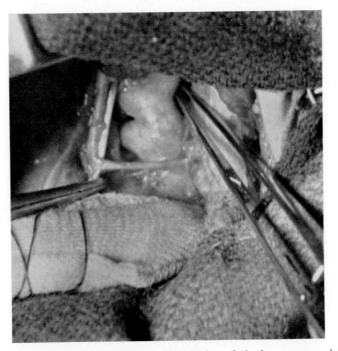

Figure 103. W.A., age six years. The right subclavian artery arising as the last branch of the aortic arch appears low on the aorta in schematic diagrams showing the embryology. However, it usually lies on the arch above the ductus and is shown under the forceps, with the ductus below in its usual position.

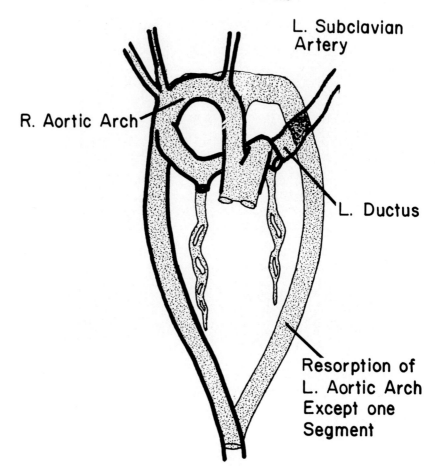

Figure 104. The left subclavian artery as a direct continuation of the ductus arteriosus. This assumes resorption of the left aortic arch except the segments involved in a common insertion of the subclavian artery and the ductus arteriosus.

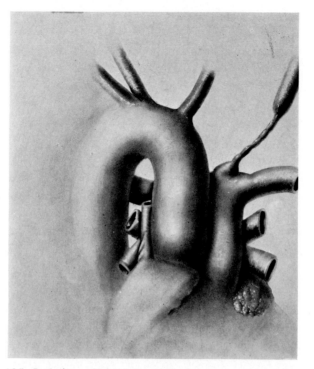

Figure 105. Isolation of the left subclavian artery from the aorta and origin from the pulmonary via a ductus arteriosus. The ductus was closed. Female, age eight years, Tetralogy of Fallot, with right aortic arch. Seen at surgical exploration.
From Replogle, R.L.: *Ann Thorc Surg, 5*:153, 1968.

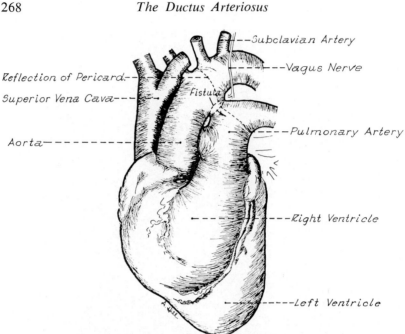

Figure 106. A window ductus occurs proximal to the left carotid artery. The embryology would appear to be persistance of the dorsal aorta segment between the 3rd and 4th arches and resorption of the proximal end of the 3rd.

Redrawn from Hara, M. and Johnson, N.: *Ann Surg, 143*:136, 1956.

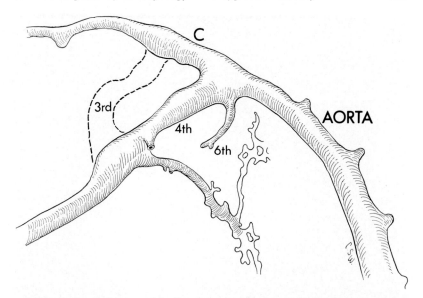

Figure 107. Scheme of possible origin of the ductus proximal to the left carotid. This involves resorption of the proximal part of the 3rd arch which is the normal left carotid and persistance of the dorsal aorta between the 3rd and 4th arches. This normally resorbs at 14 mm. The origin of the carotid moves farther along the 4th arch, the aorta. The resorbed area is labelled 3rd and the persistent area of the dorsal aorta C, indicating this has become the origin of the carotid.

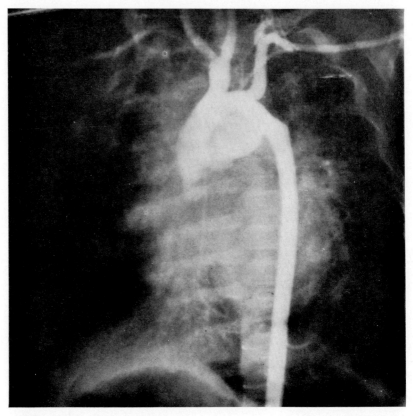

Figure 108. The aorta-pulmonary artery communication is high on the ascending aorta at the level of the innominate artery. This is distal for an aortic window. The normal innominate precludes a ductus arteriosus arising from the base of partial right aortic arch.

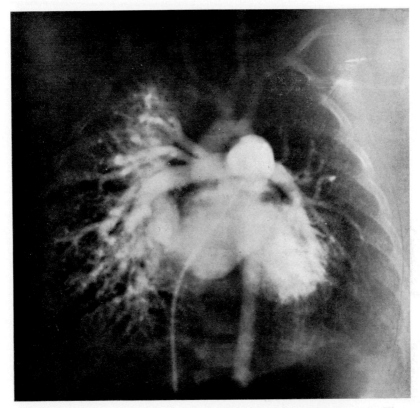

Figure 109. The vasculature of the right lung is visualized well. There
is an abnormal venous return and probably an arteriovenous anomaly.

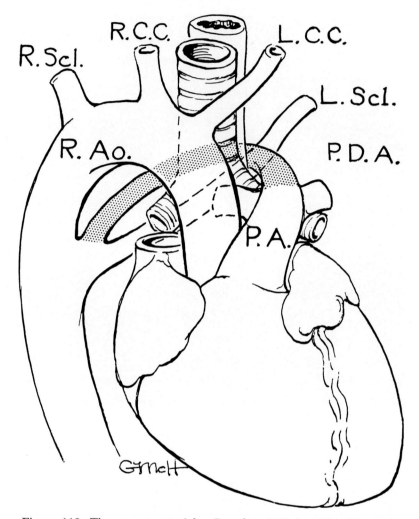

Figure 110. The case reported by Coombes (10) in 1884. The embryology is difficult. There is apparently a rudimentary root of the posterior segment of the left aortic arch and a continuation of this by the left subclavian artery. The insertion of a ductus arising in a normal position into this is not easily explained by the usual aortic arch system.

1. Quain, R.: *The Anatomy of the Arteries of the Human Body and its Application to Pathology and Operative Surgery, with a Series of Lithopraphic Drawings.* London, Taylor and Walton, 1844.

2. Turner, W.: On irregularities of the pulmonary artery, arch of the aorta, and the primary branches of the arch, with an attempt to illustrate their mode of origin by a reference to development. *Br Foreign Med Chir Rev, 30:*173, 1862.

3. Wood, J.: Two specimens of abnormal origin of the right subclavian artery. *Trans Pathol Soc Lond, 10,* 1859.

4. Stewart, J.R., Kincaid, O.W. and Edwards, J.E.: *An Atlas of Vascular Rings and Related Malformations of the Aortic Arch System.* Springfield, Thomas, 1964.

5. Potter, E.: *Pathology of the Fetus and Infant,* 2cd ed. Chicago, Year Bk Med, 1961.

6. Hara, M. and Johnson, N.: An anatomical patent ductus arteriosus. *Ann Surg, 143:*136, 1956.

7. Poynter, C.W.M.: Arterial anomalies pertaining to the aortic arches and the branches arising from them. *Univ Studies, XVI/*4:229, 1916.

8. Combes, R.H. and Christopherson, C.: Transposition of the aortic arch. *St Barth Hosp Rep Lond, 20:*273, 1884.

9. Seikert, R.G.: An anomalous human heart. *Anat Rec, 103:*761, 1949.

Sixteen

CLINICAL ASPECTS
OF ANATOMY

I T SEEMS LIKELY, IN VIEW OF THE STUDY (1) INDICATING POST-
MORTEM CONTRACTION OF THE DUCTUS, THAT RELIABLE MEASURE-
MENTS OF THE SIZE OF THE HUMAN NEWBORN DUCTUS ARE
ACQUIRED WITH DIFFICULTY. In animals, the quick freeze method
advocated by Hornblad (2) or pressure fixation as advocated by
Bakker (3) is thought to give more reliable information. This
fixation was used in the human.

The literature on the size, especially width, of the patent ductus
indicates some tendency toward increase of size with growth. The
data of Ekstrom (4) suggest that under ten years ductus width

TABLE XIV
WIDTH OF THE DUCTUS ARTERIOSUS
IN RELATION TO THE AGE OF OPERATION

Age in years Circumference in mm	a -16	b 17-25	c 26-35	d 36-45	e 46-70	Total	Percentage of Total		
Diameter in mm	- 5	6-8	9-11	12-14	15-25		a+b	c	d+e
0-1		3[a]				3	100		
2-4	8	25	15	3		50	66	28	6
5-9	11	50	26	8	1	96	64	27	9
10-14	3	22	22	12	3	62	40	36	24
15-19	1	3	13	3	3	23	17	57	26
20-29	1	5	19	11	2	38	16	50	34
30-39		2	4	4	2	12	17	33	50
40-46			1	1	1	3	0	33	67
Total	24	100	99	42	12	287[b]			

a. In a 9 month old girl the ductus circumference was 17 mm
   In a 12 month old boy and a 13 month old girl the ductus circumference was 25 mm
b. in 3 case information of the ductus width is lacking
(From Ekstrom,G.: Acta Chir Scand, supp 169, 1952.)

274

under 9 mm predominates (Table XIV). The 9 to 11 mm group
began to appear at two to four years. There was no giant ductus,
that is over 14 mm until the five to nine age group and one third of
the very large ductus appeared before fifteen years.

TABLE XV

DIAMETER OF LARGE DUCTUS ARTERIOSUS IN RELATION TO AGE

Age-Sex	Diameter of Ductus (mm)	Prior to Operation P.A. Pressure S.D. (mean)
5-F	15	90/60 (70)
6-M	16	116/59 (84)
6-F	16	86/64 (73)
7-F	16	66/34 (50)
7-F	15	74/46 (57)
8-F	16	66/38 (52)
8-F	15	77/44 (58)
8-F	15	96/65 (82)
8-F	20	—
9-F	15	—
9-F	17	61/50 (57)
11-F	16	97/61 (76)
11-F	17	107/66 (84)
11-M	16	—
12-F	23	—
12-F	15	—
14-F	20	89/46 (65)
17-M	20	87/55 (69)
19-F	15	—
21-F	15	—
22-F	25	—
23-F	15	—
24-F	16	100/49 (69)
24-F	21	65/42
26-F	15	—
29-M	25	102/56 (74)
29-M	16	80/50 (62)
30-F	15	—
31-M	24	68/39 (51)
36-M	20	—
45-M	15	115/75 (67)

Rearranged by age. (From Oldham, H.N., Jr., Collins, N.P., Pierce, G.E., Sabiston,
D.C., Jr., and Blalock, Alfred: J Thor Cardiovasc Surg, *47*:331, 1964.)

Oldham et al. (5) in a study of the large ductus 15 mm or more
in diameter showed a rather even distribution from five years with
over one-half occurring before fifteen years (Table XV). In the
younger age groups this measurement sometimes would be larger
than the aorta and could scarcely occur except on the basis of an
aneurysm. The large ductus is uniformly associated with pulmonary

hypertension, often at systemic level, and with pulmonary vascular disease. The debate whether (a) the large, high pressure aortic flow produces progressive vascular occlusion or (b) whether the vascular changes and hypertension were present since birth and merely augmented has not been settled. It seems most likely (a) and sometimes (b) occur and probably a combination of these influences are usually present.

In view of existing pulmonary hypertension, the question arises whether the ductus can be dilated by pressure. Such dilatation seems to occur in the pulmonary artery as seen both by x-ray and on dissection. Criteria for dilatation does not seem to be available either for the pulmonary artery or the ductus. The cases of Crafoord, Mannheimer and Waklund (6) did not show any pattern of increase of circumference with age as in Table XVI.

TABLE XVI

THE DIAGNOSIS AND TREATMENT OF PATENT DUCTUS ARTERIOSUS
(BOTALLO) IN CONNECTION WITH 20 OPERATED CASES

Case	Age	Width
3	2- 8/12	appr. 40
10	2- 8/12	appr. 40
12	3- 3/12	23
13	5- 7/12	21
14	5- 7/12	16
18	6- 9/12	27
8	7- 3/12	33
1	7- 7/12	43
19	8	30
17	8- 8/12	19
7	9- 1/12	appr. 10
16	9- 7/12	37
11	9-11/12	29
15	10- 2/12	24
5	11- 6/12	8
9	13- 7/12	appr. 40
2	15- 1/12	34
20	18- 2/12	51
4	18- 7/12	49
6	28-11/12	appr. 45

Rearranged according to age (From Crafoord, C., Mannheimer, E. and Waklund, Th.: Acta Chir Scand, XCI:97, 1944.)

Observations on the size of the patent ductus are of great interest in terms of theories of closure and theories of patency. The small diameter ductus which is smaller than in the newborn must have made some effort to close, but this was unsuccessful.

The very large ductus such as those over 15 mm in diameter are larger than in the newborn and consequently must have had no impetus to close and have grown in diameter.

Most ductus lie between the extremes of smaller than the newborn or over 10 to 15 mm in diameter. But the variation in size indicates closure does not follow an all or none law.

The relation of closure by physiological constriction and anatomical closure due to cellular proliferation is not known. It is often assumed that this is the normal and usual sequence. In the ductus that closes, it probably is. But this assumption does not consider (a) the prenatal histological anticipatory changes of closure

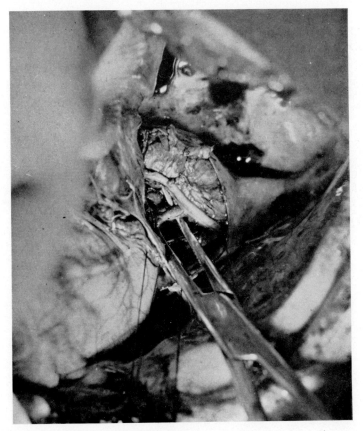

Figure 111. A small ductus 3 to 4 mm in diameter in a six year old male. There was a continuous and typical ductus murmur and surgery was undertaken without substantiating studies.

reported by some and (b) the relation of either aspect to persistent patency.

The possible combinations would seem to be:

1. Early constriction followed by anatomical closure. This is the sequence considered normal or at least usual since first stated by Gerard (7).

   a. Complete constriction with normal cellular proliferation and occlusion.

   b. Partial constriction with normal cellular proliferation and occlusion.

2. Absent or partial constriction, but normal anatomical closure regardless.

3. Early or temporary constriction but:

   a. No anatomical proliferation.

   b. Partial anatomical closure.

4. Absence of constriction with:

   a. No anatomical proliferation.

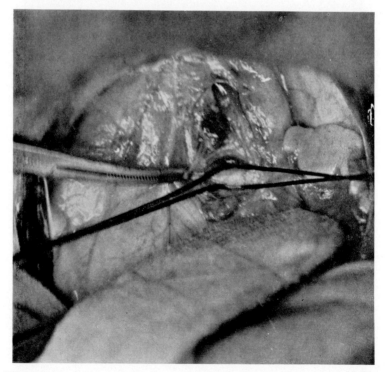

Figure 112. L.H., age eighteen months. Postrubella baby with unilateral cataract. The ductus is small 4 to 5 mm in width. The postrubella ductus is usually not especially large. The aortic angle is broad, almost 90 degrees.

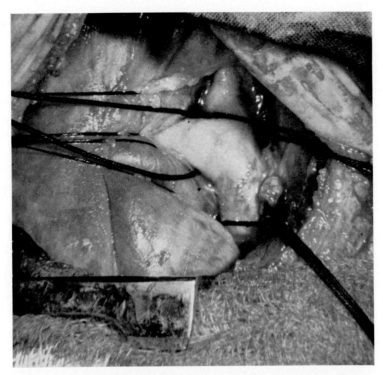

Figure 113. A large ductus in a thirteen month old mongol. The ductus bulged from the aorta almost aneurysmally. It was an isolated lesion.

    b. Slight anatomical proliferation.
    5. No functional constriction and no cellular proliferation. There has been no attempt at closure. This is the large patent ductus arteriosus.

Two smaller vessels are shown, one in a male, age six years, (Fig. 111) and the other in a female, age eighteen months (Fig. 112). Both of these had a diagnostic continuous murmur. Examinnation of the small ductus does not indicate any reason for smallness and the histology is that of the patent ductus, with no intimal mounds or evidence of partial closure.

Figure 113 is a ductus as large as the aorta and actually seemed larger, bulging aneurysmally as it entered the aorta. The patient was a mongol, age thirteen months with patent ductus as an isolated lesion.

A right aortic arch and ductus seen in a severe tetralogy of Fallot (Fig. 114), since these are rarely seen as isolated lesions.

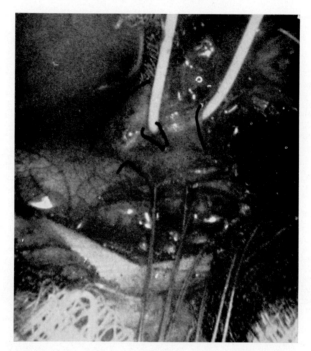

Figure 114. A right aortic arch and a right patent ductus arteriosus. Since these are rare as isolated lesions this occurred in a severe tetralogy. The ductus inserts at an angle of nearly 90 degrees. There is no discernible isthmus narrowing.

The angle of insertion is wider and there is no discernible narrowing of the isthmus.

The very large ductus whose length and width are about equal and is nearly as large as the aorta is associated with high pulmonary vascular resistance, systemic pulmonary artery pressure and in patients over three to five years of age with bidirectional flow. These patients are inoperable except in early ages and even then decisions rest upon individual circumstances. A trial closure is warranted up to five years of age if cyanosis is absent.

Figure 115 shows the large ductus in a fourteen year old female. She had dyspnea, an accentuated S_2 with no discernible split, slight cyanosis of the toes and on exercise also of the left hand. There was pulmonary hypertension at systemic level and bidirectional shunting. The pertinent questions are: (a) was the ductus larger than normal at birth, (b) did it grow in width instead of showing

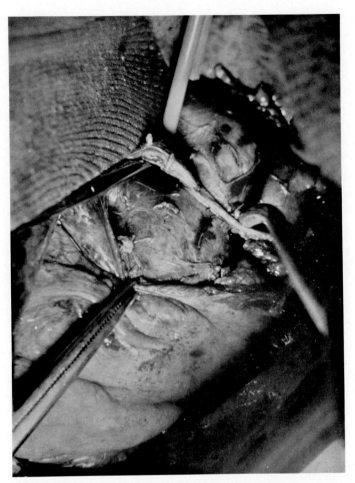

Figure 115. A ductus as large as the aorta in a girl age fourteen years. There was systemic hypertension in the pulmonary artery and reversal of flow. The toes had mild cyanosis and clubbing. The left hand became blue with exercise.

some effort at contraction or anatomical closure or (c) was it chronically distended by hypertension since birth.

In Figure 116 the ductus is very short and the superior border has no appreciable length. This could be an intermediate stage of the formation of a window ductus, the gradual approximation of the aorta and pulmonary artery.

Figure 117 is a small ductus with an aneurysmal dilatation at

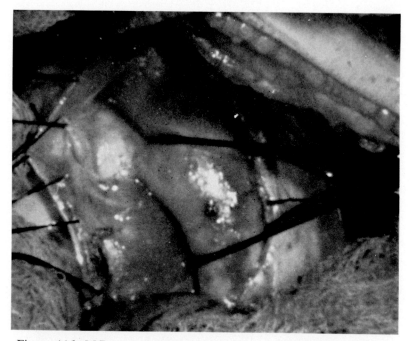

Figure 116. M.P., age thirteen months. A very short ductus arteriosus with almost no length to the superior border, but a very wide base on the aorta. This is perhaps intermediate in the formation of a window ductus— if the pulmonary artery grew and more closely approximated the aorta which also becomes larger, the ductus would have no length.

its confluence with the aorta in a six year old male. While the anatomical profile is unusual, of greater interest was a moderate degree of pulmonary hypertension, and vascular pathology as seen in a lung biospy. There was no change in pulmonary artery pressure on study six months after closure by division and suture. The possibility remains that a large ductus contributed to the pulmonary vascular pathology and this became smaller over six years.

Figure 118 is a schematic illustration of the ductus in corrected transposition. The aorta lies lateral to the pulmonary artery and arches over it.

THE WINDOW DUCTUS

There is a special anatomical category of the ductus arteriosus usually called the window ductus. This name is appropriate and

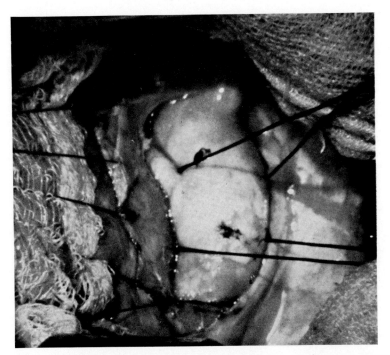

Figure 117. F.M., male, age six years. Clinically, a continuous murmur, with evidence of pulmonary hypertension and right ventricular hypertrophy in the electrocardiogram. Pulmonary artery pressure preoperatively 52/28 mm Hg with a Qp/Qs 1.7:1. Postoperatively six months, pulmonary artery pressure 44/20 mm Hg. The calculated resistance remained elevated but was reduced.

The anatomy is of great interest. (a) There is no aortic isthmus, (b) there is a suggestion of aneurysmal dilatation at the origin of the ductus, but (c) the ductus is very small in relation to the pulmonary hypertension present. A case can be made for an early large ductus with diminishing size with growth and age and a continuing effort toward anatomical closure.

descriptive since it implies a window between the aorta and pulmonary artery, an aperture without length but localized in the usual position of a patent ductus arteriosus. It is below the left subclavian and aortic isthmus. No ductus is present on the same side, the left. Although there seems to be no reason why this window could not occur on the right side when there is a right aortic arch, no instance of this could be found. However, the case reported by Garipuy (8) is suggestive since he says the communication occurred between the inferior part of the aortic arch and

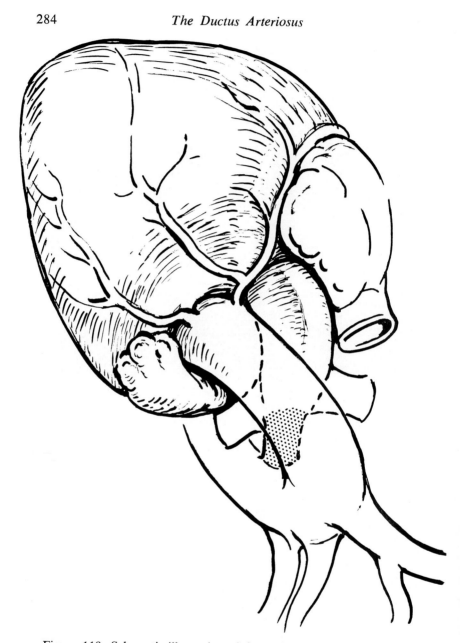

Figure 118. Schematic illustration of the position of the ductus arteriosus in corrected transposition, or ventricular inversion.

the superior part of the right branch of the pulmonary artery.
It is rather difficult to understand the embryology of this com-

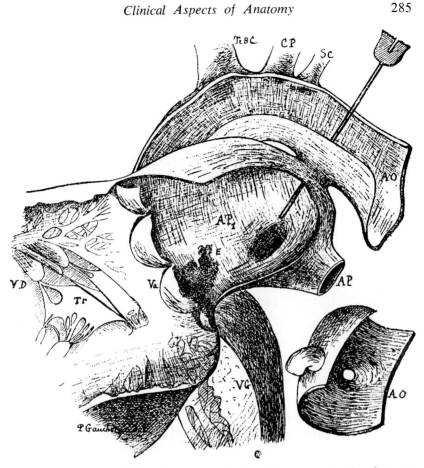

Figure 119. A window ductus—a side to side communication between the aorta and pulmonary artery at the usual site of a ductus arteriosus. There was endocarditis with vegetations on the anterior cusp of the pulmonary valve and the wall of the dilated pulmonary artery. From Gauchery, M.P.: *Bull Soc Anat Paris, 12*:252, 1898.

munication and adequate description of the histology has not been found. The possibilities seem to be: (a) the pulmonary artery lies lateral to its usual position, and the normally formed ductus merely accommodated itself to the short length required or (c) the dorsal or ventral sprout of the ductus was short or absent and the connection of the sixth arch came about by direct approximation.

The window seems to have been formed at about the usual time since, when mentioned, the recurrent laryngeal nerve lies under it as in the usual ductus.

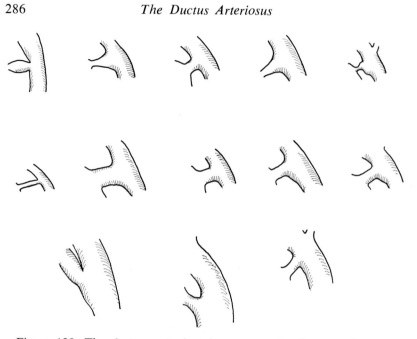

Figure 120. The ductus-aorta junction as seen in the operating room. Redrawn from sketches made at thoracotomy.

The orifice may be large, as is Garipuy, 10 mm, or may be small, 3 to 4 mm as in Olivier and Deve (9).

The window ductus is not rare. For instance these authors, in 1908, list eleven references. More recently other case reports have appeared (10).

Figure 119 shows the case reported by Gauchery (11) in 1898. She was twenty-seven years of age. A good description of the cardiac murmurs is given and it is of great interest that Potain, the great French cardiologist, made a clinical diagnosis of congenital direct aortic-pulmonary artery communication.

The opening was 6 mm. There were vegetations on the pulmonary valve and the wall of the pulmonary artery.

The variation in the ductus-aorta union is shown in Figure 120. These were redrawn from sketches made in the operating room.

1. Wilson, R.R.: Postmortem contraction of the human ductus arteriosus. *Br Med J, 1*:810, 1958.
2. Hornblad, P.Y.: Experimental studies on closure of the ductus arteriosis utilizing whole-body freezing. *Acta Paediatr Scand, suppl 190*:1, 1969.
3. Bakker, P.M.: *Morfogenese en Involutie Van de Ductus Arteriosus Bij de Mens.* (Thesis) Den Haag, Mouton & Co., 1962.
4. Ekstom, G.: The surgical treatmenrt of patent ductus arteriosus. *Acta Chir Srcand, suppl 169,* 1952.
5. Oldham, H.N., Jr., Collins, N.P., Pierce, G.E., Sabiston, D.C., Jr., and Blalock, A.: Giant patent ductus arteriosus. *J Thorc Cardiovasc Surg, 47*:331, 1964.
6. Crafoord, C., Mannheimer, E. and Waklund, T.: The diagnosis and treatment of patent ductus arteriosus (Botalli), in connection with 20 operated cases. *Acta Chir Scand, XCI*:97, 1944.
7. Gerard, G.: The theories and the facts of the obliteration of the canal arterial. *J Anat Physiol, 36*:323, 1900.
8. Garipuy, M.: Persistance du canal arteriel n' ayant entrainé aucum trouble pendant 28 ans. *Pull Mem Soc Anat Par, IX*:179, 1907.
9. Olivier, P. and Deve, F.: Communication interaortico-pulmonaire (persistance du canal arteriel) Chez une femme de 33 ans. *La Normandie Med, 23*:24, 1908.
10. Cabat. case #24222. Congenital heart disease—patent ductus arteriosus. *N Engl J Med, 218*:937, 1938.
11. Gauchery, P.: Communication congenital directe de l'aorte et de l'artere pulmonaire, an niveau du canal arteriel, avec ectasie de l'artere pulmonaire et endocardite pulmonaire. *Bull Mem Soc Anat Par, XXIII*:252, 1898.

Seventeen

THEORIES OF PATENCY

P ATENCY OR PERSISTENCE OF THE DUCTUS ARTERIOSUS might occur as the antithesis of any of the forces causing closure, chiefly medial contraction with the stimulus of oxygen and intimal and subintimal cellular proliferation. While these forces of closure are easily studied, no model exists for the study of patency. The relation of nonconstriction by oxygen and subsequent tissue proliferation is not known.

However, one study (1) suggests intimal tissue changes may take place in the absence of constriction in an environment of 10 percent oxygen. If this were true, diminished oxygenation and functional change in lumen would not assume an important role in nonclosure or patency. The major facet in persistence of the ductus would be absence of intimal or subintimal proliferation and medial involution. Delayed closure would be compatible with proliferation only.

The difference between closure and patency are seen in Figure 121 which contrasts a normal closing ductus with the nonproliferation of the intima in a section of a patent ductus.

In an anatomical classification of the patent ductus arteriosus, the facets of each category are related to tissue change and none, unless closure is expected, to constriction.

Figure 121. Photomicrograph of a closing ductus. The intimal mounds are clearly identified. The internal elastic membrane shows no evidence of infolding from vessel contraction. Right: Patent ductus arteriosus, section obtained at surgery. There is no evidence of intimal proliferation or of intimal mounds. The thin, fibrotic wall is vascularized and contain little smooth muscle and elastic tissue. (H & E, Elastin, X10).

An anatomical classification of the patent ductus arteriosus:
1. Closed within one to two months after birth (except prematures).
2. Patent but small—admits a 2 mm probe (2) or a 6 F catheter.
3. Two mm to size at birth.
4. Larger than present at birth—10 to 15 mm diameter.
5. The giant ductus—over 15 mm diameter.
6. Aneurysmal dilatation and aneurysm of the patent ductus arteriosus.

The size at birth is assumed to be the normal anatomy. A smaller ductus has made an effort to close, but closure is incomplete. A larger ductus has either grown or become dilated and aneurysmal.

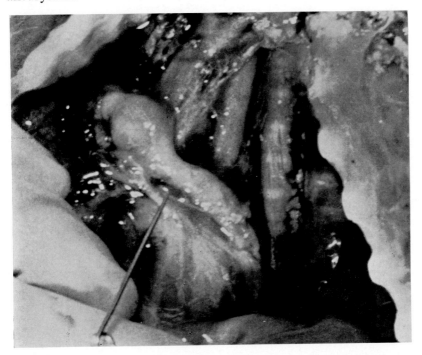

Figure 122. W.F., Unit #72-22-72, age five weeks. Full term with respiratory symptoms at three days. Radial and femoral pulses normal to palpation. Heart failure and death ensued. Pathology: right ventricle dilated and hypertrophied, pulmonary artery continued into the descending aorta. There was interruption of the aortic arch which terminated in the left subclavian. The ductus arteriosus was 8 mm long, 8 mm in circumference and was in the process of closing. The intima was wrinkled, the media thick and muscular.

But it seems clear that pressure alone will neither dilate nor prevent closure of a normal duct. This facet of the ductus problem is shown in Figure 122. This shows a closing dustus in an infant with interruption of the arch. The ductus was the only anatomical conduit for blood flow to the body below the aortic arch. Neither systemic pressure nor teleologic considerations kept the ductus patent.

Abnormalities of the ductus wall are conducive to nonclosure. This was seen especially in the absence of the media of the ductus reported by Benavides, Vela and Monroy (3). In this instance the media was absent over an area of 7 by 15 mm, and in addition there seemed to be no real media. The elastic and muscle fibers were smaller and disorganized. Rupture and hemorrhage occurred during surgery.

The next stage of wall pathology would seem to be aneurysmal dilatation or aneurysms of the ductus arteriosus.

A congenital abnormality of innervation of the patent ductus arteriosus is a feature of patency since catecholamines are consistenly absent or minimal in the media of the open ductus. While cause and effect has not been established related to administration of adrenergic blocking agents in the newborn animal, the association of absence of catecholamines and patency is, so far, a constant occurrence in nonclosure in the human.

The status of oxygen receptors in the wall is not known. But in hereditary patency in dogs diminished response to oxygen suggests an abnormality in the amount or distribution of smooth muscle and an inherited inability to constrict (10).

Maternal rubella in the first trimester of pregnancy is the one established etiologic factor in patency of the ductus. The observation of Gregg (4) in 1941 relating to congenital cataract was followed by a large literature identifying other congenital anomalies. The problem was reviewed by Lundstrom (5) who also analyzed a rubella epidemic in Sweden in 1951 and estimated a risk factor of 10 percent of the rubella syndrome in infants of mothers with the disease in the first trimester of pregnancy.

Patency of the ductus arteriosus resulting from rubella was studied by Swan (6) in 1944 in three infants ages twenty-two days, thirty-one days and twenty-eight days. Two were three weeks premature. Histological examination of the ductus, in contrast to controls of the same age, showed (a) the lumen larger and the wall thinner, (b) the internal elastic lamina was absent or poorly defined, (c) intimal proliferation was totally absent and (d) there was moderate replacement of muscle and elastic tissue by collagen.

Patency is due to abnormailty of the ductus wall.

Congenital heart disease probably occurs in about 70 percent of infants with the obvious rubella syndrome. In these, patency of the ductus arteriosus as an isolated lesion occurs in 58 percent (7).

It has been suggested (8) that the rubella ductus has an equal ratio of female to male in contrast to 3:1 in the normally occurring patent ductus. This suggests at least two factors affecting the ductus wall. An additional consideration is the recorded instances of familial occurrence.

The rubella problem has been reviewed in detail by Monif (9) in the monograph Viral Infections of the Human Fetus.

REFERENCES

1. Wilcox, B.R., Roberts, W.C. and Carney, E.K.: The effect of reduced atmospheric oxygen concentration on closure of the ductus arteriosus in the dog. *J Surg Rev, 11*:312, 1962.
2. Mitchell, S.C.: The ductus arteriosus in the meontal period. *J Pediatr, 51*:12, 1957.
3. Benavides, P.H., Vela, J.E. and Monroy, G.: Ausencia de la capa media del conducto arterial estudio anatomochnico de un caso. *Arch Inst Cardiol Mex, 26*:332, 1956.
4. Gregg, N.McA.: Congenital cataract following German measles in the mother. *Trans Ophthalmol Soc Aust, 3*:35, 1941.
5. Lundstrom, R.: Rubella during pregnancy. *Acta Paediatr Scand, 51,* suppl 133, 1962.
6. Swan, C.: A study of three infants dying from congenital defects following maternal rubella in the early stages of pregnancy. *J Pathol Bacterial, 56*:289, 1944.
7. Campbell, M.: Place of maternal rubella in the etiology of congenital heart disease. *Br Med J, 1*:691, 1961.
8. Krovetz, L.J. and Warden, H.E.: Patent ductus arteriosus. An analysis of 515 surgically proved cases. *Dis Chest, 42*:46, 1962.
9. Monif, G.R.G.: *Viral Infections of the Human Fetus.* New York, MacMillan, 1969.
10. Knight, D.H., Patterson, D.F. and Melbin, J.: Constriction of the fetal ductus arteriosus induced by oxygen, acetylcholine, and norepinephrine in normal dogs and those genetically predisposed to persistent patency. *Circulation, 47*:127, 1973.

Eighteen

THE PULMONARY ARTERY ARISING FROM THE AORTA: THE DUCTUS CONTRIBUTION

M ANY CASES OF ABSENCE OF RIGHT OR LEFT PULMONARY ARTERY HAVE BEEN DOCUMENTED and in 1955 Emmanuel and Pattinson (1) recorded forty-six instances with Tetralogy of Fallot. This malformation is seen occasionally in all clinics.

Pool, Vogel and Blount (2) reviewed the cases of congenital unilateral absence of a pulmonary artery for the purpose of exploring the role of increased blood flow to one lung as a cause of pulmonary vascular changes with consequent pulmonary hypertension.

They analyzed forty proven cases and noted: (a) a blood supply from the ascending aorta was found only in cases when the right pulmonary artery was absent (except in one case). In other instances of absent right pulmonary artery the blood supply was from bronchials or a vessel from the arch. (b) In all cases of absent left pulmonary artery the blood supply was from the bronchials or a vessel from the aortic arch. (c) Persistence of bronchial vessels or a ductuslike vessel were about equal in incidence in cases of absent left or absent right pulmonary artery.

Frequently the pulmonary artery is said to arise from the aorta, either right or left, associated with other abnormalities or as an isolated lesion. In these the ductus arteriosus may be the initial arterial segment of an aortic communication to the lung. Ductus tissue was identified in an instance of pulmonary artery arising from the aorta in the case of Wagenvort, et al. (3). There was a left aortic arch and a closing ductus on the left. The vessel was stenotic. DuShane, et al. (4) also reported a case with a normal left arch, a left ductus, and probably ductus tissue at the aortic base of the communication on the right.

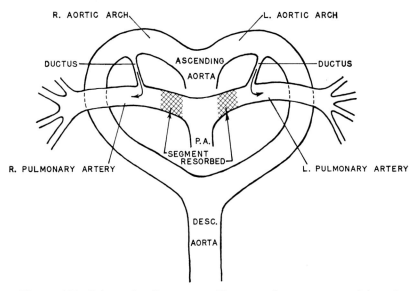

Figure 123. Schematic diagram to illustrate the apparent origin of a pulmonary artery from the aorta. The ductus originates from the aorta in the usual position but the proximal right or left pulmonary artery either does not form or is resorbed. The opposite ductus may be present either patent or as a ligament. Ductus tissue has been described in the aortic terminus of the pulmonary artery. Sometimes other mechanisms have been involved.

Figure 123 shows a basic right and left aortic arch system with a ductus to both right and left pulmonary arteries. The proximal part of either the right or left pulmonary artery may resorb or be absent leaving the ductus as the blood supply to the peripheral pulmonary artery. Since the pulmonary artery on the left is formed somewhat differently, absence of the proximal part seems to occur more frequently on the left, especially in Tetralogy of Fallot with a right aortic arch.

In addition, a residual root may be present, either in an anterior

or posterior position, either right or left. If contralateral to a
normally occurring arch, the pulmonary artery system is then:
aortic root-ductus-distal pulmonary artery.

REFERENCES

1. Emmanuel, R.W. and Pattinson, J.N.: Absence of the left pulmonary
   artery in Fallot's tetralogy. *Br Heart J, 18*:289, 1956.
2. Pool, P.E., Vogel, J.H.K. and Blount, G.S., Jr.: Congenital unilateral
   absence of a pulmonary artery. The importance of flow in pulmonary hyptertension. *Am J Cardiol, 10*:706, 1962.
3. Wagenvort, C.A., Neufeld, H.N., Birge, R.F., Caffrey, J.A. and Edwards,
   J.W.: Origin of right pulmonary artery from ascending aorta. *Circulation, 23*:84, 1961.
4. DuShane, J.W., Weidman, W.H., Ougley, P.A., Swan, HJ..C., Kirklin,
   J.W., Edwards, J.E. and Schmutzler, H.: Clinical-pathologic confer-
   ence. *Am Heart J, 59*:782, 1960.

Nineteen

THE VASCULAR RING: THE DUCTUS CONTRIBUTION

T HERE IS AN OBVIOUS VASCULAR RING ENCIRCLING THE TRACHEA AND ESOPHAGUS when a double aortic arch is present, but the ductus does not contribute to this. However, the ductus arteriosus or more likely the closed ductus, the ligamentum, contributes to a vascular ring in three possible ways. Consideration of the double aortic arch is omitted.

The basic anomaly is: (a) an aortic arch, either right or left, (b) partial arch, or a persistent aortic root of the opposite arch, either anterior or posterior and (c) a ductus or ligamentum. If the persistent partial arch or aortic root is anterior either right or left, the ductus arises from this and lies anteriorly and does not produce a vascular ring. If the posterior segment of the arch persists and the ductus arises from it a vascular ring is completed by the ductus or ligament. In the schematic diagrams, hatched vessels are posterior and open vessels are anterior.

Figure 124 shows the two possibilities when there is a right aortic arch. (a) When the root of the left arch is anterior, now probably called the innominate artery with the *ductus arising from the left innominate,* the ductus or ligament lies anteriorly and there is no vascular ring. (b) If there is a posterior portion of the left aortic root and the ductus arises from it and terminates in the pulmonary artery, a ring exists.

TYPE I. Figure 125 illustrates the anterior ring ductus as seen in an angiocardiogram. An overlay accentuates the vessels. A continuous murmur was present in an infant age eight weeks with a

295

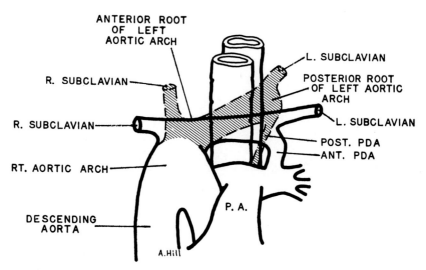

ANTERIOR ROOT
OF LEFT
AORTIC ARCH

L. SUBCLAVIAN

R. SUBCLAVIAN

POSTERIOR ROOT
OF LEFT AORTIC
ARCH

R. SUBCLAVIAN

L. SUBCLAVIAN

POST. PDA

ANT. PDA

RT. AORTIC ARCH

P. A.

DESCENDING
AORTA

A.Hill

RIGHT AORTIC ARCH WITH PERSISTING
ROOTS (ANTERIOR AND POSTERIOR)
OF LEFT ARCHES
(POSTERIOR SEGMENT SHADED)

Figure 124. The basic anatomy of the vascular ring when there is a right aortic arch. When (a) an anterior segment of the left arch persists with an anterior ductus/ligamentum no vascular ring is formed; (b) when the posterior segment of the left arch persists (cross hatch) the ductus/ligamentum produces a vascular ring.

pseudotruncus where the only blood flow to the pulmonary artery is through a persistent patent ductus. The base or segment of the left aortic arch would probably be called a left innominate artery. While the origin is the same, if a ductus arises as shown it seems desirable to use the term persistent left aortic root. If a ductus does not arise from it perhaps it could be labelled simply an innominate artery.

TYPE II. Figures 126 and 127 show an overlay against an x-ray in an instance of a vascular ring in a female age four and one-half months. The symptoms were chiefly respiratory with marked stridor.

The persistent root of the left aortic arch is posterior to the esophagus. This can usually be identified in an esophogram by the

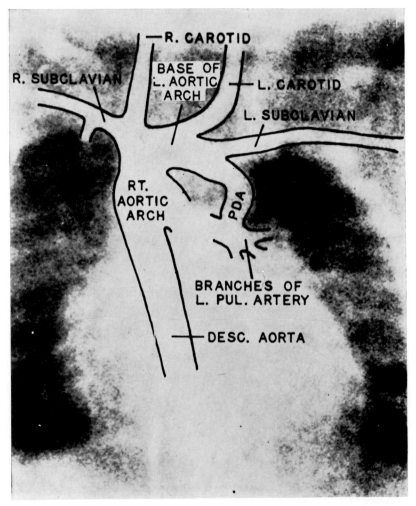

Figure 125. The anterior proximal portion of the left arch and a patent ductus are shown in an angiocardiogram in a pseudotruncus. There is no vascular ring since the root of the left aortic arch is anterior as a left innominate if this term would be preferred. No element of the vascular anomaly is posterior to the trachea-esophagus and these structures are not enclosed.

large vessel indentation. While clinically it is often called an anomalous origin of the left subclavian artery since both this and the ductus arise from it, this is not correct. When a ring is present and there is a right aortic arch and the retro-esophageal indentation is

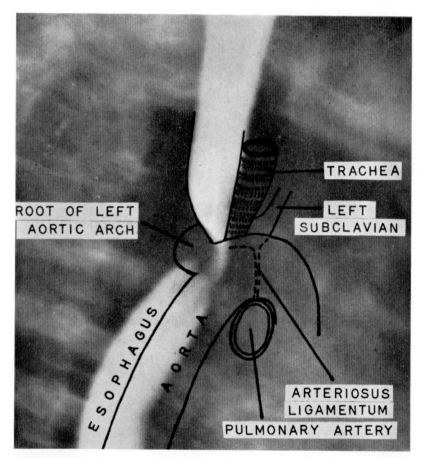

Figure 126. The lateral view shows the large diameter posterior indentation of the esophagus by a large vessel. This is too large for an anomalous subclavian artery and when present is almost pathognomonic of this anatomy as labelled.

too large for a subclavian, this anatomical pattern is present. The illustration from Bedford and Parkinson (1) is particularly informative (Fig. 128).

Figure 129 shows the relation of the vessels to the formation of a vascular ring if the aortic arch is in its usual situation, on the left. When a persistent root of the right arch is anterior, the ductus is anterior and no obstruction occurs. If the root is posterior and the ductus arises posteriorly a vascular ring is formed partially obstructing the trachea and esophagus.

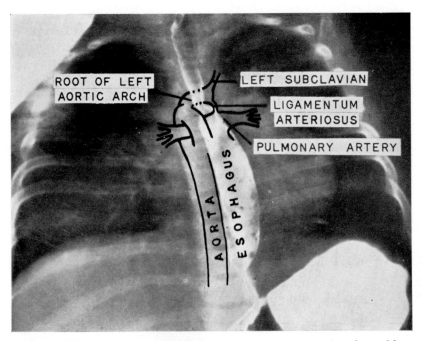

Figure 127. An overlay shows the anatomy of a vascular ring with a right aortic arch and a proximal persisting root of the left arch. Esophageal indentations are almost diagnostic.

This is the mirror image of the situation when the aortic arch is right.

A number of variations occur, especially in relation to the origin of the vessels from the arch. The possibility exists that the ductus may be both right and left although this is extremely uncommon. Either may be open or closed.

Aspects of the vascular ring including those when the ductus does not contribute to it have been illustrated in detail in the magnificent *Atlas of Vascular Rings and Related Malformations of the Aortic Arih System* of Stewart, Kincaid and Edwards (2).

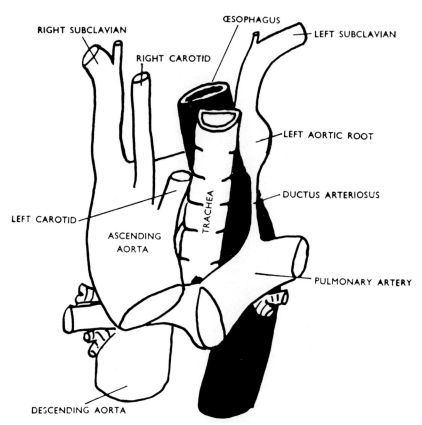

Figure 128. This diagram of Bedford and Parkinson illustrates the anatomy of the right aortic arch, persistent root of the left arch posterior to the esophagus, and the left ductus which completes the vascular ring. From Bedford, D.E. and Parkinson, J.: *Br J Radiol, 9*:776, 1936.

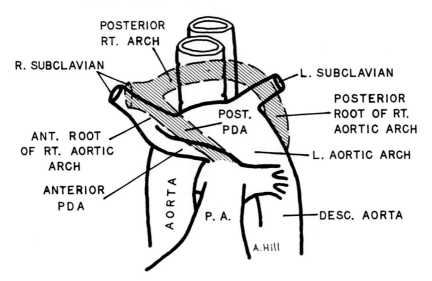

LEFT AORTIC ARCH WITH PERSISTING ROOTS (ANTERIOR AND POSTERIOR) OF RIGHT ARCHES (POSTERIOR SEGMENT SHADED)

Figure 129. This shows persistent anterior and posterior roots of the right arch in the presence of a normal left arch. When anterior there is no obstructing ring. When posterior (hatched) the ductus/ligamentum completes a vascular ring.

REFERENCES

1. Bedford, D.E. and Parkinson, J.: Right sided aortic arch (situs inversus arcus aortae). *Br J Radiol, 9:*776, 1936.
2. Stewart, J.R., Kincaid, O.W. and Edwards, J.E.: *An Atlas of Vascular Rings and Related Malformations of the Aortic Arch System.* Springfield, Thomas, 1964.

Twenty

THE SUBCLAVIAN STEAL

THERE HAVE BEEN MANY SUBSTANTIATING REPORTS and reviews of reversal of blood flow through the vertebral artery and its effect on cerebral circulation since the first report (1). This refers to occlusion of the subclavian artery proximal to the vertebral branch. Consequently, retrograde flow from the circle of Willis occurs to the subclavian artery through the vertebral artery.

The occlusion is usually atherosclerotic in adults. It may be traumatic or surgical in origin in children. Seven of twelve patients, post Blalock-Taussig surgery, with angiographic evidence of subclavian steal, had symptoms related to basilar artery insufficiency as reported by Falger and Shah (2). Massumi (3) reported instances related to congenital atresia of proximal portion of the left subclavian with late opacification of the subclavian distal to the vertebral junction. Bilateral vertebral to right and left subclavian artery flow was present in the case of Zetterquist (4), who had an atypical coarctation of the aorta.

The ductus arteriosus is involved in anatomical anomalies causing a special variety of proximal obstruction of the left subclavian artery.

In the presence of a right aortic arch, most commonly in Tetralogy of Fallot, there may be isolation of the left subclavian from the aorta. In this anomaly the left subclavian is a direct continuation of the ductus arteriosus. The ductus closes, becomes a ligament and the distal subclavian receives blood flow from the left vertebral artery.

The anomalies are shown in Figure 130, adopted from Barry (5). The left aortic arch resorbs except the portion included in seg-

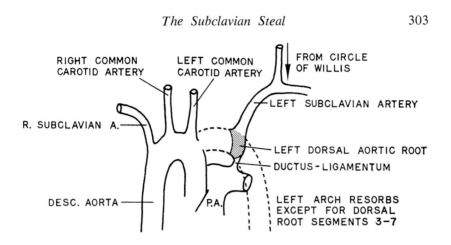

RIGHT COMMON
CAROTID ARTERY

LEFT COMMON
CAROTID ARTERY

FROM CIRCLE
OF WILLIS

R. SUBCLAVIAN A.

LEFT SUBCLAVIAN ARTERY

LEFT DORSAL AORTIC ROOT

DUCTUS-LIGAMENTUM

DESC. AORTA

P.A.

LEFT ARCH RESORBS
EXCEPT FOR DORSAL
ROOT SEGMENTS 3–7

THE DUCTUS-LIGAMENTUM ROLE IN THE SUBCLAVIAN STEAL

Figure 130. An explanation of the possible embryology when the left subclavian artery is the continuation of the ductus or ligamentum. A right aortic arch is necessary. A mirror image may occur but is unusual.

ments 3 to 7. The subclavian arises from this, and the ductus inserts into it. Retrograde flow occurs through the vertebral artery which is in its normal position.

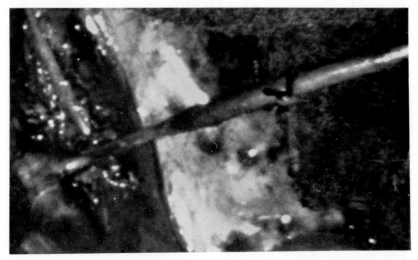

Figure 131. Photograph at surgery of the left subclavian artery as a direct continuation of a closed ductus in a female age three and one-half years. There was a tetralogy of Fallot and a right aortic arch.

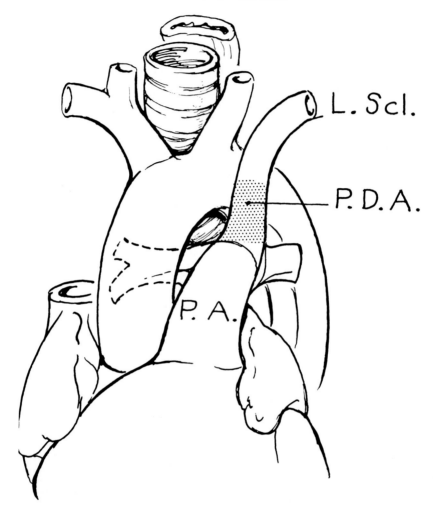

Figure 132. If the left subclavian was a continuation of the ductus arteriosus in the presence of a left aortic arch the concept that the ductus
and subclavian inserted into the same segment of the arch and the arch,
above and below resorbed, would have to be discarded. A right aortic arch
is required.

This possible anomalous status must be considered carefully
when a left Blalock procedure is contemplated, and the cineangiogram observed for absent or late opacification of the left subclavian. It can be suspected by blood pressure differential in the two
arms. Rarely the ductus may remain patent. Three cases of this

combination of anomalies have been seen in the past four years. Figure 131 is a photograph of the left subclavian artery as a continuation of the closed ductus in a three and one-half year old girl with Tetralogy of Fallot and a right aortic arch.

The usual ductus closure, with absence of (a) oxygenated blood flow through it and (b) in the presence of presumed obligatory shunting offers a further comment on the ductus closure problem.

If the aorta would be on the left and if isolation of the subclavian from the aorta should occur, a new theory regarding the embryology would be required. This hypothetical situation is shown in Figure 132.

REFERENCES

1. Reividi, M., Holling, H.E., Roberts, B. and Toole, J.F.: Reversal of blood flow through the vertebral artery and its effect on cerebral circulation. *N Engl J Med, 265*:878, 1961.
2. Falger, G.M. and Shah, K.D.: Subclavian steal in patients with Blalock-Taussig anastomosis. *Circulation, 31*:241, 1965.
3. Massumi, R.A.: The congenital variety of the "Subclavian Steal" syndrome. *Circulation, 28*:1149, 1963.
4. Zetterquist, P.: Atypical coarctation of the aorta with bilateral vertebral subclavian pathway. *Scand J Thorc Cardiovas Surg, 1*:68, 1967.
5. Barry, A.: The aortic arch derivatives in the human adult. *Anat Rec, 111*:221, 1951.

Twenty-One

ABSENCE, INCOMPLETE AND PREMATURE CLOSURE OF THE DUCTUS ARTERIOSUS

THE CASE OF STENO (1) IN 1671 TO 1672 WAS THE FIRST DESCRIPTION OF THE ABSENCE OF THE DUCTUS ARTERIOSUS. This is clearly indicated in his report of dissection of a grossly malformed infant, who also had what was later known as Tetralogy of Fallot. This is a rare occurrence but has been reported by Alpert and Bartlet (2) in association with a large atrial septal defect.

The ductus, when not present, is a finding occurring most frequently in conditions where there is another connection between the pulmonary artery and aorta which allows shunting from the pulmonary artery to the aorta during fetal life. Forms of the truncus arteriosus, for instance, do not require a ductus for aorta-pulmonary-artery communication during fetal life. Why this anatomical situation should inhibit the formation of the terminal part of the sixth aortic arch and whether the dorsal or ventral sprout of the ductus or both are lacking is not clear. Conversely, however, both a patent ductus and an aortic septal defect, an aortic-pulmonary window, may occur together.

THE INCOMPLETE OR PARTIAL DUCTUS

The ductus arteriosus arises from a dorsal sprout from the primitive aorta and a ventral sprout from a plexus originating at the aortic sac (3). Anatomical evidence suggests (a) one or the other end may not form properly; (b) the sprouts may vary in their inherent ability to close and (c) one end may persist open and the other end blindly or as a fibrous cord.

Incomplete, The Aortic End Open

The most complete report was that of Altshule (4) in a fifty-six year old male. The aortic orifice was wide and a cone-shaped sacculation 1 cm wide and 1 cm deep arose from the aorta and was connected to the pulmonary artery by a fibrous cord. Wilkinson King (5) in 1842 described the ductus in a thirty-two year old female. The aorta was wide and the *largest probe* could be passed except that at the pulmonary artery the opening was guarded by nipplelike processes. The apex was fissured and acted as a valve.

The case of Deckner (6) is more complex with a coarctation and thrombosis of the aorta. However, the ductus was 3 cm long, partially filled with a thrombus, but the aortic orifice was open and the pulmonary ostium completely closed.

Wagener (7) reported three cases, a female age thirty-eight years, a male forty-two years and a female age twenty-three years, in all of whom the aortic ostia was patent, and the pulmonary closure was by a vesicular membrane which may project into the pulmonary artery.

More current and of great interest was the report by Keith and Sagarminaga (8) of a ten year old girl in whom a typical ductus murmur would disappear completely and reappear spontaneously. At surgery a ductus 2 cm in diameter and 1 cm in length was present, but a valve or veil-like structure was found in the ductus at its entrance into the pulmonary artery and could easily occlude the ductus lumen. Apparently, this occlusion occurred intermittently. A change in left heart volume consequently occurs.

The Pulmonary End Patent, The Aortic Termination Closed

The most extensive study was that of Quiroga (9), who termed this partial persistence of the ductus arteriosus. He observed this most commonly in cardiac malformations causing reduction of pulmonary blood flow. This was seen in twenty-five instances in 735 angiocardiograms, an incidence of 3.45 percent. One half of the cases had a right aortic arch. These opacified prortuberances

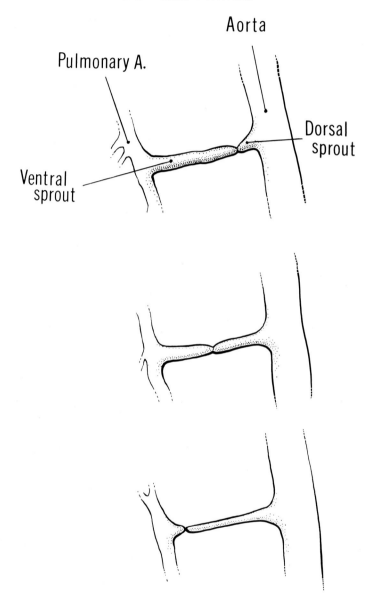

Figure 135. If the ductus originates as a dorsal sprout and a ventral sprout variation in length and behavior of the components might occur. Also see Plate 4, Huntington (18), MORPHOLOGY OF THE PULMONARY ARTERY IN THE MAMMALIA.

from the pulmonary artery are best seen in the frontal view. (Fig. 133)

Presumably premature closure of the ductus arteriosus, even partial, causes a profound disruption of the fetal circulation since aortic runoff from the pulmonary artery is prevented. Either (a) a large pulmonary flow through a high resistance area is required to produce left heart filling and reasonable peripheral perfusion, (b) a large flow at the foramen ovale is required for this purpose or (c) a combination of these would occur. This situation would be analogous in some ways to pulmonary valve atresia with an intact ventricular septum, although here a high pressure pulmonary artery circulation would not be required. However, it will be recalled that there is some evidence and some believe that if ductus occlusion occurs slowly and late in pregnancy the pulmonary vascular system can distend and accommodate a large blood flow.

An instance of possible premature obstruction at the aortic end occurred. This was a full term infant with clinical evidence of (a) severe heart failure, (b) gross enlargement of the right ventricle and right atrium, (c) electrocardiogram and vectorcardiogram compatible with this and (d) hemodynamic and angiocardiographic studies confirming the status of the ductus, obstruction at the aortic end. However, these were done at age four hours, and the possibility remains that this terminal occlusion occurred during this period. A hematocrit of 23 percent possibly contributed to the cardiac and respiratory distress. This case was reported by Arcilla, et al. (10). An angiocardiogram at age three and one half months showed no opacification of the ductus as closure continued and became complete.

Figure 134 indicates the typical finding in a six month old with Tetralogy of Fallot. The partial ductus is of considerable theoretical interest in relation to embryology and discussion of closure and is of great importance as possibly representing premature closure.

Premature Closure Of The Ductus Arteriosus

Premature closure of the fetal circulatory channels are rare. Premature closure would be defined as obstructive closure of a

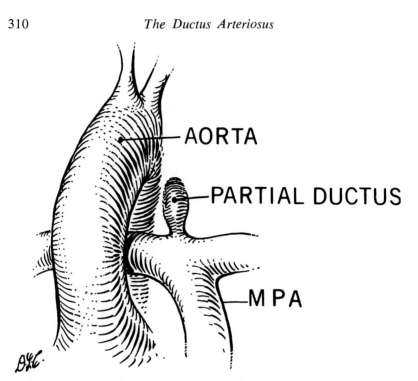

Figure 134. Drawing from an angiocardiogram, tetralogy of Fallot, age six months.

fetal channel prior to birth with prevention of the normal fetal circulation. For instance, premature closure of the foramen ovale may be compatible with live birth (11) as can premature closure of the sinus venosus.

The only instance of real full length closure of the ductus would appear to be the pathological report of Chevers (12) entitled "Remarkable Contraction of the Ductus Arteriosus in a Newborn Infant." This report concerned a seven and one-half month premature infant who lived for fifteen minutes. The ductus was almost closed, one-twelfth inch in diameter and would admit only *the shank of a large pin.* Its walls exceeded in thickness those of the other large vessels, and the interior presented a series of small pits, indicating some duration of the process of closure. The contraction of the vessel was uniform. The pulmonary arteries were wide, well developed and equaled in size the vessels of a mature fetus. The infant died of hemorrhage from the umbilicus since the cord had not been ligated.

Jager and Wollenman (13) have shown, in their detailed study of the anatomy of the ductus arteriosus in the newborn, that the vessel may be occluded in the central area by a membrane and an hourglass shape is present in a small percentage of cases.

These anatomical varieties of the ductus may be considered in relation to the embryology of the vessel. The sixth or pulmonary arch, the termination of which forms the ductus, is composed of a dorsal sprout arising from the primitive aorta and a ventral sprout arising from the primitive pulmonary artery, as illustrated by Congdon (14) in a 5 mm embryo and by Keibel and Mall (3) in a 4.9 embryo. The specimens described suggest (a) the dorsal and ventral sprouts may be uneven length, (b) the factors related to closure may affect the dorsal and ventral sprouts differently, allowing one or the other to remain open, the oppostie segment closing normally, or (c) their union may be seen as a persistent membrane. These possibilities are shown schematically in Figure 135.

Animal studies indicate surgical ligation of the ductus is compatible with fetal life if done late in gestation, but is lethal if done early. In guinea pigs surgical closure at fifty days may be done with impunity, but obstruction of the ductus at forty days had the same 100 percent mortality as ligating the pulmonary artery at forty days (15).

In animals the suggestion is strong that pulmonary blood flow accelerates late in pregnancy and the circulatory effect of premature closure of the ductus in man depends upon the period of closure. The case of Chevers (12) suggests closure may occur early innocuously, if this process is slow, since the pulmonary arteries were dilated, well developed and were equal in size to those of a full term infant.

As suggested by Fritz (16) the cases of fetal closure of the ductus arteriosus disprove the theories of closure based upon the onset of respiration, closure related to change of position, pressure from the left bronchus or even fall of pressure within the ductus as diminution of flow within it occurs. These cases emphasize more the fetal anatomical process.

He described an infant who died one hour after birth, length

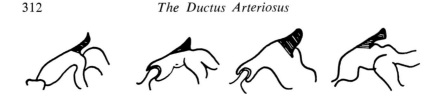

Figure 133. Partial persistance of the ductus arteriosus as illustrated by Quiroga (9). These were seen on angiocardiography and usually the pulmonary terminus opacified.
From Quiroga, C.: *Acta Radiol*, 55:103, 1961.

49 cm, weight 3,300 gm. The lungs were partially inflated and hyperemic. The right ventricle was markedly hypertrophied, the right antrium was dilated and bulged toward the left atrium and the foramen ovale was overstretched and showed small gaps.

The ductus arteriosus was completely occluded at the aortic end but open to a fine probe at the pulmonary artery terminus. Histological examination showed normal structural obliteration.

He believed the degree of obliteration indicated the process must have begun at least two weeks before birth.

Alexandrowsky (17) reported an instance of stenosis of the ductus in a premature infant, gestation seven months, length 36 cm, weight 2,100 gm. There was hydrops of the fetus and placenta, some hemorrhage in the organs and numerous erythroblasts. The lungs were greatly enlarged and the liver hyperemic.

The ductus was stenosed. It was 5 mm long, the circumference at the ostia 4 mm and 2.5 mm at the stenosed central portion. The pulmonary artery and aorta were large, 13 mm and 14 mm in circumference.

The relation of any fetal stenosis of the ductus arteriosus and the hydrops, hydramnios and erythroblasts cannot be determined.

Similar cases have been reported by others and while microscopic examination of the vessel is usually not done in instances of premature closure, the ductus is shrivelled and firm without a lumen.

The dual origin of the ductus arteriosus would seem to explain the anomalies of the ductus related to closure at either end, the vessel otherwise remaining open for varying lengths. This would presume the dorsal and ventral sprouts may act differently, the usual forces of closure may operate in one segment but not the other. There is partial closure.

REFERENCES

1. Steno, Nicholas; reprinted with a historical note: An unusually early description of the so-called Tetralogy of Fallot. Willius, F.A. *Proc Staff Meet Mayo Clinic, 23*:316, 1948.
2. Apert, E. and Bartlet, P.C.: Atheroma with atrial septal defect. *Arch Med Enf, 35*:147, 1932.
3. Keibel, F. and Mall, F.P.: *Human Embryology*. Philadelphia, Lippencott, vol II, Fig. 417, 1912.
4. Altschule, M.B.: Aneurysm of the arch of the aorta due to persistence of a portion of the ductus arteriosus in an adult. *Am Heart J, 14*:113, 1937.
5. King, Wilkinson, T.: On the open state of the ductus arteriosus after birth. *Lond Edbinb Mo J Med Sci*, no. *2*: 1842.
6. Deckner, K.: Atresie der aorta in hoehe des ductus Botalli bet 70 jalhriger. *Fran Beitr Path Anat Allg Path, 82*:172, 1929.

7. Wagener, O.: Geitrag zun pathologie des ductus arteriosus Botalli. *Deutsch Arch Klin Med, 79*:90, 1930.

8. Keith, T.R. and Sagarminaga, J.: Spontaneously disappearing murmur of patent ductus arteriosus. *Circulation, 24*:1235, 1961.

9. Quiroga, C.: Partial persistance of the ductus arteriosus. *Acta Radiol, 55/2*:103, 1961.

10. Arcilla, R., Thilenius, O. and Ranniger, K.: Congestive heart failure from suspected ductal closure in utero. *J Pediatr, 75*:74, 1969.

11. Lev, M., Arcilla, R., Rimoldi, H.J., Licata, R.H. and Gasul, B.M.: Premature narrowing or closure of the foramen ovale. *Am Heart J, 65*:638, 1963.

12. Chevers, N.: Remarkable contraction of the ductus arteriosus in a newborn infant. *Trans Pathol Soc Lond, 1*:60, 1846-48.

13. Jager, B.V. and Wollenman, O.J.: An anatomical study of the closure of the ductus arteriosus. *Am J Pathol, 18*:595, 1942.

14. Congdon, E.D.: Transformation of the aortic arch system during the development of the human embryo. *Contrib Embryol 68,* vol XIV: 47, 1927.

15. Sciacca, A. and Condorelli, M.: Involution of the ductus arteriosus. Bibliotheca Cardiologica, suppl to *Cardiologica Fasc, 10,* S. Karger, Basel, Switzerland, 1960.

16. Fritz, E.: Foetaler verschluss des ductus Botalli. *Deutsch Z Ges Ger Med, 32*:384, 1940.

17. Alexandrowsky, A.: *Stenose des Ductus Arteriosus Botalli Mit Allegemeimes Angeborener Wassercucht.* Berl 1916, (Bern) 16 p. 80.

18. Huntington, G.S.: The morphology of the pulmonary artery in the mammalia. *Anat Rec 17*:165, 1919-1920.

Twenty-Two

THE DUCTUS IN TRANSPOSITION OF THE GREAT VESSELS

A<small>N UNUSUAL EXAMPLE OF PATENT DUCTUS HEMODYNAMICS</small> was obtained in an instance of transposition of the aorta and pulmonary artery with an intact ventricular septum. There was a small atrial septal defect, and catheterization and atrial septostomy were done at age three weeks. In summary, there was systemic pressure in the right ventricle and lower pressure in the left ventricle. The pulmonary artery was not entered. There was obvious color differential between hands and feet and the right ventricle saturation was 63 percent and the femoral artery 86 percent prior to baloon septostomy. The feet were relatively pink so that clinically the differential diagnosis included coarctation of the aorta with a patent ductus below the obstruction.

During right ventricular systole (Fig. 136), the aorta and branches and the descending aorta were opacified. The site of the ductus was very apparent, but there was no opacification until the end of systole and the start of diastole, the aorta still very well opacified (Fig. 137).

The left heart was opacified by a left atrial injectiion, and the pulmonary artery consequently is not well seen. But in left ventricular systole the descending aorta opacified well (Fig. 138), and this opacification fades during left ventricular diastole (Fig. 139). Arterial or oxygenated blood enters the descending aorta during systole via the patent ductus and produces a pinkness in the feet.

315

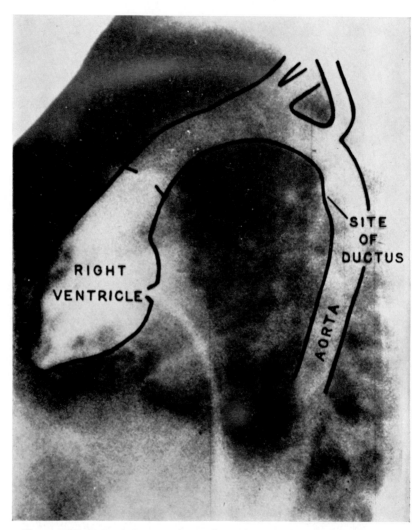

Figure 136. Frames from a cineangiocardiogram. The right ventricle has been injected. The ascending aorta, the arch and branches and descending aorta are opacified during systole, but not the patent ductus arteriosus.

This anatomy and physiology are of great interest.

1. Did hemodynamics have a role in patency. Since there was bidirectional shunt the ductus had internal systemic pressure which presumably would tend to keep it functionally open according to the theory that patency has a hemodynamic facet.

2. While there is venous shunting through the ductus during

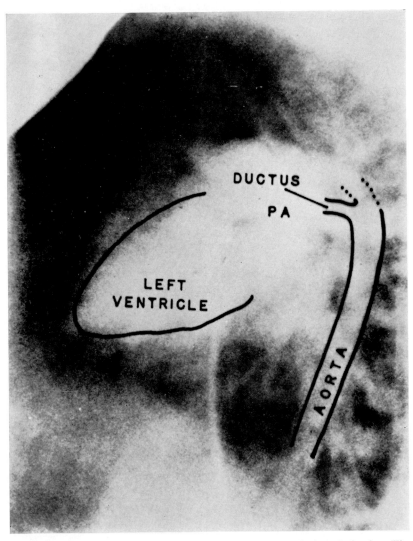

Figure 137. The ductus opacifies as systole ends and diastole begins. The aorta is still very well opacified.

right ventricular diastole, there is arterial shunting during left ventricular systole. The role of oxygen in nonclosure would have to be contrasted with the hemodynamics during intrauterine life. If the atrial septal defect allowed normal shunting of oxygen rich placental blood return to the left atrium, left ventricle, pulmonary

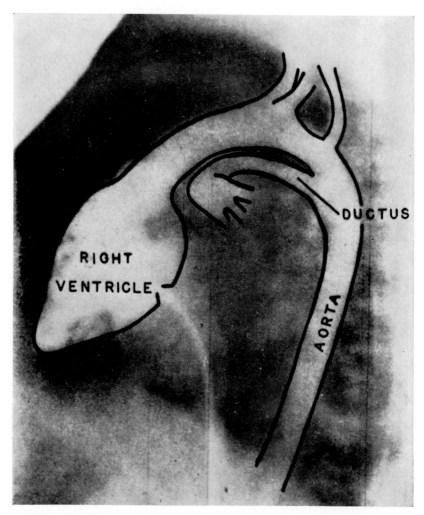

Figure 138. During left ventricular systole the descending aorta opacifies well. Since this is transposition of the great vessels, this blood is oxygenated blood from the lungs and produces pinkness of the feet. There is no real separation but incomplete functional and hemodynamic separation of venous and arterial blood in the aorta at the level of the ductus in the absence of a coarctation.

artery and ductus, then a greater than usual amount of arterialized blood could have stimulated constriction. This did not occur.

Regardless of speculation the facts are that sometimes in transposition of the great vessels with intact septum the ductus closes

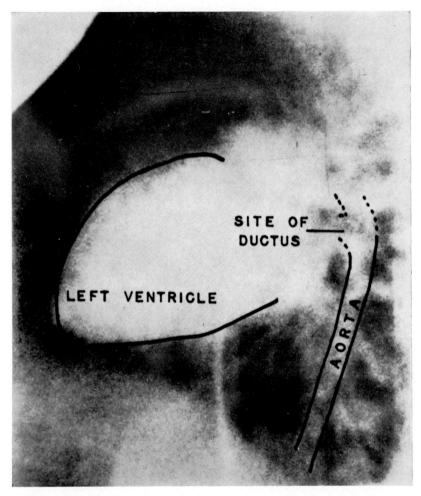

Figure 139. During left ventricular diastole, opacification of the descending aorta fades.

and sometimes it does not, 35 percent closing before age five years. Some factor other than contraction is more subtle than apparent.

Related to this problem is an instance where during surgery for coarctation of the aorta it was expedient to use part of a patent ductus to establish continuity. The vessel bore the thrust of full systemic pressure but closed in spite of this hemodynamic load and reoperation for coarctation was required.

Whether closure was due to (a) oxygen induced contraction,

although the duct had been exposed to arterial blood flow via a left to right shunt, (b) local stimulus via higher pressure or (c) an unknown stimulus activated by the surgical procedures are questions for speculation.

Twenty-Three

THE DUCTUS ARTERIOSUS IN HYALINE MEMBRANE DISEASE

Pulmonary hypoperfusion resulting from reflex vaso-constriction of pulmonary arteries and arterioles was investigated by Chu et al. (1) as the primary event in the pathogenesis of hyaline membrane disease. The physiological and pathological consequences of the respiratory distress syndrome in the newborn have been studied in great detail.

Patency of the ductus arteriosus probably is not involved in the origin of the disease. The ductus is normally patent during the period of the acute disease, the first two or three days after birth and permits either a right to left shunt into the aorta or an aortic-pulmonary artery shunt depending upon the relation of peripheral resistance to pulmonary vascular resistance. There are many factors which contribute to these.

However, in a study of the respiratory distress syndrome Rudolph et al. (2) found the group with severe symptoms all had a large left to right shunt through a patent ductus. Some also had a right to left shunt. The severely distressed infants were studied while breathing 100 percent oxygen which would tend to lower pulmonary resistance and promote shunting at the ductus level.

The structural obstruction, although functional and temporary, was shown very well by Lauweryns (3). Microradiographs of perfusion by barium sulfate showed obstruction in many small muscular pulmonary arteries 50 to 30μ, and most arterioles could not be filled in contrast to controls. The radiographs show great similarity to those obtained in advanced pulmonary hypertension where occlusion is by intimal proliferation and thrombosis.

Naeye (4) noted the small pulmonary arteries were markedly constricted in infants dying of hyaline membrane disease, especially in those examined in the first day of life.

The ductus arteriosus is patent during the acute phase of the disease. There is variable pulmonary artery pressure due to vaso-constriction and variable pressure in the aorta related to the status of (a) left ventricular function and stroke volume and (b) peripheral vessel resistance related to acidemia and hypoxemia. The shunt at the ductus level will vary, into the aorta if this pressure diminishes or into the pulmonary artery and lungs if the pulmonary disease improves.

These shunts can be documented by several procedures. It is of interest that Robertson and Dahlenburg (5) compared blood samples obtained simultaneously from the right radial artery and from the abdominal aorta through an umbilical catheter as an index of shunt. They found in twenty-seven of 139 determinations the arm sample PO_2 was higher than that in the aorta by over 10 mm Hg and only rarely does more than 15 percent of the right to left shunt originate at the ductus level.

The data indicated variable shunting, sometimes bidirectional or diminishing with 100 percent oxygen which was interpreted as indicating ductus constriction in response to increased PO_2 although increasing aortic pressure and lessening pulmonary resistance seems a possibility.

The status of ductus shunting can be identified by dye curves. In Figure 140 a left to right shunt at the ductus level in a premature is seen early in the disease which is not too severe since aortic PO_2 is 214 mm Hg with mask O_2. Injection into the left atrium appears in the abdominal aorta in one second with the long recirculation slope starting at three and one-half seconds.

This is quite different from the dye curve in Figure 141. In a severly distressed infant left atrial injection at eight hours shows no left to right shunt. The aortic PO_2 is only 55 mm Hg in mask O_2. Inferior caval injection shows a large shunt at the atrial level with a small flow through the lungs as shown by Stahlman (6).

The variable shunting in relation to oxygen administration is illustrated in Figure 142. Since O_2 produces an arterial PO_2 of

5 hour old Infant with HMD
LA Injection
Abdominal Aorta Sampling

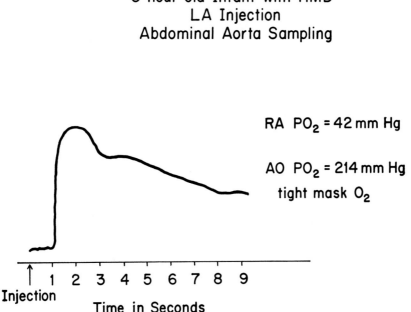

RA PO_2 = 42 mm Hg

AO PO_2 = 214 mm Hg

tight mask O_2

↑
Injection

1 2 3 4 5 6 7 8 9

Time in Seconds

Figure 140. Left atrial injection in an infant not severely affected shows a long recirculation curve of a large left to right shunt at the ductus level. Courtesy of Dr. Mildred Stahlman.

300 mm and room air 55 mm Hg, the illness is not too severe. Both dye curves are into the inferior vena cava, 0.2 ml and in the same place. In the upper curve there is only a small right to left shunt at the atrial level. The large pressure gradient aorta to pulmonary artery, the low right ventricle and thus pulmonary artery pressure gives a left to right shunt at the ductus level, pressures recorded simultaneously through separate catheters. However, on room air, arterial PO_2 drops to 55 mm Hg, the aortic pressure drops and presumably the pulmonary artery resistance and pressure increases. Physiological obstruction to pulmonary flow produces a large right to left flow at the atrial level and abolishes the left to right ductus shunt.

While the ductus arteriosus may not have a role in the pathogenesis of the disease and possibly contributes to relief of right ventricular strain by shunting into the aorta it becomes a hazard during the recovery period.

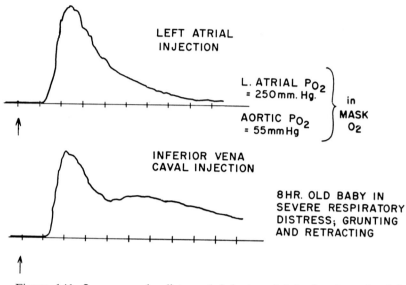

Figure 141. In a severely distressed infant and injection into the left atrium no left to right shunt through the ductus is seen. Injection into the inferior vena cava is similar to the left atrial injection, and there is almost total shunt at the atrial level. There is some flow through the lungs. Any shunt at the ductus level is minimal. From Stahlman, M.: *Pediatr Clin N Am, 11/2.363, 1964.*

Jeiger, Karn and Stern (7) reported nine premature infants recovering from the respiratory distress syndrome who required surgical closure of the ductus. Siassi et al. (8) discussed the presence of patent ductus arteriosus in three premature infants who received prolonged positive pressure ventilation but concluded that hypoxia alone is not responsible for delayed closure.

Delayed closure of the ductus in the premature infant has been noted previously (9, 10, 11) whether or not hyaline membrane disease was present. More recently McMurphy et al. (12) reported maximum ductus constriction response to oxygen developed progressively with fetal age and this physiological latency might contribute to delayed closure in the premature.

There does not seem to be anatomical and histological studies relating to a possible structural deficiency of the ductus media in the premature. Since few prematures have persistent patency of the ductus arteriosus maturation seems to produce closure. Powell (9)

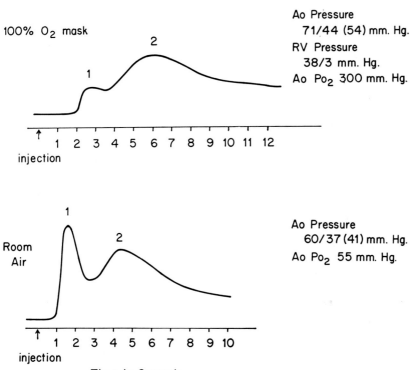

6 hour old Infant with HMD
IVC Injection
Abdominal Aorta Sampling

100% O₂ mask

Ao Pressure
 71/44 (54) mm. Hg.
RV Pressure
 38/3 mm. Hg.
Ao Po₂ 300 mm. Hg.

injection   1 2 3 4 5 6 7 8 9 10 11 12

Room
Air

Ao Pressure
 60/37 (41) mm. Hg.
Ao Po₂ 55 mm. Hg.

injection   1 2 3 4 5 6 7 8 9 10

Time in Seconds

Figure 142. The variable hemodynamics in relation to oxygen administration is seen in a six hour old infant with hyaline membrane disease. In the upper curve there is a small shunt at the atrial level and a 22 mm gradient from aorta to right ventricle and pulmonary artery allows a left to right shunt at the ductus level at room air, the arterial or aortic oxygen has dropped to a PO₂ of 55 mm Hg and lower aortic pressure and presumably increased pulmonary artery persistance and pressure. The atrial shunt is now large, and the ductus shunt has disappeared.
Courtesy of Dr. Mildred Stahlman.

notes the ductus in the premature closes when the proper gestational age is reached.

Left to right flow through the ductus occurs at some stage of the disease if the baby survives. Pulmonary vessel constriction of sufficient severity to damage lung tissues may within a few days have dilatation, causing a large shunt and heart failure. It is not clear whether this is a structural vesesl defect, and if it is, whether prolonged vasoconstriction contributes to this.

The severe failure in an infant already sick is difficult to control and surgical intervention has been proposed. However, in most instances a vigorous medical regime until the ductus diameter diminishes or the pulmonary vessels regain their tone is adequate.

REFERENCES

1. Chu, J., Clements, J.A., Cotton, E., Klaus, M.H., Sweet, A.Y., Thomas, M.A. and Tooley, W.H.: The pulmonary hypoperfusion syndrome. *Pediatrics 35*:733, 1965.
2. Rudolph, A.M., Drorbough, J.E., Auld, P.A.M., Rudolph, A.J., Nadas, A.S., Smith, C.A. and Hubbell, J.P.: Studies on the circulation in the neonatal period: the circulation in the respiratory distress syndrome. *Pediatrics, 27*:551, 1961.
3. Lauweryns, J.M.: Pulmonary arterial vasculature in neontal hyaline membrane disease. *Science, 153*:1275, 1966.
4. Naeye, R.L.: Pulmonary arterial abnormalties associated with hyaline membrane disease. *Am J Pathol, 48*:869, 1966.
5. Robertson, N.R.C. and Dahlenburg, G.W.: Ductus arteriosus shunts in the respiratory distress syndrome. *Pediatr Res, 3*:149, 1969.
6. Stahlman, M.: Treatment of cardiovascular disorders of the newborn. *Pediatr Clin N Am, 11/2*:363, 1964.
7. Jeiger, W., Karn, G. and Stern, L: Operative treatment of patent ductus arteriosus complicating respiratory distress syndrome of the premature (Abstract). *Can Med Assoc J, 98*:105, 1968.
8. Siassi, B., Emmanouilides, G.C., Cleveland, R.A. and Hirose, F.: Patent ductus arteriosus complicating prolonged assisted respiration in respiratory distreess syndrome. *Fortschr Paedol, 74*:11, 1969.
9. Powell, M.D.: Patent ductus arteriosus in premature infants. *Med J Aust, 2*:58, 1963.
10. Auld, P.A.M.: Delayed closure of the ductus arteriosus. *J Pediatr, 69*: 61, 1966.
11. Danilowicz, D., Rudolph, A.M. and Hoffman, J.I.E.: Delayed closure of the ductus arteriosus in premature infants. *Pediatrics, 37*:74, 1966.
12. McMurphy, D.M., Heyman, M.A., Rudolph, A.M. and Melmon, K.L.: Development changes in constriction of the ductus arteriosus. responses of oxygen and vasoactive agents in the isolated ductus arteriosus of the fetal lamb.*Pediatr, 6*:231, 1972.

Twenty-Four

THE EFFECT OF PATENCY ON GROWTH

T HE EFFECT OF THE DUCTUS FLOW ON GROWTH and the surgical removal of the aorta-pulmonary artery shunt has been considered in several studies. This problem also has been the subject of casual statements by those involved in the clinical problem of diagnosis and surgery. Retardation of growth in association with patent ductus arteriosus has been assumed to be related. But the problem seems more complex.

If somatic growth is controlled by a growth hormone the effect of the ductus shunt on the production of the hormone seems doubtful. However, hemodynamic study now indicates preductal aortic arch flow is augmented while postductal flow is probably diminished in any large ductus shunt. This is partly from the large shunt from the preductal arch and partly from retrograde aortic flow into the ductus and lung if the flow is considerable.

The preductal aortic arch flow has been quantitated by a flow meter probe above the ductus which confirms observations of increased forearm blood flow measured by venous occlusion plethysmography.

If the aortic arch flow and branches of the arch are augmented increased cartoid artery flow to the pituitary are perhaps increased. Thus growth should not be affected by diminished glandular blood flow.

If local abnormalities of blood flow are considered, the post-ductal area of growth probably might be affected. There does not seem to be any study related to differential torso growth, or to

327

measurements of growth hormone pre and postoperatively. There have been studies related to body growth in general, and as in so many other aspects of the ductus there is no universal pattern of growth.

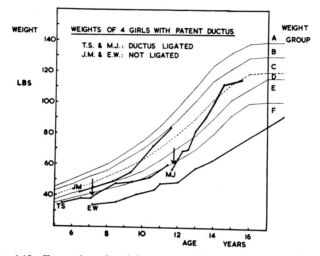

Figure 143. Examples of weight curves of four girls, two had the ductus closed and two did not. Of the two who had closure one gained weight and one did not, and those without closure also had divergent weight gain. Cosh (1) notes children with a patent ductus were underweight when compared with controls but only four of thirteen showed significant improvement after closure.
From Cosh, J.A.: *Br Heart J, 19*:13, 1957.

The growth problem is illustrated by Figure 143 of Cosh (1) which shows weight patterns of two girls without surgery and two girls with ductus closure. In the two patients without surgery, one remained underweight while one improved and became normal over the period of six to twelve years. In those with surgery one remained in the same low weight group while one improved spectacularly.

One of the very good early papers related to the growth problem was that of Porter (2) in 1947. He reported three patients in relation to various members of their family regarding height, weight and surface area. Of great interest were twins, age eleven years, one with a patent ductus and one without. The one with patency was shorter and lighter but thirty-five months after surgical care had grown 16.4 cm which was 6.1 cm more than the growth of the normal twin.

Richards (3) in 1952 reported that of nine cases of patent ductus arteriosus five were below the 67th percentile of the Wetzel grid at the time of operation. There was no definite correlation between the size of the ductus, the degree of growth retardation or post-operative acceleration. Seven showed moderate to marked improvement on the Wetzel grid. One with severe growth retardation was a maternal rubella baby.

The absence of correlation between the size of the diameter of the ductus and growth retardation was noted by Engle, et al. (4) who found the average diameter in ages three to five years and six to ten years about 8 mm regardless of the stature. Likewise there was no relation between retarded growth and familial smallness. They again noted differential growth in identical twins, the ductus twin showing diminution of growth starting at about age two years.

They noted growth retardation occurred in one third to one half of the patients and those with serious impairment remained retarded in stature.

The large series studied by Umansky and Hauck (5) had surgery before the age of eight years and the pre and postoperative growth patterns and all variables studied were based on 327 patients.

They concluded: (a) patent ductus arteriosus patients tended to be shorter and to weigh less than normals of similar age and sex, and over three times the expected numbers were at or below the 10th percentile in height and weight; (b) Marked postoperative acceleration was seen in a number of patients, 20 percent for height and 28 percent for weight; (c) the poor growth in patients below the 10th percentile had no explanation other than that prenatal influence, rather hemodynamic aspects of the shunt, seemed responsible. (d) Maternal height was not a genetic determinant of stature prior to surgery in the group below the 10th percentile in height but correlated following surgery; (e) Postoperative acceleration of growth and height-weight status at age thirteen years were not impaired if surgery was done before the age of eight years.

However, the total group of patients studied was not restricted to isolated patent ductus arteriosus, but it was felt that other factors involved exerted minimal influence. There ware only four patients with noncardiac anomalies which might be growth retarding, and the associated cardiac anomalies were probably of minor importance. The rubella syndrome group was less than 10 percent.

It was emphasized that the ductus shunt did not seem to be the most important cause of smallness in those with retardation at or less than the 10th percentile for height and that other factors were involved in these.

There are many reports which note retardation of growth preoperatively in some patients and postoperative absence of rapid growth, especially in those with more marked growth failure. Some other factor causing smallness is present. In some patients the shunt factor predominates. These will usually be those with large shunts, enlarged hearts and some symptoms. It is common to observe, however, that increase of growth and spontaneous physical activity occurs in many patients considered well and symptom free by their parents.

The role played by (a) preductal increase in aortic flow and (b) postductal diminution of flow in total or differential growth is not clear. The influence of moderate or marked pulmonary hypertension from an early age, when the arteriovenous shunt is not large and may be small, may be a factor in smallness although adequate data is not available.

In general, congenital heart disease of any kind tends to be associated with smallness, and following successful surgery this is frequently overcome by adolescent growth.

1. Cosh, J.A.: Patent ductus arteriosus. A follow up of 73 cases. *Br Heart J, 19*:13, 1957.
2. Porter, W.B.: The effect of patent ductus arteriosus on body growth. *Am J Med Sci, 213*:178, 1947.
3. Richards, Mary R.: Pre and postoperative growth patterns in congenital heart disease as shown by the Ketzel grid. *Pediatrics, 9*:77, 1952.
4. Engle, M.A., Holswade, G.R., Goldbert, H.P. and Glenn, F.: Present problems pertaining to patency of the ductus arteriosus. I. Persistance of growth retardation after successful surgery. *Pediatrics, 22*:70, 1958.
5. Umansky, R. and Hauck, A.J.: Factors in the growth of children with patent ductus arteriosus. *Pediatrics, 30*:540, 1962.

Twenty-Five

AGE AND THE PATENT DUCTUS ARTERIOSUS

THERE ARE NUMEROUS REPORTS OF PATENCY of the ductus arteriosus in older patients (1, 2, 3, 4) and even in the eighth decade (5, 6, 7, 8, 9). These reports are clinical or clinical-pathological, and there are few instances of older patent ductus patients who have had proper physiological studies to identify the severity of the disease. The patent ductus is an incidental finding at autopsy, or the murmur is an incidental finding on physical examination and heart disease of any severity is excluded by a heart relatively normal in size by x-ray and with slight electrocardiographic abnormality. When present this abnormality is usually indicative of hypertrophy of the left ventricle, a result of moderate aorta to pulmonary artery flow through a small or moderate size patent ductus.

While it is not possible to accept the concept that their health had not been impaired, many have no complaints referred to the cardiovascular or pulmonary systems. They have survived miscellaneous infections and dental caries without having bacterial endarteritis of the ductus. They have lived what they consider a normal life. While being free of real symptoms, they probably have never experienced the spontaneous energy of good health. Closure of even the modest asymptomatic ductus in a very active child achieves a change in usual vigor often surprising to parents. The vague but increased fatigue associated with substantial left to right shunts through the ductus and increased cardiac work of 30 or 40 percent is readily overcome by determination and increased effort, especially in childhood.

A smaller group have the ductus manifested by more substantial symptoms. Cardiac decompensation has been reported at sixty-six years (2), seventy-five years (6), seventy years (6) and there are other such reports (7 ,8). In this age group the role of arteriosclerosis and age and the effects of the patent ductus are cumulative. The oldest patient with patent ductus arteriosus would appear to be the case reported by White, Mazurkie and Borschetti (10). This man was followed for forty-three years and died at the age of ninety years (eight months and eleven days). He had led an active life until age ninety when he complained of shortness of breath on exertion. The contribution of the patent ductus to serious heart disease or decompensation in the forty to sixty year age group is more evident.

In the older patient, dilatation and atheroma of the pulmonary artery becomes a prominent facet of increased flow or pressure and elapsed time. The contribution of the increased left ventricular output to the aortic atheromatous change is not clear.

Likewise, the influence of increased cardiac output in the absence of systemic hypertension upon the coronary arteries is not clear. There are a number of reports of angina and coronary artery disease in the presence of a patent ductus, but these cases occurred in ages when this could be anticipated in the absence of a ductus. White (11) in 1884 reported a male, age fifty-three years, who had vertigo and pain in the chest and died during a paroxysm. The ductus was the size of an anterior tibial artery. Other clinical observations (12) report similar cases. Since the diastolic systemic pressure is lowered in the medium sized patent ductus and since maximum coronary flow occurs during diastole, the relation between hemodynamics and coronary ischemic symptoms seem possible. Recent hemodynamic studies show forward flow in the aortic arch in diastole, and in some patients T wave inversion in V5 and V6 disappeared after surgery suggesting the presence of a *coronary steal*. There is increased left ventricle work, and often dilatation and hypertrophy. In the same way, if pulmonary hypertension is initiated by pulmonary vascular changes, the relation of right ventricular hypertrophy to the indigenous coronary supply has not been elucidated, except as Shipley and Wearn (13) indicated capillary ratios in relation to muscle mass did not increase with hypertrophy.

The application of surgical closure of the patent ductus in the patient over forty depends upon the philosophical point of view. The question whether the (a) benign small shunt lesion, (b) the larger ductus with moderate or large shunts and mild to moderate symptoms or (c) the frankly ill older patient fifty to seventy years, should undertake risks of thoracic surgery represent decisions with many facets. The larger the ductus, the more clinical symptoms are evident and the greater the advantage of having the ductus closed. The approach applicable to a preschool child should be the same—a patent ductus arteriosus should be closed surgically unless there is some specific contraindication.

The technical surgical problems are related to manipulation of atheromatous or partly calcified vessels, and individual decisions are required.

It is of interest that a medium sized ductus with a large or at least an average aorta-pulmonary artery flow with probably a Qp/Qs ration of 1.5 or 2 to 1 should not develop increasing arteriolar resistance over fifty to seventy years. Rather than accelerated acquisition of pulmonary hypertension there has been decelerated pulmonary vascular changes. There are few reports of hemodynamic and histological studies in the older patent ductus patient.

REFERENCES

1. Luys, M.: Persistance du canal arteriel chez une femme de cinquante-deux ans. *Bull Soc Anat, 30*:227, 1855.
2. Josephson, A.: Offenstehender ductus Botalli nebst atherom in den asten der arteria pulmonalis. *Nord Med Ark, 10*:1, 1897.
3. Horder, T.J.: Infective endocarditis. *Q J Med, 2*:289, 1909.
4. Keys, A. and Shapiro, M.J.: Patency of the ductus in adults. *Am Heart J, 25*:158, 1943.
5. Aiken, J.E., Bifulco, E. and Sullivan, J.J., Jr.: Patent ductus arteriosus in the Aged. Report of this disease in a 74 year old female. *JAMA, 177/5*:330, 1961.
6. Fishman, L. and Silverthorne, M.C.: Persistent patent ductus arteriosus in the aged. *Am Heart J, 41*:762, 1951.
7. Fishman, L.: Patent ductus arteriosus in patient surviving to 74 years. *Am J Cardiol, 6*:685, 1960.

8. Storstein, O., Humerfelt, S., Muller, O. and Rasmussen, H.: Patent ductus arteriosus in a woman age 72 years. *Br Heart J, 14*:276, 1952.
9. Bain, C.W.C.: Case reports: Longevity and patent ductus arteriosus. *Br Heart J, 19*:574, 1957.
10. White, P.D., Mazurkie, S.J. and Borschetti, A.E.: Patency of the ductus arteriosus at 90. *N Engl J Med, 280*:146, 1969.
11. White, W.H.: Patent ductus arteriosus. *Trans Pathol Soc Lond, 36*:182, 1884.
12. Kapp, L.A.: Patent ductus arteriosus with coronary arteriosclerotic heart disease. *Med Bull Vet Admin, 19*:93, 1942.
13. Shipley, R.A. and Wearn, J.T.: The capillary supply in normal and hypertrophied hearts of rabbits. *J Exp Med, 65*:29, 1937.

INDEX

335

insertion prevented flow, 84
Increased cardiac work, 332
Increased fatigue, 332
Increased pulmonary venous return, 118
Increasing resistance, 120
Infant type, 173
Infarction of the left lung, 233
Infection, 218, 227
Inferior cervical sympathetic nerve, 66
Inferior surface of the ductus, 59
Infolding of the media produces a
  diaphragm, 167
Ingham, 170
Initiate closure, 92
Innervation, 66
  innervation of the ductus arteriosus,
  66
Innominate artery, 58
Insertion into the aorta, 47
  insertion of the ductus, 46
Internal elastic lamina, 41
  internal elastic membrane, 5, 47
Intima, 39, 46
  intima is thicker, 40
  intima thickened by fibrous,
    collagenous and elastic tissue, 223
  intimal and subintimal areas, 41
  intimal mounds, 40, 42, 207
  intimal placque, 189
  intimal proliferation, 40
  intimal tissue changes, 287
Intimal occlusion may arise from
  portion of smooth muscle cells of
  the media, 201
Intrapulmonary venous shunt, 151
Inversion of the two types of
  coarctation, 176
Involution, 4
Involution of ductus tissue in the
  aorta, 166
Irregular forms of coarctation, 176
Irreversible vascular disease, 201
Isthmus of the aorta, 29

J

Jacobi, 234
Jaffe, 225
Jager, 40, 219
Jarmakani, 152
Johnson, 177
Jones, 4, 228
Jordan, 163
Junction of the ductus and pulmonary
  artery, 47

K

Karn, 324
Keiger, 324
Keith, 10, 99
Kellogg, 19
Kennedy, 3, 90, 91, 95
Kerwin, 225
Kesson, 170
Kilian, 17
King, 82
Kovalcik, 71
Kromer, 167
Krovetz, 115, 132

L

Lambs, 91, 98
Lamella, 46
Langer, 38
Late fetal circulatory physiology, 124
Lateral bulge of the ductus, 59, 60
Lauweryns, 322
Leape, 235
Leatham, 139
Lees, 151
Left aortic arch with persisting roots
  of right arches, 301
Left atrial injection, 322, 323
Left atrial maximal volume, 152
Left atrium, 130
Left bronchus, 59
Left subclavian, 29
Left vagus nerve, 57
Left ventricular ejection fraction, 152
Left ventricular end-diastolic pressure
  and volume increased, 153
Left ventricular muscle mass, 154
Left ventricular stroke volume, 152
Left ventricular systolic index, 152
Left ventricular wall mass, 152
Left ventricular wall thickness, 152
Ligamentum arteriosum, 14, 15, 43
Light microscopy, 48
Lin, viii
Lind, 17, 21, 92
Littman, 133
Lobar emphysema, 235
Longitudinal muscle layer, 46
Longitudinal muscle mass, 45
Lundstrom, 290

M

Mackler, 220
Magnified arteriogram, 189

Ramkin, 151
Randell, 226
Ranges, 3
Ranniger, 309
Rascoff, 234
Rat, prenatal changes in ductus, 98
Rathke, 25
Ratio of flow through ductus, 20
Rauchfuss, 88, 218
Recanalization, 189
Recurrent laryngeal nerve, 57, 220, 285
Reduction of pulmonary diffusing
    capacity, 152
Rees, 163
Regurgitant retrograde flow into the
    ductus, 145
Rehman, 52, 57
Relation of age to voltage in V1 and
    V5, 134
Relation to the pericardium, 52
Relation to the thymus, 59
Replogle, viii, 267
Respiratory gas transfer, 151
Response after exercise, 112
Response of isolated ductus arteriosus
    to oxygen, 72
Reversal of adult R/S progression, 130
Reversal of blood flow through the
    vertebral artery, 301
Reversible pulmonary hypertension, 136
Reynaud, 163
Reynolds, 41
Reynolds number, 116, 117
Richards, 329
Right aortic arch and ductus, 279
Robertson, 322
Rodbard, 197
Rokitansky, 38, 163
Rosenthal, 197
Ross, 151
Rouiller, 5
Rowe, 99, 101
Rubella, 67
    risk factor 10 percent in the rubella
    syndrome, 290
Rudolph, 112, 322
Rupture and hemorrhage of the
    ductus, 218
    rupture into a bronchus, 225
    rupture into the lung, 222
Rupture, in the newborn, 220
Rychter, 36

S

S2, loud, 195
Sabatier, 17
Samek, 226
Scammon, 78
Scharfe, 86
Schlaepfer, 220
Schroetter, 220
Schultze, 89
Sciacca, 4, 95
Senac, 76
Servetus, 15
Shah, 301
Shape of the ductus, 51, 61
Shepard, 120, 202
Shift in the position of the heart
    with respiration, 82
Shipley, 332
Short, 189
Siassi, 324
Silva, 48, 66
Silver impregnation methods, 67
Simultaneous V1-V6, 139
Size and shape of ductus, 60
Size of the ductus arteriosus in
    twin fetus, 52
Size of the human newborn ductus, 273
Skoda, 162
Slitlike lumen, 43
Smooth muscle cells, 5
    smooth muscle fibers, 42
Soderlund, 69
Spencer, 202
Spherical dilatation, 219
Spontaneous healing of endarteritis, 232
Sprout from the dorsal aorta, 28
Stahlman, 322
Staphylococcus infection of ductus, 229
Status of ductus shunting, 322
Steno, 305
Stenosis above left subclavian, 176
Stenosis of the esophagus, 234
Stephens, 179
Stern, 21, 324
Stillbirths with contracted ductus, 62
Stillborn, position of pulmonary end, 59
Strassman, 84, 86
Streptococcus viridans, infections of
    ductus, 229
Structural changes in lung vessels, 187
Structural deficiency of the ductus
    media, 324
Structural obstruction, 322